Dr. Nieca Goldberg's
Complete Guide to
Women's Health

Dr. Nieca Goldberg's
Complete Guide to
Women's
Health

Nieca Goldberg, M.D.

with *Alice Greenwood, Ph.D.*

BALLANTINE BOOKS / NEW YORK

Copyright © 2008 by Nieca Goldberg

Published in the United States by Ballantine Books, an imprint of The Random House
Publishing Group, a division of Random House, Inc., New York.

BALLANTINE and colophon are registered trademarks of Random House, Inc.

Library of Congress Cataloging-in-Publication Data
Goldberg, Nieca.
Dr. Nieca Goldberg's complete guide to women's health /
by Nieca Goldberg, with Alice Greenwood.
p.   cm.
Includes bibliographical references and index.
ISBN 978-0-345-49212-8 (hardcover)
1. Women—Health and hygiene—Popular works. 2. Gynecology—Popular works.
3. Obstetrics—Popular works. I. Greenwood, Alice. II. Title.
III. Title: Complete guide to women's health.
RA778.G62 2007
613'.04244—dc22   2007030470

Printed in the United States of America

www.ballantinebooks.com

2   4   6   8   9   7   5   3   1

First Edition

Book design by Susan Turner

I dedicate this book to my parents, Minda and Leonard Goldberg, whose love and support inspired me to help others.

CONTENTS

PART I

The Best Health Care 101

ONE

Step into My Office

I T'S VERY HARD FOR MANY OF US TO TAKE CARE OF OURSELVES. WE are busy and stressed out and managing the care of the people around us and working ridiculously long hours and . . . I bet I don't need to tell any of you who have picked up this book about juggling twenty things at once. But what happens when you don't feel quite right, not quite your normal self? Do you know what to do and when to do it? Do you know what to watch out for and what to wait out? As I know from firsthand experience, women in midlife are often busy taking care of their families, young and old, as well as advancing in their careers, and they often feel as though their bodies are changing overnight. They may lack stamina, have difficulty sleeping, find themselves gaining weight, suffer from backaches and headaches, or have other symptoms of stress. Many of us are part of the so-called sandwich generation, responsible for caring for both children and elderly parents while we work at demanding jobs. It's no wonder we don't take good care of ourselves. When you're trying to do it all and taking care of everybody else, it's very easy to neglect your own well-being.

Every day in my practice, I meet women who have gone from doctor to doctor with symptoms of exhaustion, sleeplessness, and low back pain. They have had enough blood tests and X-rays to last a lifetime, yet they have no diagnosis to explain their symptoms or any help in reducing them. None of the physicians seems to have taken the time and trouble to ask these women how they were feeling or to discuss what was going on in their lives. Maybe the physicians were pressed for time or didn't have the communication skills to elicit the information from these patients. But these women were left high and dry, without help. This is not okay! Stress takes a physical as well as emotional toll on us all, which is why it's extra important to stay fit and be healthy.

I also juggle too many things at once, and I have a family history of heart disease. I learned the hard way about how stress could lower my resistance to illness. Shortly after the publication of my first book, *The Women's Healthy Heart Program* (originally published as *Women Are Not Small Men*), I was admitted to the hospital with a fever of 104 degrees and blood pressure of 70/50—signs of a serious infection. Now, looking back on that time, I realize I was doing too much: lecturing in the evening, seeing my patients by day, constantly responding to my cell phone and e-mail, and not getting enough sleep because there was so much to do. Hindsight is always 20/20, as they say.

But at the time, all I knew was that I had a lot to do in very little time, and that everything I had to do was very important—everything, that is, except taking care of myself. Finally, one Saturday morning I found that I couldn't get out of bed. I had a severe case of the flu and was unable to fight it off because I had such low resistance. Even though I know (I'm a doctor, after all) that stress lowers your immunity, I had to feel it first-hand to make some real changes in my life. After that experience I have become much more alert to what stresses me out and how my body reacts to being on overload. I want to share that information with you—before you too collapse and end up in the hospital.

But it's hard to get good information, and it's even harder to know whom to get it from. Yet unless we have reliable and accurate information about our bodies and our health care, we won't have the basis to make good decisions for ourselves. Everyone I talk to, including my friends and my patients, wants advice from someone they can trust. They want to hear straight talk, with clear explanations. Let's say your arm hurts. Where do you go? To an orthopedist? Is that really the right specialty? Maybe, maybe not. How do you know? Or you are managing your elderly mother's care and she faints. What do you do? Whom do you call? Or you realize after leaving the doctor's office that there were terms you didn't understand and you want to know what they mean.

I have many friends who end up calling on me for help, and I am really glad that they do. I can interpret symptoms, explain treatments, translate medical jargon, and give them the information they need to make good decisions. I want to do the same for you in this book: teach you about your body and about good health. I want to alert you to those symptoms that should send you running to your doctor, and distinguish those from the ones that are less serious and easily treatable. Knowledge is indeed power, but only if the information is good. And it's perfectly reasonable to be confused and not know what to think. All the controversy around hormone therapy is a good example. One day estrogen is touted as the cure for everything under the sun, and the next thing you know, it's in the news that it could cause serious harm. Clearly, common sense, intelligence, and experience are needed to interpret what is being reported.

But most doctors give patients just enough time during an office visit to figure out what specialist to send them on to. My friend Genevieve complains about the forty-five minutes her doctor makes her wait, only to spend six minutes with her. She says it takes her more time to get her clothes off. The venerable old-fashioned family doctor who took you from birth to death and literally knew you inside and out is becoming a mythic figure from the past. In this era of specialists, we have trouble finding someone to filter the barrage of sometimes confusing information about medicines, treatments, and diseases that seems to be coming at us from all directions. What I hope to do in this book is to give you the inside track on how to effectively handle this information so as to better negotiate the system and improve your health.

A good friend of mine called me when her mother, Beth, was hospitalized because she needed a pacemaker. Beth had been told to stay in bed, and the doctors kept asking her if she was short of breath. My friend didn't understand why they were asking about that, and the doctors were not quick to return her phone calls. After listening to her, I asked her if anyone had said the word "pneumothorax." When she said yes, I was able to tell her that her mother's lung had collapsed. I then explained the typical course of treatment, what she could expect, how long it would take, and so on, and she was comforted. Why didn't her mother's doctors give her this information? How hard is that to do? I want to be able to provide that comfort to all women.

Because of patient confidentiality, I have not used the actual names of my patients in these stories. I hear story after story after story, and I believe that by sharing them, I will be able to reassure and educate women about how to take good care of themselves. The sister of one of my patients had been recently diagnosed with breast cancer, and my patient wanted me, her cardiologist, to examine her breasts. She asked me to do it because she was afraid that another (male) doctor might think she was being hysterical. Nothing, after all, was wrong with her; it was her sister who was sick. But she sensed that I wouldn't judge her or find her fear ridiculous, and of course, she was right. I was happy to examine her and reassure her that she was fine.

Another of my patients, who had had a heart procedure, was experiencing pain in her groin. She was convinced the pain was the result of the cardiac procedure—which had occurred two years previously. When I examined her, I had an idea, and I asked her if she had had her legs waxed recently. She was amazed that I should ask about that. But when I removed the ingrown hair and she felt better, we both laughed. I wonder if a male doctor would have been able to help her. I am happy to be a woman's doctor who's also a woman.

Providing women with good health information is part of my job. It's one of the reasons that I established the Total Heart Care Clinic for Women in New York City. As I became increasingly aware that women with heart disease were underdiagnosed, undertreated, and underrepresented in the medical profession, I got upset and wanted to do something about it. I wanted to ensure that women get the treatment they deserve and that barriers come down so that women have the same access to good health care as men do. It's not just in relation to heart disease that women are getting short shrift but in many other areas as well.

I know something about feeling marginalized. After graduating from a women's college (Barnard in New York City), I found myself knocking at the door of the world's largest fraternity—medical school. And I was not always met with open arms. Since I felt uncomfortable and uneasy, despite all my training and determination, certainly it's not surprising that many women might feel that way too when they interact with doctors.

I remember being an intern and sitting with several other female interns on the stairs at the medical college, all of us angry, frustrated, and upset because there was so little empathy for the lives and concerns of the women in the medical system. With Cyndi Lauper singing about girls having fun in the background, we realized that we definitely were not having fun. One of my friends was sure that her three-year-old daughter wouldn't recognize her since she was absent so much of the time. I couldn't imagine finding the time to have dinner with my new husband two days in a row. As we sat together, I vowed then and there that one day when I had my own practice, I would remember that my patients had lives and that they were complex human beings, not merely sets of symptoms or diseases.

Yet after twenty years in practice, I still find myself frustrated by the politics of medicine. As my friends point out, I have serious trouble acknowledging the power of the white male establishment. In fact, anger at what I see going on around me is why I am writing a *women's* health book. For too many years the health care system ignored 50 percent of the population, and never even recognized that this was the case. With this book, I hope to provide some of the necessary guidance to help you handle that fraternity, and at the same time to share information with you that will improve your health.

As a champion of women's health and an advocate for wellness, I want to provide you with the ammunition you need to be armed and dangerous when meeting with a doctor. I want to help you become informed, educated, knowledgeable, and cautious about medical care. I want to help you understand your body—what's normal, what's common, and what's suspicious—and to "talk" to you, woman to woman, friend to friend. I want to share my expertise about the health challenges we women face as we go into midlife and beyond. I want to make sure that women enter these years healthier than ever before. I hope that this book will be an accessible and clear reference guide for understanding how to keep yourself in good health.

However, this is not a one-woman job. I can't do it alone. You have to join me—learn what to watch out for, what to ask about, how to ask good questions and insist on good answers. I can help. It's what I do: work hard to keep women healthy.

In the following chapters, I'll give you some of the basics, a kind of crash course: Dealing with Your Doctor 101. I'll tell you what to look for in a doctor and how to be an effective patient. I'll outline what to expect from an office visit, what questions to ask, and what answers to get. I'll let you know what's normal and what might signal a problem. And I'll give you an insider's perspective on what your doctors are thinking. I want to be the doctor going to the doctor with you.

The chapters that follow outline how the body functions, what can go wrong, what tests should be done to establish a correct diagnosis, what the results of the tests mean, what questions you should expect your doctor to ask you, what information you need to provide in order to be an effective patient, and what treatments are associated with different physical conditions. I'll also explain some fundamentals about alternatives to traditional medicine and what to beware of if you are contemplating plastic surgery.

The final section of the book is a "get healthy" plan, a diet and exercise program that you can actually stick with, and one that will maximize your energy, lower your stress, and allow you to maintain good health.

So step into my office and let's start getting healthy!

TWO

How to Make Your Visit to the Doctor Work for You

YOU KNOW HOW YOUR FRIENDS TELL YOU THAT THEY HAVE A GREAT doctor to recommend? Well, don't believe them. When people recommend their doctors, they very often confuse good communication skills with good medical skills. Both are required for the doctor to be good. Being a nice person and knowing how to manage a conversation—wonderful attributes, for sure—don't necessarily mean that someone is the right doctor for you. A good doctor evaluates the entire person, not simply the small piece of the body that fits into her area of specialization. I'll never forget when I was listening to a patient's lungs and saw a mole on her back that I didn't like the looks of. I asked her if she had been evaluated by a dermatologist, and she said, "What for?" I realized that the mole was where she couldn't see it and none of her other specialists had noticed it. This makes me wild.

On the other hand, sometimes a patient has so many specialists that she gets into trouble. The problem is that each specialist is specializing and no one is coordinating the care. Talk about the right hand not knowing what the left hand is doing. Although my practice focuses on women and heart disease, I deal with all kinds of health concerns, and I either treat the problem or recommend an appropriate specialist. But it is really important that someone keep track of what's going on. I always make sure that I talk to the specialist and discover the results of the consultation; I also need to know if any medication or other treatment was prescribed. Sometimes there are potential interactions with medications, and often specialists don't know what other drugs the patient has been prescribed. As I say, someone has to be watching out for the whole patient.

Some women I know spend more time choosing what to wear for dinner than they do finding an appropriate doctor. But a little time and attention to the project could prevent a great deal of frustration and dissatisfaction. In this chapter I want to tell you what to look for in a doctor, how to find the right doctor for you, how to manage the office visit, how to talk to the doctor, and how to make sure that your doctor talks to you. I think of this as a primer for the practical patient.

To help make the process easier, here are five rules to follow to find the right doctor for you.

RULE NUMBER ONE

Tell Your Doctor Everything

One of my patients, Jean, who has high blood pressure, felt light-headed and dizzy. She went to the emergency room, and the doctors there told her she needed a brain biopsy. When she came to see me for her regular checkup, she told me about it, and also mentioned to me that since her arthritis had flared up, her rheumatologist had put her on steroid medication. I found that her blood pressure was low, and thought that might be caused by her reducing the amount of fluid she was drinking. When I asked her, she told me she was trying not to drink too much because her ankles had become swollen and she thought she was getting "too waterlogged." I explained to her that the swelling was a typical reaction to being on steroids and that her low blood pressure was what was making her feel faint and dizzy.

I adjusted her medication, but for safety's sake, I sent her to see a neurologist, who confirmed my diagnosis and assured her that she had no need of a brain biopsy. With all her doctors and all the medications, no one was in charge. No one was talking to anyone else, and no one knew what anyone else was doing. Happily, I took the time and trouble to ask her about her other symptoms and so avoided the unnecessary and frightening prospect of a biopsy.

Rule Number Two

If You Don't Feel Comfortable Talking to Your Doctor, Change Doctors

As far as I am concerned, if a woman has the opportunity and the encouragement to express her symptoms, her visit to the doctor is efficient. The patient is the doctor's greatest ally in figuring out what, if anything, is wrong. My patients know when something isn't right. I trust them.

Therefore, you absolutely have to be comfortable talking to your doctor about how you are feeling, about your fears, about embarrassing or unpleasant symptoms, about your stresses and frustrations, and about your bad habits. If you feel as if you are being silly or imposing on a busy physician or not really that sick—all things I have heard women say—you are not with the right doctor for you. I have had the opportunity to meet and talk to thousands of woman across the country and internationally, and I realize that women want to feel that they can talk to their doctor and ask the questions that concern them. Quite often they don't feel as if they can. That's most likely the doctor's problem, not yours.

Communication between doctor and patient is all-important for health care to be effective. That's just common sense, but I am surprised at how many times my patients tell me that they couldn't talk to or understand their previous doctor. If you don't feel comfortable explaining your problems to your doctor, or if you feel intimidated by his or her manner, you won't be able to provide the type of information required for a proper diagnosis. If you don't tell your doctor all your symptoms because you are frightened and want them to go away, your doctor can't help you. Poor communication causes harm.

I give out referrals all the time, and not only do I suggest physicians whom I trust and know to be intelligent and caring, I also have a sense of their personality and if it will be a good match for my patient. Not everyone communicates the same way; not everyone has the same bedside manner. And as knowledgeable as a doctor might be, if he or she can't communicate or respond to the needs of a patient, the patient will not be happy.

Rule Number Three

If Your Doctor Doesn't Ask All About You, Find One Who Does

If your doctor rushes you out of the office, it is not only bad manners, it is bad medicine. You don't have to have an advanced degree to realize that if you don't listen, you don't hear. What you want is a doctor who takes a very thorough background history about you and your family and gives you a complete—that is, not superficial—physical examination. This process of getting to know the patient is called taking a history and physical and is sometimes referred to as an "H and P." Without a proper H and P, a doctor runs a real risk of missing something important.

It's also important to know, and to tell your physician about, the health history of other members of your family. None of us is able to change our genetics, and a great deal of our medical and physical life is inherited. Sometimes if you are aware of your genetic load, you can take steps to mitigate what is in store for you. For example, if there is heart disease in your family background and you are healthy, you can diet and exercise.

Your doctor should do baseline blood work—that is, analyze your blood for electrolytes, glucose, kidney function, thyroid function, and liver function and do a complete blood count to check for anemia and potential infection. A lipid panel involves a check for cholesterol. A urine specimen is taken to check for the presence of sugar (a sign of diabetes) and protein (a sign of kidney damage that may be due to high blood pressure). If any of these tests is abnormal, further testing should be done.

Rule Number Four

*If Your Doctor Does Not Explain What Is Wrong with You
and What the Treatment Is, Get Another Doctor*

I am a small woman with a big mouth. I once fired my mother's doctor because he was such a poor communicator. My mother had been hospitalized and needed a procedure that required a consent form. Neither my mother nor my father understood what was written on the form— and why should they? They didn't go to medical school; they owned a

THE HISTORY AND PHYSICAL

The history part of the history and physical should be a series of detailed questions designed to allow the doctor to get to know you. The doctor should ask:

- Questions about your general health.

- Questions about any particular physical problem. If you have one, you should be able to tell the doctor:
  - When it began
  - What brings it on
  - What relieves the symptoms

- Questions about your medications. It's a good idea to bring a complete list of your medications and supplements, including dosages, or just throw everything you take into a shopping bag and bring it with you.

- Questions about any allergies you have.

- Questions about your family's medical history.

- Questions about your medical history. Even if you go to a specialist, you need to explain your whole history because your body is a series of interconnected systems (like individual instruments that together make music in an orchestra).

The physical exam involves a direct examination of your body. Most doctors usually begin with a check of your vital signs.

- The doctor will take your blood pressure. Both arms should be checked (although many doctors don't) because certain heart conditions can cause a difference in blood pressure of as much as 15 percent between arms.

- Your pulse should be checked. Normal is between 60 and 80 beats a minute.

- Your height and weight should be recorded. Many women are not happy to be weighed, but in fact it's important information for your doctor and should be checked at each visit.

- Your lungs should be checked for respiration rate—how fast you are breathing. Normal is between 10 and 16 breaths per minute.

Your eyes, neck, and throat should be examined.

- The doctor should look in your eyes with an ophthalmoscope. This is an instrument that allows the doctor to see the blood vessels in your eyes. She is looking for any potential damage to the arteries from high blood pressure, high cholesterol, or diabetes.

- The thyroid gland and the lymph nodes in the neck should be felt (the medical term is called "palpated"). The doctor is checking for enlargement or swelling that might indicate an infection, inflammation, or a tumor.

- The doctor should listen to the blood flow in the neck, using a stethoscope, to hear if there is any obstruction in the carotid arteries. If they are narrowed, you might be at increased risk for stroke.

- The doctor should look at your mouth and your throat to see if you are dehydrated. If your tongue color is not normal, it can be the sign of a vitamin deficiency.

The exam should also include listening to the lungs and the heart. What I usually do is listen to the lungs and the heart while the patient is sitting and then again when the patient is lying down. I listen for any abnormal heart sounds that may indicate a problem. I check the pulses in the arms, legs, and groin, behind the knees, and in the foot and ankle. If I hear any diminished pulses, it may signal a narrowed artery to one of these areas. I also look to see if there is any swelling or discoloration of the skin.

I also make sure to check the psychological condition of my patient because stress, anxiety, and depression have a negative impact on health. I talk with the patient and try to observe if she is anxious, angry, scared, or teary.

restaurant. This doctor had the nerve to call me and say, "Hi, Nieca, I left the consent form in the chart. When you get to the hospital, please have your mother sign the form."

As far as I am concerned, that was unprofessional. If he was too busy to explain the procedure to my parents, why would we let him do it? I left a return message on his voice mail: "Hi, Jerry. My mother won't need your services anymore." My friend Mary, a nurse, helped me to find my mom a new doctor, one who thought it part of the job to interact effectively with her patients. She explained the procedure and answered my parents' questions with a great deal of patience and kindness. She had the procedure and still sees the same doctor to this day.

RULE NUMBER FIVE
Find a Doctor Whose Style Works for You

Everyone, patients and physicians, has his or her own individual style of communicating. Every office has a style of operation. What you are looking for is a match, something that works for you. Some of my colleagues and patients like e-mail. For me, e-mail is appropriate only for very quick and nonclinical messages, such as missing an appointment. You don't want to leave an e-mail message that you think you may be having a heart attack. I try to discourage e-mail because I find that talking to a person, even over the telephone, can tell me a great deal. I pick up cues about her health, such as whether she is panting for breath, and I am able to ask follow-up questions when I need to. But what works for me and in my office may not work for everyone. Ask questions to determine whether there's a good match between you and your doctor.

It's also wise to understand the kind of office staff associated with the doctor's office. A good friend of mine had to interact with someone who served as gatekeeper to a specialist, and this woman, whom my friend nicknamed Godzilla, was difficult, unapproachable, and unfriendly. My friend finally took herself elsewhere—not because anything was wrong with the care the doctor gave her, but because of the difficulty Godzilla created about appointments and getting information from the office. Medicine is a service business. You can demand good service or take your business elsewhere.

HOW TO BE AN EFFECTIVE PATIENT

There's a reason they call it a "doctor-patient relationship": like other relationships, it requires something from both parties. Good care involves a good patient going to a good doctor and having good communication.

TIPS ON HOW TO CHOOSE
THE RIGHT DOCTOR FOR YOU

- Ask a doctor you trust for a recommendation.
- Remember that when you choose a doctor you are also choosing an office staff and policy.
- Is the office open when you can go—evenings or weekend hours?
- Ask whom you call in an emergency if the doctor is unavailable.
- Find out what hospital affiliation the doctor has. Is that convenient for you?
- Ask about communication. Are there phone hours? Does the doctor respond to e-mail?
- Find out if your insurance plan is accepted by the doctor.
- Look up the doctor's credentials on hospital websites or medical society websites.
- Is the office conveniently located for you?

The doctor-patient relationship is a two-way street. That means to get the best care possible you have to do your part too. If you do, your care will be better than if you don't. You should be honest with yourself about why you are consulting a doctor. If you are hoping that if you go for enough opinions you'll eventually hear what you want to hear, rather than what each doctor has agreed is your problem, you may want to re-think the visit.

You should know why you have come to the doctor and be able to explain. Seems obvious, right? But way too often patients come to me because their internist wanted them to consult a heart specialist, and when I ask why they have come they say, "Because my doctor told me to." Or worse, "Because the doctor's secretary gave me your name."

If your doctor tells you to have a test or to take medication and then return for a follow-up visit, and you haven't yet had the test or have never filled the prescription, call the doctor before the appointment and tell him or her why you haven't done so. There are lots of reasons people don't take their medication as prescribed: they can't afford it, they forget, they are scared of side effects, they had a side effect. We all do that. Even I forget to take my full course of antibiotics from time to time. Don't be reluctant to tell your doctor; it's important information for your doctor to have. Make sure to tell your doctor if you haven't complied with her or his advice, for whatever reason. Good health care is based on good information. Garbage in, garbage out, as they say.

If you are going to a specialist for a second, third, or even eighth opinion, it's also a good idea to bring whatever past medical information is relevant and make clear to the specialist why you are there. You should be sensitive to the fact that not all specialists are comfortable practicing outside their specialty. Don't ask a cardiologist to treat your foot fungus.

WHAT YOU CAN DO TO ENSURE AN EFFECTIVE CONSULTATION WITH YOUR DOCTOR

When you see your doctor, come with information. If you are going to a specialist, come with lab results or radiology films. You should carry with you a list of the medications you take and the dosages. It's easy to forget something that you take routinely, including supplements and over-the-counter medications.

It's also a good idea to write down the questions you want answers to. I find that many people develop amnesia when they come to see a doctor, and because they are nervous, they have trouble taking in information. If you think you might not remember what the doctor said in answer to your questions, it might be wise to bring a friend or a family member to the office with you. Many of my patients take notes, which is a great idea. After they leave the office, people often can't remember what they were told.

When your doctors ask you how you have been feeling, this is not social chitchat. Tell them everything, even if you think it is nothing or silly. Don't be your own doctor; don't screen information. And most important, don't be afraid of sounding stupid.

Also, it isn't a good idea to try to interpret your symptoms yourself. Just state the facts. When patients come to me and say their stomach hurts, that means something to me. I know the follow-up questions to ask to rule out, for example, a heart attack. But when a patient says she

TIPS ON BEING
AN EFFECTIVE PATIENT

Remember that the doctor works for you. You are the paying customer and are entitled to information and attention. In order to get the best care possible:

- Tell the doctor why you have made the appointment. Is the visit your annual checkup, or is there a specific concern that worries you, or is the visit a second opinion consultation?

- Bring a complete record of any previous tests and charts and a list of your current medications, including dosage and how often you take the medicine.

- Tell the doctor about any vitamins or supplements you are taking.

- Ask for clarification if you don't understand what the doctor is saying.

- Ask for a definition if you don't understand a word or an expression.

- Ask the doctor what any tests or medications are for.

- Ask the doctor to write down how often and at what time of day to take the medication, and whether it should be taken with anything (food, water).

- Ask the doctor if there are any side effects.

- Ask the doctor whether the generic form of the drug is appropriate. Don't decide by yourself.

- Remember that if you are going to see a specialist, you are seeking out her expertise for a certain condition. Don't assume that a specialist will take care of all your medical needs.

has indigestion, I have to find out what she really means. The clearer the communication about physical symptoms, the better able the doctor will be to diagnose properly what is going on. The more specifically you can describe your symptoms, the better. If you can tell me where it hurts, what kind of pain (sharp, dull, sporadic, constant), when it occurs (when you lie down, after meals), and for how long, it helps me make a valid diagnosis.

Sometimes a little knowledge really is a dangerous thing. When a television personality had a CT (computer tomography) scan to see her coronary arteries, my patients called me saying they wanted one too. But of course these radiological tests are not for every problem, and they're certainly not appropriate for everyone. Your doctor should be able to evaluate what tests you need, if any. For example, if you complain of back pain, don't be frightened if the doctor recommends an MRI (magnetic resonance imaging) rather than a simple X-ray. If your description of the problem suggests bone or joint problems, an MRI is entirely appropriate. Lots of patients think tests are magic. But they have limited and specific uses and reveal only certain types of information. Some tests even carry some risk. You can't have a CT scan if you're pregnant because it involves X-rays. The latest CT scan of the heart requires a dye that some people are allergic to and which should be avoided if you have kidney problems. Your doctor needs to evaluate if a given test has more benefit than risk for you.

WHEN TO CALL YOUR DOCTOR

Call your doctor whenever you don't feel good. Call when you don't feel "right." Let the doctor decide if you need to be seen.

This is not a definitive list, for sure, but if you experience any of the following, get checked out.

- Although some hair loss is normal, if you see your hair coming out in clumps, talk to your doctor. It could indicate a hormone imbalance, thyroid dysfunction, too much testosterone, or stress. All these conditions require intervention.

- Although some weight gain or weight redistribution is expected in middle age, watch out for excessive gain or loss, especially if you haven't changed your diet.

- If you find yourself terribly thirsty and craving sweet foods, it may be a symptom of diabetes. Talk to your doctor.

- If you feel faint or experience shortness of breath or light-headedness, don't decide it was just something you ate. Call the doctor.

- If your periods are associated with very heavy bleeding, tell your doctor. It may be a sign of fibroids or an underactive thyroid gland.

- If you have chest pain, call your doctor because you need to be evaluated for heart attack, blood clot to the lung (pulmonary embolism), pneumonia, or problems with the stomach, esophagus, or gallbladder. It could also be a muscle pain.

- If you are extremely tired, check with your doctor. It might be a sign that you are anemic or have an infection. Your thyroid could be not functioning at the right level. You could be depressed. You might simply be overworked.

- If you find yourself feeling faint or dizzy, you should be checked for a heart problem, dehydration, anemia, and infection. It might also be a neurological problem in the brain.

- If you discover lumps in your neck, breast, groin, or anywhere else, check with your doctor. It could be a cyst, a tumor, or an infection. Don't ignore it and hope it goes away.

- If you have palpitations, it could signal that something is wrong with your heart or thyroid gland, or that you are having hormonal changes associated with your menstrual cycle or menopause.

Sometimes I am amazed by patients who come in with their diagnosis all figured out, usually because they have discussed their symptoms with their friends or read about it on the Internet. Elly, who is fifty years old, is a good example. She scheduled an appointment with me because she had chest pain and had read on the Internet that I take women and their health seriously. She thought she might be having a heart attack. Yes, it's true that all women are at risk for heart disease, but it doesn't mean we all will get it.

When we met, I took a history, did a physical exam, and made recommendations about further testing. I tried to reassure her that based on the history she gave me, her symptoms were not likely to be from heart disease. Only then did she confess that she had had a test done by another doctor a few weeks previously and the results showed that her heart was normal. It turns out that her chest pain occurred regularly once a week, just after she took her medication for osteoporosis. She never had chest pain at any other time. When I told her I thought her chest pain was coming from her esophagus and that the medication she was taking was known to irritate the esophagus, she said she didn't believe me.

In medical school we were taught to keep an open mind. Patients need to keep an open mind too. When a patient tells me her symptoms, I think about a range of conditions that could cause them, and I decide, based on their severity, what kinds of tests are appropriate. Elly already had had a test for heart disease, but she was sure she knew better than both her doctor and the test. In order to convince her that she might be wrong, I suggested she stop her medication and see what happened. To her amazement, after she stopped, the chest pain went away.

BEWARE OF MEDICAL INFORMATION THAT YOU GET FROM THE INTERNET AND TV

Many women are too busy to go to the doctor and, seeking information and being used to taking care of themselves, they research their problem on the Internet. But this is not always a good idea. How do you determine whether the information is scientifically grounded and objective? And how do you really know the author's agenda? Recently I went to a website advocating the widespread use of CT scans to screen for heart disease. The website was sponsored by a pharmaceutical company and the doctors involved all had financial incentives to perform these scans. This makes me somewhat suspicious of the information. You should be too.

Health care information on the Internet is geared toward everyone, not to you specifically. It is designed to address most of the people most of the time, but you are unique. Also, the information can be outdated. Unless you read the fine print, you may not notice when the information was posted. In medicine and health care, every day brings new information. Surf the Web wisely. Find sites that are sponsored by organizations that bring together recognized, unbiased experts in the appropriate fields. Some organizations that provide reliable information are the National Institutes of Health (NIH), the Centers for Disease Control and Prevention (CDC), WebMD, and specialty organizations such as the American Heart Association and the American College of Obstetricians and Gynecologists. I have included these and other reliable sites in the

Resources section at the end of the book. What you don't want to rely on is something like "Debi's Tips on Gallbladder Disease."

TV advertising should also be used carefully. Remember that what TV ads are looking to do is use a zippy sound bite to make a profit. So when a TV commercial or other media ad promises improved health from one medication or another, remember it's not about good medicine but rather about good marketing. Your doctor knows what's better for you than an advertiser.

One of my patients heard an advertisement that convinced her that progesterone cream can be used to prevent heart disease. Do I even need to tell you that it doesn't? This kind of silly claim is actually dangerous because many people believe what they hear and read in the media. Good genes and a good lifestyle, with occasional assistance from medications, prevent heart disease. Progesterone does not play a part. In fact, progesterone cream can actually cause various problems, such as blood clots, gallstones, or breast cancer. Although these side effects are rare, why put yourself at risk unnecessarily?

FROM THE DOCTOR'S POINT OF VIEW

Here are some insider tips on how doctors react to certain patients. When someone comes to me and says she hated her last three doctors, I become somewhat suspicious and maybe even defensive. All three? Hmmm. I have to think that maybe something is going on that is preventing a good doctor-patient relationship from forming, and it may not be all the doctors' fault. When someone comes to me for a third or fourth opinion and explains that all the previous doctors said the same thing and she hopes I'll have another answer, I worry about that too. Is she just coming to hear what she wants to hear? If so, do I want to participate in this game?

When I want to do a complete history and physical on a new patient and she says, "Why bother? Another doctor has already done one," I explain that I like to do my own in order to come to my own conclusion. I am happy to explain, but I hope I am understood. For some patients, insurance is a consideration and they worry whether their insurance will pay for a second opinion. It's wise to check.

It also bothers me when a patient is not up-front with me and doesn't tell me that she had a series of high-tech tests a week ago because she wants them repeated. It's unnecessary, and talking to me about it would let us evaluate why she didn't trust the results the first time around. Many of these tests are incredibly expensive, and most often the insurance company won't pay for repeated tests (especially at close intervals). There's no point in not disclosing information.

Finally, if a patient comes to me and says that several months ago she was told to have a heart procedure but she didn't want to and so didn't have it, it makes me nuts. She might have a life-threatening disease, and yet she ignored her doctor's advice. That is not a good idea, period. If you find a lump and a breast biopsy is recommended, it's dumb to wait six months, hoping it will go away. Even if you are frightened, you want to be a good patient. There's nothing wrong with being scared. We're all scared when we're sick. But it's not good for you not to listen to sound medical advice. So my advice to you is follow your doctor's recommendations. If you are confused by the advice, ask for a better explanation. Just don't ignore it.

THREE

If You Have to Go to the Hospital

WHEN DO YOU GO TO THE HOSPITAL? WHEN YOU'RE SICK. THIS may seem entirely obvious or even silly, but I see many patients who are really sick but somehow manage to ignore it. They think it will pass and get better, or they are too afraid of being in a hospital to acknowledge how sick they feel. Nothing is gained by ignoring your sickness; in fact, usually, it makes matters much worse than they need to be. If you don't feel well, if something seems wrong to you, call your doctor. If your doctor says you need to be in a hospital, go to the hospital.

My husband, a radiologist, is always amazed by my late-night conversations with patients as he listens to me plead with them to go to the hospital. For example, Joan called the answering service on a Saturday night to discuss the sudden loss of vision in her right eye. When I spoke to her, she said it only lasted for a few minutes. I told her those were symptoms of a ministroke, called a transient ischemic attack (TIA) (see page 152), and she needed to go to the hospital right away. She was in Chicago and told me she would get on the next plane. I told her there are hospitals in Chicago, but she was reluctant to be seen by a doctor she didn't know. Finally I convinced her to go.

No one likes to go to the emergency room (ER). I have heard every excuse imaginable to avoid it, from "It takes too long to be seen" to "They don't take care of me like you do, Dr. Goldberg." I know that these excuses reflect fear or past bad experiences. The bottom line is if you trust your doctor, then follow her advice. If she tells you to go to the ER, go, because it may save you from a life-threatening condition.

For example, a patient of mine who had diabetes called me to say that her cat had scratched her arm and that her arm had suddenly blown up and was swollen, red, and painful. She said she was also getting chills. I told her to call 911 and go to the ER right away. She said, "Why? My heart is feeling great." I explained to her that because of her diabetes she had to be really careful about infection. I didn't want to panic her, but I suspected that she might have what is called cat-scratch fever, a serious infection. The doctors in the ER found that she had a high white blood cell count, indicating infection, and a fever of 102 degrees. It's better to take care of a problem while it is still manageable, before it becomes a full-blown crisis. So don't argue with your doctor if she tells you to get moving.

You also go to the hospital if you need a procedure or an operation. Certain procedures require equipment, medication, and monitoring that cannot be provided in a doctor's office. There are one-day outpatient procedures, such as endoscopy, colonoscopy, and hernia repairs, and other procedures that require being admitted to the hospital and staying overnight (inpatient). How long you need to stay is determined by your doctor, the nature of your problem, and the procedure, not by your schedule.

When I had to have knee surgery, I was able to schedule it at my convenience because it was not an emergency; rather, it was an elective procedure. I was able to prepare myself and put my life in order, knowing that I would be unavailable for a number of days. But if you have an emergency, you can't wait.

HOW TO PREPARE FOR YOUR HOSPITALIZATION

Usually for an elective procedure—which means you can choose to have it or not—your doctor will give you preoperative instructions. It is most important that you follow them exactly. Also, it is important to tell your surgeon who your other doctors are and whether you are being treated for chronic problems, such as high blood pressure, heart disease, diabetes, or breathing difficulties. If the preoperative instructions are to stop taking your blood thinners a week before surgery, for example, make sure you speak to the doctor who prescribed the blood thinners before you stop. Blood thinners, such as aspirin, clopidogrel (Plavix), or warfarin (Coumadin), are prescribed for a variety of conditions, including stroke, heart attack, atrial fibrillation, artificial heart valves, and deep vein thrombosis (see Chapter 8). You need to be sure that it is safe for you to stop taking the medication. Don't make that decision for yourself or trust the Internet for information. Not every surgery requires that blood thinners be stopped. For instance, patients don't have to go off their medication for cataract surgery. Just check everything out with your doctor.

QUESTIONS YOU SHOULD BE ASKED BEFORE SURGERY

- Do you have allergies?
- Do you have diabetes?
- Do you have any history of heart disease, stroke, or high blood pressure?
- Do you have any bleeding problems?
- Do you suffer from breathing difficulties?
- Do you have kidney problems?

If you take herbal supplements, you need to inform your doctor about that as well. Sometimes there are interactions among medicines and supplements. If you have sleep apnea (see page 367), mention this too, because the anesthesiologist needs to know how to prepare for you.

Most doctors require a broad array of preoperative tests to ensure that you are physically prepared for your procedure. Usually blood work is done to make sure you don't have an infection. Your blood's clotting factor is checked. Your blood count is done to assess for anemia. Electrolytes are tested to check liver and kidney function. A urine analysis is done to check for infection and kidney function. If you are male and over forty or female and over forty-five, an electrocardiogram (see page 163) is performed. Depending on the nature of your procedure, a chest X-ray may be taken. If you have a heart condition, you may need an echocardiogram or a stress test (see page 164).

All of these tests are ordered to ensure your safety, not make the hospital or doctor rich (which I sometimes hear). You wouldn't race your car without checking the oil filter or get into a plane that hadn't been checked out for five years; in the same way, your body needs to be thoroughly evaluated before the procedure.

WHAT SHOULD YOU TELL YOUR DOCTOR?

Everything! And I mean every single thing you can think of. Your life may depend on it. If you take any medication or supplement (including vitamins), if your diet is in any way abnormal (you drink twenty cups of coffee a day), or if you have any medical condition, even a chronic one that you never think about, you need to tell your doctor about it.

I remember a woman I was caring for while I was an intern. She had not been completely honest about her alcohol intake. Two days after surgery her heart was racing and she was delirious. When a concerned family member told me that my patient drank a lot, I realized that she was suffering from alcohol withdrawal. If I had known about her alcohol intake at the start, I could have prevented her complications with medication.

A young woman I know died having plastic surgery in a doctor's office because she forgot to inform the doctor that she had a heart condition. She didn't think plastic surgery was a big deal, and she didn't understand that fixing her face could have a relationship to her heart. Don't second-guess your doctor. Don't make decisions about what information is relevant and what isn't. Tell everything, and let the doctor decide if it is important or not.

WHAT YOUR DOCTOR TELLS YOU

When you tell the doctor all about yourself, your medications, and your conditions, the doctor will determine if you need to do anything special to prepare for your procedure or surgery. Most doctors will check with your specialists, if you have any, to make sure you will be safe.

One of my patients was planning on cosmetic surgery to have her eyelids done. Her doctor told her that she had to go off the aspirin she was taking for her heart for two weeks before and after the surgery, but that she should check with me. I told her that she could not go off the aspirin, that it would be dangerous for her. She was upset and said she would take the responsibility. I said no, and I knew her surgeon would agree with me. As far as I was concerned, this was a choice between her eyelids and her life. Even if she had some conflict, I didn't. Eventually she saw (from under slightly droopy eyelids) that I was right.

WHAT TO BRING WITH YOU TO THE HOSPITAL

Obviously, if you are in crisis and having a medical emergency, such as acute abdominal pain or bleeding, you call 911 and get to the hospital quickly—without wasting time to pack your makeup. If you can, however, it is a good idea to take your insurance card, a list of your medications (or just put them all in a bag and take them with you), and a list of any allergies you may have.

CALL 911 FOR ANY OF THESE SYMPTOMS

- Unusual bleeding
- Breathing difficulty
- Chest discomfort
- Sudden abdominal pain
- Sudden problems speaking or seeing
- Sudden paralysis of some part of your body

If you are having same-day surgery or an outpatient procedure, make plans for how to get home. It's best to bring someone with you because if you have an anesthetic you may be woozy. Also, it's a good idea to have someone along who has not had any sedation to listen to the doctor's discharge instructions.

Don't bring anything valuable to the hospital, such as your watch or other jewelry. Leave your wallet at home too (but it's not a bad idea to have a few dollars with you for the TV or phone charge).

WHAT TO EXPECT IN THE EMERGENCY DEPARTMENT

Especially in big cities, emergency departments (EDs) are busy places and usually very crowded. When you get in, a triage nurse will ask you some questions. The point of triage is to prioritize the severity of your condition and thus determine how fast you'll be seen. I often hear complaints from my patients that they are kept waiting too long. Although everyone wants to get treated and get out, the most dangerous and serious problems are dealt with before the less life-threatening conditions. If you have a sprained ankle, you won't be seen before someone coming in with chest pains. Therefore, if you are kept waiting, you're relatively lucky.

TAKING MEDICATIONS

The issue of medication is often confusing to people who are used to taking their own medication and now are being given different medications in the hospital. Most often, the hospital gives out medication, which means you don't take your own in addition. It's always a good idea to go over medications with your doctor. A good friend of mine was hospitalized and needed medication for her blood pressure. Her normal medication was a small pink pill, and so when the nurse brought her a blue pill she didn't want to take it. It is a good idea to question what you are taking, and certainly medication errors happen all the time. But if the nurse or physician assures you that the medication is the same, don't worry. Sometimes generic forms or alternatives may look different from what you usually take.

WHO'S WHO ON THE STAFF?

Lots of people will come and talk to you, and often they will ask you the same question over and over. That's their job; try to be patient.

The attending doctor is your personal doctor. Generally the person responsible for admitting you to the hospital is your regular doctor. If you come in through the ED as an emergency, you might have an attending assigned to you. If you know anyone in the hospital, you can ask for that person, or call your own doctor to get a name. The attending physician functions as the captain of the ship, ensuring that there is some coordination among the many people involved in treating you. Someone has to manage what's going on. One of my patients was recently on a trip to Wisconsin and started to experience chest pain. When she called me, I told her to go to the nearest ED, and I called the ED doctor to inform her of my patient's medical history.

Some hospitals have hospitalists. These are physicians whose function is to supervise your hospital care, functioning as your doctor and ensuring that your care is timely, efficient, and effective. They communicate with your attending physician, who will see you as an outpatient.

The house staff (the hospital is sometimes referred to as the "house") are interns, residents, and fellows—doctors at various levels of training. They all may interview you and ask you questions. This is how they learn, and they have to do it. Interns are newly minted doctors, usually one year out of medical school. They do not decide your plan of care but are extremely instrumental in updating your doctor about your condition and care. Sometimes my patients minimize the importance of interns and residents, but I always remind them that this is how I started. Residents are one to three years out of school and are learning a specialty, such as internal medicine or surgery. Fellows are past residency and are what are called subspecialists—for example, cardiology is a subspecialty of internal medicine. The house staff has no other responsibility than to care for hospitalized patients. Someone is always there and on call.

The nurses are the people responsible for actually administering the care and educating patients about their treatment. Many patients find that the nurses are their favorite people in the hospital. (They are my favorite people in the hospital too.) This makes good sense, since nurses deal most directly with the hourly, daily routines of care. Nurses also can serve as your advocate. They know everything! They call the physicians and ensure that you get what you need.

Other people with whom you may interact during a hospital stay are consultants, such as dieticians, social workers, specialists in one field or another, and what we call ancillary staff, such as technicians and the people involved in transport.

KNOW YOUR RIGHTS AS A PATIENT

It's so easy to feel like a passive victim in a hospital, and so easy to assume that you are helpless. But although being a patient is not in the least an empowered position, there is no need to give up your expectations about how you will be treated. First of all, you are entitled to privacy—which means more than just having the curtain closed around the bed when you are being examined. The privacy of your name and your condition is actually protected by a set of federal regulations called HIPAA (for Health Insurance Portability and Accountability Act). Medical records are also protected under HIPAA. In fact, you should know that doctors are not allowed to discuss your condition with anyone at all unless you give express permission. So if you want your significant other or a family member to be able to talk to your doctors, you have to explicitly give permission.

If you are having surgery or a procedure, most likely you will be asked to sign an informed consent form. This is a document that explains to you what will be done to you, and any associated risks. Read it carefully. You might be surprised to know that these documents can contain errors. If it is your right knee that requires surgery, make sure you see the word "right" on the form. If the form is confusing, don't sign it. Wait for your doctor to explain it to you. Someone might pressure you to sign the consent form, maybe even try to bully you, but stay tough here. If they are in a hurry, it is not your problem. If you can't understand it or have any questions, it is your right (and it is actually smart) to wait until you have answers.

ADVANCE DIRECTIVES, LIVING WILLS, HEALTH CARE PROXIES

Many people do not like to deal with the possibility that they may not be able to control what happens to them if they are incapacitated by an illness. That's perfectly understandable. Living wills and advance directives are designed so that you determine what you want done—and, more important, not done—in the event you are unable to make such decisions on the spot. Assigning someone the role of health care proxy means that if necessary, that person can make decisions for your care. Although the subject may be unpleasant to think about, it's a good idea to have such documents prepared in advance of an emergency and to know where they are.

MEETING THE SURGEON

Most commonly, patients are admitted to the hospital by their regular doctor. If they have had the opportunity, sometimes patients choose their surgeon and meet with him or her before admission. Often, though, patients meet their surgeon just before the procedure. The surgeon should answer your questions and explain to you what the procedure will be, what you can expect by way of recovery, and so on. Surgeons have had a bad reputation as being poor communicators, but I find them to be men and women of few words who really get to the point. The surgeons I recommend to my patients are both talented and good communicators. Your doctor should pick a surgeon who is not only a good technician but also someone who fits your personality.

MEETING THE ANESTHESIOLOGIST

The anesthesiologist is also critical to a successful result for your surgery or procedure. You should have a conversation with him or her before your surgery and ask questions about what will happen and what to expect. If you have sleep apnea or any other airway disorder, chronic lung disease, or allergies, tell the anesthesiologist. If you have any previous procedures and have had reactions to medications, tell the anesthesiologist.

TIPS TO KEEP YOU SAFE

Over the past few years, the media has brought public attention to the fact that hospitals and doctors make mistakes. My parents' generation thought doctors infallible; the boomer generation knows better. The government and various professional organizations have been lobbying for improved patient safety and mandating specifics of care. Nonetheless, it's still a very good idea to be careful and watchful and to bring someone with you who can ensure that your care is the way you want it to be.

> When you visit someone in the hospital, use your common sense.
> - Don't go if you have a cold.
> - Don't bring children if they are not well.
> - Don't bring food or drink without explicit permission.
> - If you are asked to put on a gown and gloves and wash your hands (this is normal procedure in an intensive care unit), do so.
> - Go during normal visiting hours.

You will be given an ID bracelet with your name when you are admitted to the hospital. Sometimes your birth date or other information will also be included. Some hospitals even go so far as to put bar codes (like in the supermarket) on the ID bands because it is easy to make an identification mistake. It is the law that before you are given medication or any other intervention, someone is supposed to ask you your name and to properly identify you. It seems a little silly when a doctor you've known for twenty years asks you your name, but the process is in place for your protection. You want to get your medication, not the one meant for someone whose name is similar. You want to get the right procedure for you, not one that has been noted on the board for someone else.

In addition to ID bands, regulations demand that the site of the surgery be marked with ink. Again, this is to avoid errors. If you are having a right-side surgery, you want your right side marked. Mistakes happen.

Before surgery, and before you have any anesthetic, you are supposed to confirm what is going to happen to you. Someone will ask you (probably for the fifth time) why you are there. And you will say "For a right lung biopsy" or "For a left hip replacement." Again, don't be impatient with what might seem endless repetition; it is for your safety.

Keep It Clean

There are sick people in hospitals. Duh, right? But that means that special precautions need to be taken in order to avoid spreading infection and disease. The most obvious safety precaution, washing the hands, seems to be the hardest for health care workers to remember. If anyone comes at you without washing their hands, remind them, even if you feel awkward about it. This is not a time to be polite.

What to Expect After Surgery

Your recovery depends on what kind of procedure or surgery you have. Your doctor should be able to explain to you what you can expect and what kind of pain you may experience. There are many medications available to reduce pain, especially after surgery, including medication drips that you can control yourself. If you are in pain, tell the nurse. The nurse will get extra medication for you from the house staff or your doctor. It is actually not good for your recovery if you are in pain, so don't be a hero.

Nowadays, we know that if you start moving as soon as possible after surgery, even if you don't feel like it, it is better for you. That's the reason the nurses will try to get you up and sitting and even walking the same day as your surgery. The more you move, the fewer complications you'll have. You may have physical therapists assisting in this process.

LEAVING THE HOSPITAL

Your discharge planning should begin as soon as you are admitted to the hospital. Seriously, it may take days to prepare, and starting early means there won't be any unnecessary delays. Depending on what you have had done, you may need special care at home, or a stay in a rehab facility, or special medications. The social service team should be involved and helping you for the next step. You want to make sure you are safe and comfortable and able to heal.

You need to be officially discharged from the hospital by a physician. You are supposed to receive written discharge instructions as well, which should have the types and times of medications you should take, the names and numbers of the doctors to call, and a follow-up appointment. If you need prescriptions, make sure you have them in hand before you leave.

Most people have good experiences in hospitals and in fact are grateful that their problems have been taken care of. Planning ahead of time, knowing what to expect, taking good care of yourself, and having patience for your recovery should make the hospital stay okay.

FOUR

What You Should Do
to Take Good Care of Yourself

L ET ME TELL YOU THE STORIES OF TWO WOMEN. LUCY IS FORTY-seven years old and in good health, she thinks. She walks several miles every week and takes tango classes. Sometimes when she finds herself short of breath and easily tired, she assumes that she is simply overdoing her exercise. A friend of hers told her about an herbal remedy for shortness of breath, ginseng, and she has started taking it daily. Although she doesn't really feel better, she thinks that this is simply the price one pays for being a middle-aged woman.

Jennifer, forty-five, is afraid that she is not in good health. She has noticed that her hair is thinning, and although she has been eating exactly as she always has, she is beginning to put on weight and get thick around the middle. Even though she feels somewhat foolish, she calls her internist quite often to ask about one symptom or another. She thinks a new mole has appeared on her arm and she is anxious about it being cancer; sometimes she finds it difficult to drive at night because her vision is blurry (a brain tumor?); her knee hurts when she exercises, which she fears is the harbinger of a knee replacement. In response to her anxiety and her symptoms, her internist refers her to various specialists. The specialists assure her that nothing is wrong.

These two women manage their health very differently: one never seeks medical help and assumes everything is normal, while the other anxiously seeks medical advice and believes that her health is compromised.

Which one do you most closely identify with? With similar symptoms—all normal for midlife changes—people react very differently. These responses are more than the half-full or half-empty perspectives of different people. They reveal various attitudes toward knowing one's body and interacting with the medical establishment.

Both are important: know yourself and know the system. For women to manage their well-being and their health issues, they need an awareness of what is normal or usual both for their age group and for themselves, and they need to evaluate how, when, and for what they should interact with a health care professional.

In this chapter I want to explain to you what's normal and what's not, and tell you what you can do to keep yourself healthy through the normal changes of midlife.

WHAT'S NORMAL

As our bodies change, it is natural to have many questions about what is normal and what isn't. Many of my friends and my patients want to know if what they are experiencing is okay. They want to know why they have stopped sleeping well or why they are running to the bathroom so frequently and even sometimes leaking. Many of my patients tell me that they find themselves unable to remember things and that they don't like the way their skin looks and feels. Some find themselves gaining weight although their diet hasn't changed. Some of my friends and patients ask me if there is a physical reason why they feel less interested in sex. Some complain that their hands and feet are always cold. All these symptoms are normal, and I will explain the reasons for them in more detail in the following chapters.

Women also want to know what to do to maintain good health. They want advice about whether estrogen therapy is really dangerous and if they should be taking calcium supplements to maintain bone strength.

They want to understand menopause. They ask how often they should go for a mammogram and a Pap test, and whether they should have an electrocardiogram every year. They want to know when they should have a colonoscopy, what kinds of blood tests should be done at a yearly physical exam, and of course what the results mean. My patients ask which symptoms warrant a hysterectomy and which are normal for growing older. Others want information about birth control and sexually transmitted infections. Some want information about where to go if a partner is abusing her sexually or physically. Some ask me if it's normal to feel their heartbeat when they're resting.

So let's talk about what physical changes are normal for women in midlife. I want you to have accurate and adequate information and to be reassured about what you can expect.

Changes You Can Expect in Midlife

Weight Gain

Let's start with a common complaint: putting on weight, even when we eat exactly the way we always did and exercise as often. After thirty, our metabolism begins to slow down, and a slower metabolism means that we don't burn off the calories we take in the way we did when younger. Why does our metabolism slow down? The answer is hormones. Hormone levels get lower as we approach middle age and beyond, which causes us to become more insulin-resistant. Insulin is a hormone (see pages 262–263) that helps us convert the different types of sugars we eat into energy. Being more insulin-resistant means that the sugars and carbohydrates we take in are less efficiently processed into energy. The result is often weight gain and getting thicker around the middle.

What can you do about it? I am certainly not suggesting throwing in the towel on maintaining your once-girlish figure. You just need to work a little harder at it. And that's normal. You need to eat a little less than you used to and exercise a little more. That doesn't mean you need to go on a strict diet or exercise hours every day. Not at all. When I say work harder, what I mean is maintain a reasonable exercise regimen and eat a reasonable diet. Note the word "reasonable." I don't want you eating seven almonds and four carrots for a meal. Balance and common sense are the best techniques to manage normal weight gain in middle age.

PERIMENOPAUSE

I don't hear a lot of talk about perimenopause, or at least not enough, and I think the lack of information does women a disservice. Perimenopause is defined as the time before the onset of menopause, and you know you have it if you begin to have symptoms of hormone fluctuations. Some clinicians believe that women experience more symptoms during perimenopause than during menopause, symptoms that may be overlooked, ignored, or even ridiculed because no one is looking for them or helping women understand them. Some women even experience these perimenopausal symptoms for up to fifteen years. Every woman is different—and that's normal. There is no "right" way to enter menopause; there are no "better" or "worse" symptoms.

What are some of the symptoms? Some lucky women don't even notice either perimenopause or menopause symptoms because they are nonexistent or very mild. For others, there may be many symptoms, such as hot flashes, vaginal dryness, sleep problems, mood swings, and breast tenderness. You may menstruate fewer days, or the number of days between your periods may increase. Some women's symptoms are so severe that physicians recommend hormone therapy—pills or patches (see page 87).

Some women experience heart symptoms, such as rapid fluttering or skipped beats. If you do, don't assume this is normal. You don't want to ignore unusual heart symptoms, and you should always check with your doctor if you feel anything unusual. One of my patients called me because she was experiencing racing heartbeats and she was understandably frightened that something was wrong with her heart. When she described her symptoms, I realized that there was a periodicity to them. They always occurred a few days before her period started. Other than those occurrences, she was fine, with no symptoms at all. I asked her if she was due to get her period in the next day or two. She thought I was a soothsayer! But no, just a careful listener. So before you run for open-heart surgery, breathe in and out, check the calendar, and review your symptoms with your doctor.

OTHER NATURAL CHANGES

Typically as we enter midlife and beyond, our skin quality changes and becomes less elastic (see page 326). It is also normal for hair to become thinner due to hormonal changes as well. Our joints are not as lubricated as they were when we were younger, and many women begin to experience joint pain that is associated with arthritis (see page 203). Other changes that are entirely normal are changes in vision. Haven't you had a meal with friends your age and no one's arms are long enough anymore to read the menu? Many times I have shared a meal with a group of friends who pass around those little magnifying reading glasses you can get in the drugstore.

Although these changes are not generally met with delight, being middle-aged has its upsides. You can enjoy the increased freedom that comes when the early child-rearing years are over. Many of us have managed careers and finances for so many years that we have enough money to enjoy ourselves from time to time. Besides, there is little anyone can do about the normal process of change, so we might as well accept it.

WHAT YOU NEED TO DO TO KEEP FIT AND HEALTHY

If you want to enjoy these years and feel energized, fit, and healthy, I have a few words of advice: get regular exercise, don't smoke, eat a healthy diet (see page 339), get regular medical checkups, and if you have been prescribed medication for anything, take it and follow your doctor's advice.

EXERCISE IS GOOD FOR YOU— MAKE TIME EVEN IF YOU DON'T HAVE ANY

No one I know has a lot of spare time, and most of the women I know are busy from morning till night and then some. I'm busy and plenty stressed too, but I find that exercising keeps my energy up and my spirits lifted. So I make the time, even when I don't have any to spare. I try to do an hour a day, which means getting up a bit earlier or going to bed later. I find it makes me feel good. In fact, when I get really cranky, my husband sends me off to the gym because he knows I'll come home in a much better mood. Make time for exercise. It pays off in a number of ways: physically, emotionally, and psychologically. And you might find new friends at the gym.

There are different kinds of exercise, and each type affects the body in special ways (see Chapter 18). For example, swimming is great exercise for your heart, but it doesn't do much for your bones. To maintain bone health, you need to do what's called weight-bearing exercise, which means being upright, on your feet, so that your bones bear your weight. Walking is great weight-bearing exercise. Walking on a treadmill works too, as does dancing or any other kind of upright aerobic activity.

No one is too old to exercise. An eighty-year-old woman who lives alone and is in good health came into my office. She exercises three times a week, and the benefits are obvious. When I examined her, I found a robust and a healthy woman, in fact healthier than many younger women I see. In addition to regular exercise and regular doctor visits, she spoke about how much social support she had, and what an active social life she engaged in.

Her experience is actually confirmed by research. Because I am interested in women's cardiac health, I wanted to study how effective cardiac exercise programs were for women who had had heart attacks. Most men who have had heart attacks are recommended to cardiac exercise programs by their doctors, and most follow their doctor's recommendation. However, very few women are referred by their doctors to such programs (your guess is as good as mine as to why not). But even those women who had joined exercise classes were more likely than men to drop out after a short while. The programs had been designed for men in the 1960s, when heart disease was thought to be a man's issue, and the women I interviewed said that they didn't like the exercise format and that they found the gym atmosphere not in the least nurturing.

It was important to me to find a way to keep these women in their exercise program. I thought that if the program was redesigned and not too taxing physically or if the women did not have to compete with the men for the machines in the gym, they might stay on longer. I divided a group of women (those who were actually referred by their doctors) into two groups: one was an all-female low-impact aerobics class, and the other group did a standard gym exercise program with machines. I found that the women in the aerobics class really enjoyed their experience, especially the camaraderie and friendship. The women in the regular gym class did not enjoy the experience as much, but they were in better physical shape. The moral of this story is that to maximize the benefits of a cardiac exercise program and to remain in the program, women need to have social support, companionship, and a regular exercise schedule.

SMOKING IS TERRIBLE FOR YOUR HEALTH

There is absolutely nothing good about smoking. It causes all kinds of harm at any and all ages. It takes its toll on your heart, your lungs, and anyone who comes near you. Throughout this book, you'll see countless references to the damage that smoking does. Smoking triples a woman's risk of having a heart attack. It increases the risk of lung and throat cancers. Smoking raises blood pressure, causes the arteries to constrict, and increases the likelihood of blood clots and stroke. Women who smoke have higher levels of bad cholesterol and lower levels of good cholesterol. Women who smoke reach menopause three years earlier than those who don't, and their symptoms, such as hot flashes, are often more severe. If you smoke, you are at greater risk for osteoporosis. Smoking during pregnancy and being exposed to secondhand smoke are associated with increased fetal mortality and behavioral problems in children.[1]

Although I have never smoked, I have a sense of how difficult it is to stop because I see how challenging it is for my friends and patients to quit. My friend Clara was a longtime smoker, although she is a nurse and knows better. She had been trying to quit for years, and sometimes she even succeeded for a short time. But then she would start again. Even though she didn't smoke when we were together, the smell of her cigarettes remained on her clothing and made it difficult for me to breathe. My nose got clogged, my eyes got puffy, and I started to wheeze. Clearly I was allergic to my friend's smoking. Finally I told her that it was hard for me to be with her and that she had to stop. For some reason, this made an impression on her. She went to her doctor, a colleague of mine, got a prescription for one of the smoking cessation medications (see page 43), and has not smoked for several months. When her doctor asked her why now, Clara said, "Because Nieca said I smelled."

TIPS ON QUITTING

Here's the good news: if you stop smoking, after two years your risk of heart disease is cut in half. After ten years your risk is the same as if you had never smoked.

When I begin a smoking cessation program with my patients I start by assessing and asking questions. The last question I ask is, What is the date you plan to quit smoking?

Why do you smoke? I want to know why my patient is smoking. Sometimes women explain that they smoke because they are stressed, anxious, depressed, or trying to lose weight. If we can determine the underlying reason for smoking, I can recommend appropriate support, such as counseling and an exercise program to accompany the quitting program. Low-calorie healthy snacks such as carrots and sugar-free candy to help satisfy food cravings are also useful.

When do you smoke? It also helps to know what the triggers are. I can't tell you how many times my patients tell me that they are only social smokers. My response to that is to tell them that's like being a little bit pregnant.

How addicted are you? This is a most important question. In order to assess the level of addiction, I ask how soon you smoke a cigarette after getting up in the morning. If the answer is within the first five or ten minutes, I know you are highly addicted and probably will need nicotine replacement.

Who is in your support network? It's very hard to quit when all your social connections continue smoking. Clara and her husband quit smoking together. Support is associated with success. I have patients who have joined smoking cessation groups and found them useful.

Do you need medications? I recommend a variety of smoking cessation medications to the women I see. I also recommend counseling, because studies have shown that a five-to-ten-minute interaction with a health professional improves quit rates. Quitting cold turkey is difficult, particularly if you are a heavy smoker. If you are, you are likely to have nicotine withdrawal symptoms such as headaches, nausea, fatigue, depression, and anxiety.

WHAT CAN BE DONE ABOUT NICOTINE ADDICTION

Medications are used to address nicotine addiction and to diminish the urge to smoke. Many insurance companies are covering smoking cessation medications.

Nicotine replacement, whether patch, gum, or spray, is prescribed for nicotine addiction and reduces withdrawal symptoms associated with smoking. The dose of the nicotine replacement is based on how many cigarettes you smoke. It is really important not to smoke while using the nicotine replacement because you will receive too high a dose of nicotine. Nicotine replacement should not be used immediately after a heart attack, but it can be started a few weeks later.

Zyban or Wellbutrin are brand names for bupropion, an antidepressant medication that decreases nicotine withdrawal symptoms and cravings for cigarettes. Bupropion has been relatively successful in reducing relapse rates and has a more sustained quitting rate compared to nicotine patches alone. A new drug, Chantix (varenicline), has been proven successful in removing the urge to smoke. People who took varenicline were more successful in quitting than those on bupropion.

One of the women I treat didn't want to use bupropion because it was an antidepressant. I explained that in her case it was being used to help her to quit smoking. She had failed on nicotine patches and I recommended dual therapy to work on the nicotine addiction and urge to smoke. She eventually agreed and was most successful. She is now approaching her third anniversary as a nonsmoker.

KEEP HEALTHY WITH REGULAR CHECKUPS

Other than exercising, not smoking, and eating right, what can you do to ensure good health? Do reasonable health care maintenance. Go to your internist yearly and have blood work, a good history taken, and a physical (see page 13). Have a yearly mammogram and Pap smear. If you are over fifty, or if you're younger and have a history of colorectal cancer in your family, ask your doctor about scheduling a colonoscopy.

TAKE YOUR MEDICINE

I always dread initiating the medication discussion. No one wants to take medication, but sometimes it's necessary. Whenever I bring up the M-word, I see the look of dejection and disillusionment on my patients' faces. Invariably the women I see want to know if they can try lifestyle changes before starting medication. Although such changes sometimes work for gastrointestinal problems, mildly elevated cholesterol or blood pressure, or pre-diabetes, very often lifestyle changes are not enough. Many common conditions, such as thyroid disease, require medication, and although a healthy diet and an exercise regime are always good, they can't fix everything.

When I have the medication discussion with my patients, I start off by saying that the medication prescription really involves more work for both of us. It's not a quick or easy fix. Once you are on medication, it is important that you have a clear line of communication between you and your doctor. It is my responsibility to explain to you what you are taking, to alert you to any side effects, to explain how to take the medication, and to ensure that you understand. You have the responsibility to take it as prescribed and to let me know if you have any side effects. It is my job to monitor whether the medication is actually working and making you better.

When Mindy, who is a fifty-seven-year-old artist, was diagnosed with high blood pressure, she was very reluctant to start medication. She thought she was too young. I told her that she was too young to have a heart attack or a stroke. She agreed to take the medication. The good news is that her unhappiness about taking medication has provoked her into switching to a healthier lifestyle—she has started to lose weight, is eating a better diet, and is doing a regular exercise program. Because she has started to take her health seriously and is doing what she can to improve it, she's been able to make a difference in her health status. I was able to reduce her medication. Both of us were pleased. Sometimes a prescription can be a great motivator to pick up healthier habits.

WOMEN AND MEDICATION

There is limited information about whether there are gender differences in medication side effects, and if so, what they are. Pharmaceutical companies have recently started to study and report gender-related differences in the effectiveness of drugs, and we know some things and not others. For example, we know that statins (a class of drugs for lowering cholesterol) have a similar impact on the cholesterol of women and men, but we don't know if women are susceptible to side effects different from the ones known to affect men.

This is what we do know about women and medication:

- Women use more medications than men.
- Women's response to medication may change with age.
- Hormonal changes may influence the effectiveness of medication.
- Hormonal changes may make certain drugs more toxic.
- During pregnancy, increased water retention may reduce the efficacy of certain drugs.
- If you're pregnant, drugs should be chosen to reduce fetal side effects.
- Dosages have to be carefully adjusted for women's smaller average body stature and increased body fat compared to men.

With all these things in mind, my philosophy on prescribing medication is to use the lowest effective dose to get the medical condition under control.

KNOW THE ANSWERS TO THESE QUESTIONS BEFORE YOU START YOUR MEDICATION

Before swallowing a single pill, ask your doctor the following questions:

- What is the medication for?
- What are the benefits of the medication?
- What are the side effects of the medication?
- What symptoms should make me call the doctor?
- Is there information available about interactions with the other medication(s) I am taking?
- How long will I have to take the medication?

- Are there generics available? Is the generic equivalent to the name brand?
- Do I have to take it with or without food?
- What time of day is best for taking the medication?
- What should I do if I forget to take a pill?
- How long before I should feel better?

If you don't plan on filling the prescription, or can't get to a pharmacy easily or conveniently, discuss it with your doctor.

DO'S AND DON'TS ABOUT TAKING MEDICATION

Follow directions about what you should or shouldn't do. For example, if you take an antacid with your medication, then your medication won't be absorbed. If the label says to take the medication with or without food or with a full glass of water, do so. These directions are recommended to improve the effectiveness of the medication and to reduce side effects.

You may not know that medication can be affected by food and supplements—even something as ordinary as grapefruit. In 1989, researchers who were testing the effects of alcohol on felodipine (Plendil), a blood pressure medication, used double-strength grapefruit juice to disguise the taste of the alcohol. They found that the study subjects' levels of felodipine were much higher than expected, and concluded that there was an interaction between the drug and grapefruit that increased levels of felodipine in the body.[2]

Grapefruit and grapefruit juice are great food choices because they

---

A TIP FOR SAVING MONEY

If you have a prescription plan that allows you a ninety-day supply at a time, ask the doctor to write a ninety-day prescription. Ordering a ninety-day supply may save you some money. Ordering medicines by mail can often be cheaper too. If you opt for this, it's a good idea to ask your doctor for a two-week prescription that you can give to your local pharmacy. That way you can be sure to have enough medication until your ninety-day supply arrives in the mail.

contain vitamin C and healthy flavonoids. But the flavonoids and another component of the grapefruit, furanocoumarins, interact with proteins in the intestine that are responsible for the metabolism of many drugs. This interaction may also occur with pomelos and Seville oranges. When the metabolism is inhibited, the level of the drug in your body is higher for a longer period of time—which means there's a potential for increased side effects. For example, if you are on felodipine for high blood pressure and you drink grapefruit juice, your blood pressure may be lower than expected. You should avoid grapefruit and grapefruit juice if you are taking felodipine, the antibiotic erythromycin, and certain cholesterol medications (see page 186). It doesn't matter if you eat grapefruit or drink the juice hours before or after the medication—the interaction is still possible. As I said, there are always alternatives. Your doctor can reduce the dose of the medication or prescribe alternatives that are not affected by grapefruit juice. But first your doctor has to know what's going on. That's your job.

Grapefruit is not the only substance to avoid when dealing with certain medications. Supplements such as St. John's wort also need to be carefully monitored. Remember, just because you can get something over the counter or even in natural form doesn't mean it is a good idea or right for you. If you are taking oral contraceptives, for example, St. John's wort may reduce the amount of estrogen available to your body, possibly leading to vaginal bleeding. St. John's wort also may have an impact on the blood-thinning properties of certain medicines, such as warfarin (Coumadin), putting you at increased risk of blood clots.

I always tell my patients that medications and supplements are chemicals that you are adding to your body; all of them can cause side effects. Be responsible and bring a list of all your medications and supplements to your doctor's office. You want to do everything you can to maximize the benefits of your medical regimen and to minimize your risks.

RECOGNIZING ALLERGIES AND SIDE EFFECTS

It's important to know the difference between an allergic reaction to a medication and a side effect. An allergic reaction usually involves a rash, hives, or even shock symptoms, such as collapsing or fainting, soon after beginning the medication. Allergic reactions can be life-threatening, which is why you are asked (or should be) about allergies when your history is taken. It's even a good idea to have your allergies to medication written down in your wallet. If you are allergic to penicillin, sulfa, other antibiotics, or any other medication, make sure to always tell the doctor.

The symptoms of side effects are different from allergic reactions. Typically people complain of headaches, muscle aches, or stomach upset. Even though side effects may be less extreme than allergies or even predictable, they should not be ignored. Tell your doctor about them. Some side effects may alert your doctor that you may have an adverse reaction to the medicine or a poor tolerance for it. That's good information for your doctor, who can then prescribe something else. There are always alternatives.

A patient of mine, Meg, learned this the hard way. Once she was prescribed codeine for some ailment and she got a stomachache and constipation. These are known side effects of the medication, but Meg decided she was actually allergic to it and told everyone, including her doctors, who responsibly noted it on her medical record. What she effectively did, however, was eliminate a whole class of drugs for pain control for no good reason.

I learned about what she had done when I was called to the hospital after Meg fell off her bicycle while she and her daughter were riding in Central Park. When I arrived at the emergency room, Meg's daughter ran up to me upset not only about the fall but about how much pain her mother was in. I finally figured out what happened with her previous pain medication and explained to Meg, the ER doctor, and the nurses that no, Meg was not really allergic to codeine. She had never had allergic symptoms such as a rash or hives. She had never collapsed or passed out after taking the medication. Then I did a lot of paperwork to correct the medical record, and Meg got morphine for the pain. Since the pain medication was used for only a short period, she didn't even have the unpleasant side effect of constipation, and she was certainly more comfortable.

If you have a side effect, call the doctor. Don't just decide to stop the medication; doing so may indeed resolve the side effect, but without the appropriate medication your medical condition may be left untreated. You don't want that.

If you have any doubt about the way you are reacting to the medication, call the doctor who prescribed it for you. Some of my patients are overly influenced by what they see on television. If they see a pharmaceutical commercial that details a long list of side effects, they often get scared and stop taking the medication. Worse yet, they don't tell their doctor until two weeks later. A more productive and safer way to handle this problem would be to call the doctor's office immediately if you are worried and let her know you have some concerns. Too many women are afraid of annoying the doctor. I make it a point to discuss potential allergies and side effects, and the difference, with my patients. Make sure your doctor does the same for you.

HOW HEALTHY ARE YOU?

The more you know about your health, and your health habits, the better able you will be to take good care of yourself and recognize when something is "not right" and should be attended to. Why don't you start now by checking out your Women's Health IQ to see where you are on the spectrum of women's health?

WHAT'S YOUR HEALTH IQ?

Take a moment to answer the following questions. Your score will tell you where you are in the spectrum of good health.

1. Who is your primary health care provider?
     a. My gynecologist (1 point)
     b. My internist/family physician (0 points)
     c. I usually see only specialists (2 points)
     d. I don't have one (3 points)

2. When was the last time you had a checkup?
     a. Within the year (0 points)
     b. 5 years ago (1 point)
     c. 10 years ago (2 points)
     d. I don't go to the doctor (3 points)

3. How well do you communicate with your doctor?
     a. I find it hard to say what I need to say in my allotted time
        (2 points)

   b. I generally do whatever the doctor tells me to do without asking questions (1 point)
   c. I tend to ignore my doctor's recommendation (3 points)
   d. I bring a list of questions and my physician responds to my concerns (0 points)

4. How well does you doctor communicate with you?
   a. It's hard to judge because my doctor does all of the talking (1 point)
   b. My doctor keeps getting interrupted during my visit (2 points)
   c. My doctor listens very carefully and is responsive to my concerns (0 points)
   d. My doctor seems to ignore or belittle my questions (3 points)

5. How much do you know about your family's medical history?
   a. My family has a "don't ask, don't tell" policy when it comes to health matters (2 points)
   b. I know my family's medical history (0 points)
   c. I don't know my family's medical history (1 point)
   d. I don't see why it is important (3 points)

6. Which of the following medical conditions do you think is considered the leading women's health concern?
   a. Heart disease (0 points)
   b. Breast cancer (1 point)
   c. Osteoporosis (2 points)
   d. Thyroid disease (3 points)

7. Do you exercise?
   a. I try to exercise 1–2 times per week but am not regular (1 point)
   b. I do vigorous exercise for at least ½ hour per day 3–4 days per week (0 points)
   c. I am a couch potato (3 points)
   d. I don't currently exercise but have great plans to do so (2 points)

8. Do you smoke?
   a. Yes, and I have no plans to quit (4 points)
   b. I quit smoking less than 1 year ago (3 points)

      c. I quit between 1 and 5 years ago (2 points)

      d. I quit more than 10 years ago (1 point)

      e. I never smoked (0 points)

9. How would you describe your eating habits?
      a. I eat primarily fast food (4 points)
      b. I eat 3 balanced meals, but my snacks are candy, chips, and soda (2 points)
      c. I seem to be a yo-yo dieter, constantly alternating between a healthy diet and fast food (3 points)
      d. I try to eat healthy meals and snacks (0 points)

10. How would you describe your menstrual status?
      a. I am still menstruating (0 points)
      b. I think I am in perimenopause because of changing menstrual periods (1 point)
      c. I am in menopause; my last period was 1 or more years ago (2 points)
      d. I have never been regular, so I don't really know and never had a checkup (3 points)

11. Have you gone through menopause and are you taking hormone therapy?
      a. I am not in menopause (0 points)
      b. Yes, I take hormone therapy for menopausal symptoms (0 points)
      c. Yes, I take hormone therapy for heart disease prevention (3 points)
      d. Yes, I take hormone therapy for osteoporosis (1 point)

12. What do you do when you are angry?
      a. Suck it in and smile (3 points)
      b. Rant and rave (3 points)
      c. Withdraw (3 points)
      d. Identify the problem and act on it (0 points)

WHAT'S YOUR SCORE?

0–6   You are well informed, and by reading this book you will become a more discriminating health care consumer.

7–12   Almost there, but you need to learn more about your personal health care needs. Focus on the women's normal health exam, learn how to navigate the system, and participate in the women's healthy lifestyle plan.

13–24   This book will show you the way to a healthier you by helping you to understand your personal health care issues and developing a plan for a healthier life.

25–36   You are clueless right now, but don't despair. You are capable of overcoming the obstacles to get to a healthier heart, mind, and body. Use this book as your guide to good health.

PART II

What to Do About
How Your Body Is Changing

FIVE

The Hormones That Make Us Uniquely Female

HORMONES ARE A VERY BIG DEAL, PHYSIOLOGICALLY SPEAKING. They are primarily responsible for making girls different from boys. From before puberty through menopause and beyond, hormones have an impact on how we feel every day of our lives. The sex hormones estrogen, progesterone, and yes, even testosterone are released by the ovaries and prepare our bodies for pregnancy, childbirth, and lactation. They also promote sexual desire—as well as give us PMS, cramps, mood swings, and hot flashes. You might say that the hormones that make us uniquely female are both a blessing and a curse.

Do you remember what it was like to be an adolescent, all those thundering moods? I can remember when I first got my period: my mother called it being "unwell," while my school pals and I would ask each other if we had our "friend." Why, I wonder, were there so many euphemisms around this most natural phenomenon, one that is shared by the sorority of women? Just as girls who are first starting to menstruate are in thrall to their hormones and suffer "symptoms" to a greater or lesser degree—cramps, pimples, food cravings, sore breasts, crying jags—women who are approaching menopause, the period of time called perimenopause, have symptoms too.

Like puberty, perimenopause and menopause are a time of hormonal change. (This change too used to be spoken of in whispers, as if it were some kind of female disease.) The hormones that sparked our puberty and took us through our childbearing years are the same hormones that in their fluctuations and absence are responsible for perimenopause and menopause, leading to an entirely different set of physical issues.

In addition to the symptoms noted above, during the years leading up to menopause many women experience headaches, sleeplessness, mood swings, weight gain, vaginal dryness, and irregular periods. Perimenopause is a process of hormonal change that can take from six to ten years. Most commonly, women begin to experience changes in hormone levels about eight years before menopause. When you have missed your period for an entire year, you are officially in menopause. Generally women experience menopause between the ages of forty-seven and fifty-three, but that's just an average. Women have menopause at much earlier and later ages as well. To understand the processes involved in hormonal changes, let's start at the beginning and outline how the sex hormones function as we go through our life cycle.

THE REPRODUCTIVE YEARS

Here are some nuts-and-bolts facts. The ovaries, the female sexual or reproductive glands, are located on either side of the uterus. They are normally almond-shaped and about one and a half inches long. The major function of the ovaries is to produce eggs (ova) for fertilization.

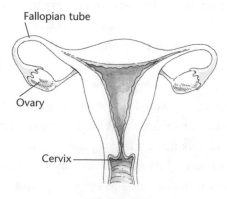

Fallopian tube

Ovary

Cervix

NORMAL UTERUS

The hormones released by the ovaries influence sexual characteristics such as breast development, regulate the menstrual cycle, and enable conception and pregnancy. Estrogen and progesterone are also responsible for the vaginal secretions that make us comfortable during sexual activity. Our little bit of testosterone goes a long way too; it's good for our sex drive and is sometimes even labeled the hormone of desire. Testosterone also helps to maintain bone and muscle strength.

Our Monthly Preparation for Reproduction

Just a quick refresher course on how our bodies cycle through the monthly preparation for reproduction. It's truly an intricate and remarkable system.

The ovarian cycle starts in the brain—specifically, in the hypothalamus, which secretes gonadotropin-releasing hormone (GnRH) into the pituitary gland. When the GnRH alerts the pituitary that the cycle is about to begin, the pituitary releases follicle-stimulating hormone (FSH), which helps immature follicles in the ovaries to mature. The maturation process causes the release of estrogen, which prepares the endometrial lining of the uterus to receive a fertilized egg. (This part of the process is called the follicular phase.)

When the pituitary gland, serving as "command central," receives information that there is a heightened level of estrogen in the blood, it decreases the amount of FSH and produces luteinizing hormone (LH). Ovulation, the release of the egg from the follicle, occurs about thirty-six hours after the onset of LH production. The burst follicle (which is now called the corpus luteum) signals that an increase of progesterone is called for (the luteal phase).

The egg travels through the fallopian tubes into the uterus. If the egg is not fertilized and conception does not occur, the level of progesterone falls and the endometrial lining of the uterus is sloughed off, which results in menstrual bleeding. The fall of the progesterone level sends a signal to the brain to start the entire cycle again.

Pregnancy

HORMONES AND PREGNANCY

If a fertilized egg is implanted in the uterine lining, another hormone kicks in, human chorionic gonadotropin (HCG), which triggers the production of progesterone. Progesterone helps to develop and maintain the placenta, an organ that develops during pregnancy and helps to nourish the fetus. But progesterone is also responsible for some of the unpleasant symptoms associated with the early weeks of pregnancy, such as nausea, heartburn, breast tenderness, and fatigue. If you have asthma, the higher levels of progesterone during pregnancy can worsen your respiratory symptoms.

The placenta itself produces estrogen, which increases blood flow—that's good for the developing baby. Increased levels of estrogen kickstart another hormone, prolactin, which readies the breasts for lactation. For many women, all this hormonal upheaval is associated with heightened emotions. After delivery, hormones decrease to normal levels, but the precipitous drop may contribute to postpartum depression. (There is simply no free lunch in this business.)

Occasionally I see pregnant women because of signs or symptoms of heart problems that often turn out to be pregnancy-related symptoms of a normal heart. This was just the case with my patient Charlotte.

Charlotte, a real estate executive, became pregnant for the first time at age forty-one. She and her husband came in to see me early in her pregnancy because her obstetrician had recommended that she see a cardiologist for a consultation. The obstetrician was concerned because she had heard a heart murmur (a term that refers to an extra heart sound) and wanted expert corroboration. Charlotte and her husband were worried that something would affect Charlotte's health or the health of their baby.

After examining Charlotte, I agreed that she indeed had an extra heart sound. But since she didn't have any symptoms of heart trouble, I suspected that the extra heart sounds were due to her pregnancy. It is actually quite common to hear extra sounds, even early in a pregnancy. They are caused by an increased flow of blood due to enlarged blood vessels in the breast that prepare the mother for breast feeding. An ultrasound of the heart proved that her heart was normal. Although there are women who do develop heart conditions in pregnancy (see Chapter 8), this was not the case for Charlotte.

I reassured Charlotte and her husband that everything was fine and that the heart sounds would not in any way hurt the baby. I also told them that the sounds would go away after the delivery. When Charlotte returned with her beautiful, healthy baby six months after her delivery, there were no extra heart sounds at all.

AVOID THE OSTRICH APPROACH TO YOUR HEALTH

Few people like running to multiple doctors or seeing various specialists. In fact, most people are scared and even phobic about discovering that something may be wrong with them. This is the ostrich approach to health care: If you don't go to the doctor, the doctor can't give you any bad news. But I want you to avoid this behavior. It is sometimes useful and reassuring to seek out specialists, especially when you're frightened. In this case, the obstetrician was absolutely correct: there *were* extra heart sounds, and it is responsible doctoring to recommend that those sounds be checked out by a cardiologist. Because Charlotte came to me, I was able to reassure her that all would be well, and prevent her from taking unnecessary and perhaps harmful medication. If you are pregnant, make sure you ask the doctor if any medications or tests that may be prescribed will pose any harm to you or your unborn child. As women, our health care needs should be considered in the context of whether or not we are pregnant or plan to become pregnant.

SOME THINGS TO EXPECT WHEN YOU'RE EXPECTING

You probably know that we are born with a finite number of eggs. That number gradually decreases, especially as a woman gets into her thirties and beyond. Hormone levels also begin to decrease, which is why it is more difficult to become pregnant as you get older. As we age, our periods begin to be irregular—certainly less regular than when we were in our twenties. But middle age is no time to become complacent about birth control if you don't want to conceive. In fact, many women are surprised to find themselves pregnant just when they were beginning to think they wouldn't have to worry about it anymore.

Normal symptoms of pregnancy, such as mild shortness of breath and palpitations, generally are not problematic. Of course, no matter what your age, smoking and drinking alcohol should be avoided. And if your legs, hands, and face get swollen, tell your doctor. If you are on medication for any chronic conditions, such as thyroid disease, high blood pressure, high cholesterol, or heart disease, or if you are taking blood thinners, it's a good idea to discuss the medications with your doctor *in advance* if you are thinking of becoming pregnant. Some medications can affect the fetus even in the first few weeks, so planning is a wise precaution. For example, if you have diabetes and take oral medications to control your sugar, you should switch to insulin because it is safer. Blood pressure medications and blood thinners may need to be changed. I always ask my patients if they are planning to have a baby so that I can make safer medication choices for them. I think it is most important for women in midlife, who have a higher likelihood of having diabetes or heart disease, to be screened for these conditions before becoming pregnant.

There are some health conditions (such as lupus, kidney disease, and some forms of congenital heart disease) that may cause complications in pregnancy. If you have chronic medical problems, you should talk to your doctor about the safety of becoming pregnant, for you and for the fetus.

WHAT TO WATCH FOR WHEN PREGNANT

Pregnancy in midlife carries more risk than when you are younger. A woman in her forties faces a 50 percent risk of miscarriage as compared to a 12–15 percent risk for a woman in her twenties. Therefore many obstetricians consider pregnancies in middle-aged women to be "high risk"—which means they watch you more carefully than younger women. There is nothing wrong with being watched carefully.

Middle-aged women who become pregnant have an increased risk for several pregnancy-related conditions, such as preeclampsia, gestational diabetes, and gestational hypertension.

Preeclampsia. This condition, signaled by high blood pressure (over 140/90) and protein in the urine, can appear around the twentieth week of pregnancy. Sometimes there are other symptoms as well, such as headaches, swelling of the hands and face, weight gain, or vision problems. Preeclampsia can inhibit blood flow to the placenta and potentially harm the fetus. However, if you get regular prenatal care, your doctor will monitor your blood pressure and urine for signs of preeclampsia and recommend treatment if necessary. Most doctors suggest bed rest, which lowers your blood pressure, and sometimes aspirin to improve blood flow. Most women with preeclampsia have normal, healthy babies, but you don't want to allow your blood pressure to get too high, which is why your doctor checks it at every visit.

Gestational diabetes. Although no one knows what causes gestational diabetes, which is a condition of high blood sugar during pregnancy, many believe that the hormones that support the placenta may cause insulin to be poorly metabolized (a condition called insulin resistance). Therefore the mother does not have sufficient insulin to convert the glucose from food into energy, and her blood sugar levels become elevated. The extra glucose can cross the placenta and affect the baby, causing it to have a higher-than-normal birth weight. Babies who have been affected by gestational diabetes have a greater risk for obesity and type 2 diabetes (see page 264) as adults. Mothers who have gestational diabetes are also at increased risk for developing type 2 diabetes in later life. Treatment for gestational diabetes is designed to lower blood sugar levels through diet, exercise, and insulin if necessary.

Gestational hypertension. This refers to high blood pressure (greater than 140/90) that occurs during pregnancy, usually after the twentieth week. Your doctor will monitor your blood pressure and may suggest bed rest. If your blood pressure is not controlled, you may require medication. If gestational hypertension is untreated, your baby could be born prematurely or with a low birth weight. Usually, once the baby is delivered, the mother's blood pressure returns to normal.

Genetic abnormalities. The presence of Down syndrome, spina bifida, Rh incompatibility, and other genetic problems can be determined through amniocentesis. Amniocentesis, a prenatal diagnostic test in which a needle is inserted through the abdominal wall and a small amount of amniotic fluid is withdrawn and analyzed for genetic abnormalities, is usually recommended for pregnant women over thirty-five. However, in January 2007, the American College of Obstetricians and Gynecologists revised its professional recommendation, saying that pregnant women at any age should be screened for Down syndrome (a genetic abnormality which causes mental retardation and is associated with other health problems) and other genetic abnormalities. That doesn't mean that everyone has to have amniocentesis. There are various less-invasive screening tests that are available, and younger women can be screened with blood tests and ultrasound. If the initial screening is in any way abnormal, then amniocentesis would be recommended.

MEDICATION AND PREGNANCY

The older you get, the more you have to balance, or maybe I should say juggle. Carol, who is forty-six and pregnant for the first time through in vitro fertilization (see page 65) and an egg donor, came to me for a consultation. She suffers from heart arrhythmias and some time ago had an unsuccessful procedure to try to correct her condition. Carol had looked up her medications on the Internet and read that beta-blockers, the medication she was taking to treat her arrhythmias, may have some fetal side effects—although this has never been proved for humans. Without consulting me, she stopped taking her medication when she became pregnant.

It is *never* a good idea to stop taking medication without discussing it with your doctor. When Carol stopped her medication, her heart started racing. Because her heart was racing, she began to feel light-headed and dizzy.

Balance, balance, balance. We have to balance the health of the baby with the health of the mother. With medication, the fetus may indeed have a slower heart rate, but without medication, the baby may not get enough oxygenated blood, especially if Carol's heart starts beating too fast. The same conflict and need for balance is involved in Carol's decision to breast-feed the baby. In order to breast-feed, she should stop the medication because it could have a negative impact on the baby. However, if she stops the medication, she could become so light-headed that she might drop the baby.

We have to wrestle with decisions such as these all the time. The best advice I have for you is to balance risks and benefits, and not be rigid about a single point of view. Also, be sure to talk everything over with your doctor. Be especially accurate about describing all your symptoms. Then you and your doctor can decide what to do.

ANTIDEPRESSANTS IN PREGNANCY

There have been very few drug safety studies in pregnant women because of understandable concern about potentially endangering the fetus. However, a recent study in the *New England Journal of Medicine* on the use of selective serotonin reuptake inhibitors (SSRIs) in pregnancy showed a small increase in birth defects.[1]

Another antidepressant, bupropion (Wellbutrin), is commonly used in pregnancy; however, it has never been studied. This is one of many cases where the benefit of the drug to the mother has to be weighed against potential harm to the fetus. I urge all women to discuss their medications with their doctors.

HAVING TROUBLE GETTING PREGNANT?

According to the American Society for Reproductive Medicine, about one-third of women between the ages of thirty-five and thirty-nine and two-thirds of women over forty have trouble becoming pregnant. "Trouble" is defined as not being pregnant after one year of unprotected sexual intercourse. After age thirty, the probability of having a baby decreases 3–5 percent per year, and after forty, the rate is even faster. Yet 20 percent of women in the United States have their first child after the age of thirty-five, according to the American Fertility Association.

There are many reasons for infertility, with increasing age certainly a factor. This makes sense because as you age, your eggs age as well, and if your male partner is also middle-aged, his sperm is less robust and plentiful than when he was younger. Also, your hormone levels are not as high as they used to be, and you may not be ovulating as consistently as you once were. There may be structural or physical problems that require surgery, such as the fallopian tubes being blocked, or fibroids in the uterus (see page 67). There can be many reasons, alone or in combination, for infertility; sometimes there is no explanation at all.

WHEN SHOULD YOU GO TO AN INFERTILITY SPECIALIST?

If you are over thirty-five and have been trying to conceive for a year without success, you might want to consider consulting an infertility specialist. As part of the history, the doctor will ask about your lifestyle. That's because lifestyle factors, such as smoking, being overweight, taking high doses of nonsteroidal anti-inflammatory drugs such as ibuprofen (Advil, Motrin), and stress can have an impact on hormone production, and hormone production has an impact on fertility. The doctor will do a physical exam to check the reproductive organs and also to determine if there are any physical signs of hormone depletion, which can be seen in the vagina and cervix.

If the physical exam and history suggest that there may be hormone problems, the doctor might schedule an imaging test, such as a CT scan, of the pituitary to check for tumors. If the results are normal, a course of hormone therapy may be indicated. If there are structural issues, surgery may be recommended to correct the problem, or the doctor may suggest in vitro fertilization to bypass it. Infertility treatments today hold out hope for many people who would not have had a chance at conceiving even a few years ago.

HORMONES FOR INFERTILITY PROBLEMS

If infertility is due to lack of ovulation from low levels of estrogen, the first line of treatment is usually a course of hormones, such as clomiphene citrate (Clomid), which is an oral medication that stimulates ovulation. It works by blocking estrogen so that the hypothalamus signals the pituitary to release FSH and LH into the bloodstream. A week after stopping the Clomid, there should be a surge of LH as a response to the increased levels of estrogen in the blood, which then triggers ovulation. Some women who take Clomid suffer from mood swings, headaches, and nausea. There is also a 10 percent increase in the rate of multiple births (twins, triplets).

If, after repeated attempts and adjustment of the dosage, there is no success, the next step might be injections of more heavy-duty hormones, called gonadotropins, to artificially induce ovulation. But you should be aware that although couples treated with gonadotropins have a 60 percent rate of pregnancy, over half of those pregnancies result in miscarriage.

Candidates for gonadotropins are women who have very low body fat, perhaps because they exercise excessively or have an eating disorder such as anorexia. You need to have some fat on you to have regular periods and normal hormone production. Women who have polycystic ovary syndrome (see page 66) may have irregular ovulation and benefit from gonadotropins, but their risk for multiple births is increased. Women who are undergoing in vitro fertilization are often given gonadotropins to stimulate egg development, but there too the chance of a multiple pregnancy increases.

If you are taking gonadotropins, you have to be carefully monitored because there is a slight risk of developing ovarian hyperstimulation syndrome, a condition where the ovaries are overstimulated and multiple eggs are produced. The condition can be mild to severe, with symptoms ranging from abdominal pain to vomiting and potentially dangerous fluid buildup around the heart and lungs.

IN VITRO FERTILIZATION (IVF)

IVF, once rare, is now relatively commonplace and often recommended for older couples. In addition to hormone medication, if you undergo IVF you can expect to have ultrasounds to observe the follicle and ovary. The way it works is this: an egg that has been harvested from a woman (you or a donor) is united in a lab environment with sperm that has been donated from a man. The resulting embryos are then transferred into the uterus. Don't be upset if it doesn't work the first time. Many couples repeat the procedure for several months. The success rate is approximately 25 percent.

The older you are, the more trouble you will have conceiving with IVF. IVF pregnancy rates are 50 percent lower for women older than thirty-nine compared to women younger than thirty-five. A woman of thirty has a 35 percent chance of having a baby through IVF, but at forty the success rate is only 15 percent.

WHAT ELSE CAN INTERFERE WITH GETTING PREGNANT?

Thyroid disease. Your body is a mass of interconnected systems, and some reasons for infertility may have nothing to do with your reproductive system but may be related to other health issues. For example, if you have thyroid disease (see page 256), you have an increased risk for infertility as well as a lowered libido. Once the thyroid disease is recognized and treated and thyroid function is normal, fertility is usually restored.

Polycystic ovary syndrome. About 10 percent of the women who are seen in infertility clinics have polycystic ovary syndrome (PCOS), which means that they have multiple small cysts on their ovaries. These cysts are caused when an egg follicle matures but the egg isn't released. PCOS is associated with abnormal hormone levels and can cause irregular or absent menstrual periods and infertility.

There is some research that suggests that infertility associated with PCOS can be caused by insulin resistance and that when this is treated with medication and a low-carbohydrate diet, ovulation may improve.[2] Supporting this is the observation that PCOS is also associated in the long term with higher-than-average rates of diabetes and heart disease. Therefore, even if you don't want to become pregnant, the insulin resistance should be treated. In addition, PCOS can cause heavy menstrual bleeding, increased hairiness (called hirsutism), and weight gain.

Ovarian cysts. Cysts, which are benign (noncancerous) fluid-filled sacs, can develop in the ovaries at any age. Your doctor can feel a cyst during a normal physical exam. Sometimes these cysts cause no symptoms whatsoever and disappear after menopause, or sometimes they can be painful or cause a feeling of fullness or bloating. Some cysts can simply be watched, while others should be removed surgically, depending on your age, the size of the cyst, and its makeup, as revealed by an ultrasound. Large and solid cysts should be examined to rule out ovarian cancer.

Ovarian cysts differ from PCOS in a number of ways. As noted in the preceding section, PCOS is associated with other clinical findings besides cysts, but an ovarian cyst is just that—a cyst on the ovary.

Sometimes it is possible to remove the cyst without removing the ovary; sometimes the ovary has to be removed. If so, the good news is that you can still get pregnant with only one ovary.

Endometriosis. More than five million women in the United States are diagnosed with endometriosis every year; it is a major cause of infertility. The condition occurs when endometrial tissue, which normally lines the uterus, builds up outside the uterus, growing on the ovaries, the fallopian tubes, or the uterine walls. But just like endometrial tissue within the uterus, this tissue needs to be shed. The problem is that there is no exit, and therefore the tissue is trapped in the abdominal cavity, which results in pain, heavy menstrual periods, adhesions, and infertility. It is not clear what causes endometriosis—probably a mix of genetics, menstrual fluid backup, and problems with the lymph system.

Since the most common symptoms of endometriosis are pain and/or heavy periods, which can be due to many causes, endometriosis may be difficult to diagnose without an ultrasound or laparoscope. The condition can be treated with medications, from over-the-counter pain medication to hormone therapy, and, if necessary, surgery.

Fibroids. Fibroids, which are benign (noncancerous) tumors, are very common in women of reproductive age, but most fibroids (77 percent) are undiagnosed because they are not large enough to feel and often they produce no symptoms. They can be small, less than an inch in diameter, or large, up to eight inches. Large fibroids can cause discomfort, pressure on the bladder, and heavy periods. Heavy menstrual periods can lead to anemia. Fibroids can occur within the uterine wall, on stalks (called peduncles) that grow from the surface of the uterus, or within the uterine cavity. It's not clear what causes them.

African American women are more likely to develop fibroids than women of other racial groups and more likely to develop them at a younger age. Women who are overweight are more prone to fibroids because fat cells release estrogen, which can stimulate fibroid development. Women who have fibroids may have more difficulty becoming pregnant because the fibroids may interfere with implantation. They also may have a higher rate of miscarriage and can go into premature labor. The first step in diagnosis is an ultrasound or other imaging test to confirm the presence of fibroids.

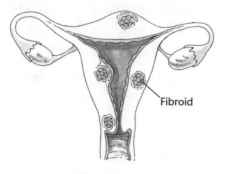

UTERUS WITH FIBROIDS

If your fibroids are not causing you problems and you are not planning to become pregnant, you may want to do nothing at all about them, especially if you are close to menopause, when fibroids usually shrink. But if you have symptoms, such as heavy bleeding to the point where you are anemic, or if you want to become pregnant, there are several treatment options (see chart opposite).

Not every one of these interventions is appropriate for every woman. Treatment depends on many factors, including your age, the size and number of the fibroids, the severity of the symptoms caused by the fibroid, and whether or not you want to have children. For example, gonadotropins are effective in the short term to relieve symptoms, but the fibroids return after the therapy is stopped. Some doctors prescribe the drugs before surgery because they help to shrink large fibroids. You need to discuss the options with your physician to determine the right treatment for you.

CONTRACEPTION

Many women today don't remember a time before the pill became widely available, but there are, and have always been, many alternative methods of birth control. As with any medication, there are pluses and minuses to consider.

Andrea came to see me because she was scared. Everyone in her family had died early, in their forties, of heart disease. She considered herself healthy and never had to see her doctor except for her yearly checkup. The only medication she was taking was birth control pills. She had just turned thirty-seven and wanted me to assess her risk of heart

OPTIONS FOR FIBROIDS

Treatment	Where/How to Get It	What It Does	Side Effects
Pain medication (nonsteroidal anti-inflammatories such as Advil or Motrin)	Over the counter	Temporary pain relief	Stomach upset, bleeding, high blood pressure
Birth control pills	Prescription	Reduces bleeding, thus reducing pain and pressure	Raises blood pressure Causes weight gain Increases risk of blood clots to leg or lung Causes gallstones Warning: avoid smoking while taking birth control pills
Gonadotropin-releasing hormone agonists (GnRHa)	Hormone medication Injection or inhaler	Reduces size Improves anemia	Causes depression, insomnia, reduced libido
Myomectomy	Laparoscopic surgery	Removes fibroid Restores normal menstrual flow Better option if pregnancy is considered in future	Risks of surgery are infection and bleeding
Hysterectomy	Surgery to remove uterus	Controls heavy bleeding Reduces anemia	Can't become pregnant Onset of menopausal symptoms
Myolysis	Electrical needle through the abdomen	Cuts off blood supply to fibroid, causing it to shrink Reduces bleeding	A new procedure; not clear if it affects fertility or if it is more effective than hysterectomy and myomectomy

Treatment	Where/How to Get It	What It Does	Side Effects
Uterine fibroid embolization (UFE)	A catheter is threaded into the blood vessel feeding your fibroid and an artificial clot is introduced to block blood flow to the fibroid like a plug	Cuts off blood supply to uterus Shorter down time compared to surgery Pregnancy possible, more likely to be by C-section Considered better for women who are in their postpregnancy years	New procedure May need hysterectomy if it doesn't work Vaginal discharge, infection
Radiofrequency ablation (MRI and ultrasound used to locate fibroid)	Radiological procedures Less invasive than hysterectomy, myomectomy	Uses heat energy to destroy fibroid	New procedure Still being evaluated for risks

disease so that she could take evasive action. This is exactly the kind of patient I, as a cardiologist, like to see—someone who is ready to prevent heart disease.

Her laboratory testing indicated that her cholesterol was elevated. A level as high as Andrea's is usually treated with medication, but my recommendation to her was not to panic. I told her that the elevated cholesterol might be inherited, or from the birth control pills, or a combination of both. I suggested a change in birth control and told her to repeat cholesterol testing in three months' time.

My experience with Andrea reminded me how important it is to treat the whole person, not simply the symptoms the person presents. Although I repeatedly reassured her that she would be okay, her fear overrode everything I said. She didn't tell me directly how frightened she was, but she called and called and asked the same questions over and over. Finally I realized that she needed more direct reassurance, so I asked her to come in for another discussion of her test results. I could hear the relief over the phone. Sometimes it's important to talk to patients face-to-face—even to tell them that nothing is wrong.

When she came in, I told her how good it was that she had been proactive, checking herself out because of her family history. I also told her how common her symptoms were in women on birth control, and since hormones can elevate cholesterol, someone with her history probably should not take them. We talked for a while, and I told her that by simply stopping the birth control pills, she was doing everything she could to keep herself in good health.

In fact, when the tests were repeated after three months, her cholesterol was normal.

TYPES OF CONTRACEPTION

There are many choices for contraceptives, and most are very effective when used properly. However, there are risks and side effects, and as always, these should be considered. There are some general principles, however. If you have multiple sexual partners, or if your partner has multiple partners, you may want to use one of the barrier methods (condoms, diaphragms) in order to protect yourself from sexually transmitted infections and HIV. If you are over thirty-five, smoke, and have any history of heart disease or stroke, or any of the risk factors that might predispose you to these conditions, I would recommend that you avoid hormone-based contraceptives because the combination of risk factors and hormones increases the risk of heart attack and stroke. Talk to your doctor.

Birth control pills. These must be prescribed by a doctor. They work by tricking the body into thinking it's pregnant, thereby suppressing ovulation and thickening cervical mucus. The pills, combinations of estrogen and progestin, are taken orally for a number of consecutive days, stopped for a short interval, and then started again. If taken properly, the pill is 99 percent effective against pregnancy.

There are some risk factors associated with taking oral contraceptives. As I said, women who are over thirty-five, women who smoke, and women who have conditions associated with heart attack such as diabetes, high blood pressure, high cholesterol, or certain conditions that increase the risk of blood clots should discuss the risk and benefits of taking the pill with their doctor. There is research that shows that taking oral contraceptives increases the risk for heart attack eightfold in women over thirty-five who smoke. That's why it's a good idea to have a complete physical workup before you decide what form of birth control is right for you. Some women experience side effects, such as water retention, breast tenderness, depression, and nausea.

Birth control patch. Also called a transdermal patch because it is applied to the skin, the patch works by releasing hormones (estrogen and progesterone) to prevent ovulation and thicken cervical mucus. The patch is changed weekly and is worn for three weeks consecutively; after a break of a week, the patch is reapplied for another three weeks. It must be prescribed by a physician. When used correctly, it is 99 percent effective.

However, you should be aware that in November 2005, the FDA published a warning that women wearing the patch might be exposed to higher levels of estrogen than they would be on most birth control pills. High levels of estrogen put some women at increased risk for blood clots, strokes, and heart attacks. Women who smoke are at greater risk for these complications and should find another form of birth control. Discuss these risks with your doctor.

Implants. As the name suggests, implants must be surgically implanted by a physician, usually in the upper arm. They are tiny capsules that release hormones (progestin) to prevent ovulation and to thicken cervical mucus. They must be replaced every five years and can be removed at any time. This method is almost 100 percent effective but may have side effects, such as irregular bleeding.

Hormone injections. Like the other hormone contraceptives, the injections suppress ovulation and thicken the cervical mucus. A physician injects hormones into the arm, thigh, or buttocks at regular intervals. If properly administered, injections are almost 100 percent effective. However, once the injections are stopped, fertility may not return for up to eight months. The injected hormones may lower HDL (good) cholesterol and increase the risk of contracting a sexually transmitted infection.

Vaginal ring. A vaginal ring must be prescribed by a physician. It is a soft, flexible ring that releases hormones (estrogen) to prevent ovulation. A woman inserts it herself, and it is worn consecutively for three weeks and removed for one week each month. When used correctly, it is 95 percent effective.

Diaphragm. A diaphragm is a physical rather than hormonal means to prevent pregnancy. It is a soft cup of synthetic material that has to be properly fitted by a physician to be effective. You insert the diaphragm into the vagina when you need protection. Not only does it physically block sperm from entering the uterus by covering the cervix, but it also holds a spermicidal jelly or cream so that any sperm that may make it past the rim are killed. You should leave the diaphragm in place for six hours after intercourse but not longer than twenty-four hours because there is a risk of toxic shock syndrome (a rare but sometimes fatal bacterial infection). Some women who use a diaphragm develop urinary tract infections. When a diaphragm is properly fitted and used correctly in combination with a spermicide, it is about 94 percent effective.

Male condom. A male condom is easily available and can be bought without a prescription. It is a sheath designed to fit over an erect penis so that when ejaculation occurs, the semen is collected inside the condom. It is important to remove the condom carefully so that the semen doesn't spill. Condoms provide protection against sexually transmitted infections (STIs). A recent study showed that women who had not had previous sexual partners and whose male partners used condoms consistently were 70 percent less likely to acquire the highly contagious STI caused by the human papilloma virus (HPV). Women whose partners used condoms half the time had a 50 percent decrease in risk. This shows the importance of using condoms regularly.[3] When used correctly, they can be 97 percent effective at preventing pregnancy.

Female condom. A female condom is also available without a prescription. It is a lubricated sheath that lines the vaginal walls and has rings on each end. One ring remains outside the vagina; the other is closed and covers the cervix like a diaphragm. Since the female condom provides a physical barrier, it protects against STIs. When used correctly, it can be 95 percent effective.

Spermicides. Spermicides do not require a prescription and come in several forms: foams, creams, jellies, or suppositories. Used alone or with barrier methods (condoms, diaphragms), they function to kill sperm on contact, thereby preventing fertilization. However, when used alone, they are only 26 percent effective in preventing pregnancy; therefore it is best to couple spermicides with other contraceptive methods. Also, they do not reduce the risk of infection.

Intrauterine devices (*IUD*). An IUD must be inserted into the uterus by a physician. It is made of soft plastic material, is about one and a half inches long, and has two strings attached. IUDs contain either copper or synthetic hormones. Those with synthetic hormones should be avoided by women over thirty-five, women who smoke, and women with risk factors for heart disease and stroke, just like other hormone-based contraception. Both types of IUD prevent conception by affecting the lining of the uterus and the cervix, although it is not entirely clear why or how. IUDs are about 99 percent effective when inserted correctly. You should check that the string is in place after each period, but don't pull on it. IUDs should not be the choice of birth control for women who have a history of unexplained vaginal bleeding or who have an STI. There is an increased risk of pelvic infections and of cramping.

GROWING OLDER WITH YOUR OVARIES

Although the reasons are unknown, hormone production changes during your mid-thirties. By the time you reach your late forties, this hormone fluctuation usually results in shorter menstrual cycles (less time between periods) and lighter flow during menstruation. Typically, in your early to mid-fifties, your ovaries begin to shrink and hormone production decreases until eventually your periods end.

Doris, who is forty-nine, came to see me because she was having palpitations every night, and they were accompanied by hot flashes. She was sure something was terribly wrong. She had read my previous book about women and heart disease and so knew that very often women's heart symptoms are misdiagnosed.

I asked her if the palpitations made her feel faint, and she said no. I also asked about the amount of caffeine that she drank, and while taking her history asked about any thyroid disease and if she had any history of heart disease. I also asked whether her menstrual periods were unusually heavy or irregular.

Although she was still menstruating, her periods had been irregular for several months. Since I suspected that her symptoms were related to perimenopause and she hadn't seen a gynecologist in a while, I recommended that she go for a routine checkup, including a Pap smear. As I say, it's always important to rule out physical causes other than meno-pause before making the diagnosis.

As it turned out, Doris's palpitations were the result of natural hor-monal changes, consistent with perimenopause. One option for her would be hormone therapy, which would reduce the palpitations, even out the hormone levels, and mitigate the hot flashes, which would help her sleep. But because of a family history of heart disease and cancer, she was reluctant to take hormones.

The biggest help for Doris was to realize that her heart was fine and that her symptoms were normal and not dangerous. Women, so often trained to be "good" girls, may not complain about symptoms; if they do seek medical attention, the doctor (especially if he's male) may tell them that their complaints are simply a result of getting older. The implication is that they should get over it and deal.

But it is dangerous to assume that every problem is just a part of aging. You don't want to dismiss a heart issue, such as palpitations, as normal without going to check out the symptoms with a doctor. Once you get plugged into the medical system, you'll have your heart, blood pressure, cholesterol, thyroid levels, and other indicators monitored. That is a good thing.

Are You Moving Toward Menopause?

As I explained in the beginning of this section, the changes that herald menopause, called perimenopause, usually begin about six to ten years before menstruation finally ends, typically in a woman's late forties. Vari-ations in estrogen and progesterone levels cause irregular periods. Not only is the timing of menstruation different from one month to the next, but the flow may be very inconsistent—heavy one month and very light the next. Spotting can also occur. Also, during these years, as estrogen levels begin to decline, weight, blood pressure, and cholesterol levels may increase. (These symptoms may not be as pronounced if you are on the pill.) Perimenopause can also be associated with the symptoms of menopause, including hot flashes, sleeplessness, and night sweats, and may even be more severe than after menopause. Or as many of my friends say, they simply don't feel like themselves. My friend Gail calls it "going to the dark side." Some women who want to know whether their symptoms relate to perimenopause have their FSH level tested. A high FSH level usually coincides with low estrogen levels. Tests for levels of progesterone, luteinizing hormone, and estrogen are not always helpful in clinching the diagnosis because the numbers can go up and down on a daily basis.

HOW TO ASSESS YOUR MENOPAUSAL STATUS

The World Health Organization has a classification system for determining where you are in relation to your menopausal status. These definitions are what your doctor uses to determine where you are in this progression:

- Premenopausal: women over the age of thirty-five who are having regular menstrual periods

- Perimenopausal: women who have irregular menstrual cycles with at least some menstrual bleeding during the previous year

- Menopausal: women who have had no menstrual periods in the past year

How to Manage Your Menopause

Every woman I speak to, either professionally or otherwise, has a unique experience of menopause and reacts to that experience entirely individually. When I conducted an informal poll of my friends, one said she had only muscle cramps, another said she was hot on rare occasions, and another was still menstruating at the age of fifty-eight. With so much individual experience, it's difficult to talk about menopause as if it were a single definable medical phenomenon.

The tendency to medicalize and pathologize this perfectly normal physiological change has unfortunately suggested to American women (and more than thirty-two million women in the United States are menopausal) that something is wrong with them. Nothing is wrong. On the contrary, menopause is as natural and expected as puberty. Sometimes, however, hormone fluctuations result in unpleasant symptoms. Depending on intensity, you and your doctor can decide if your symptoms are tolerable or require some treatment. Don't think that everyone suffers; 15 to 20 percent of women experience no physical symptoms at all other than the end of their menstrual periods.

For the boomer generation, often so competent and in control of their lives, the unfamiliar and sometimes extreme symptoms of menopause can be unsettling, to say the least. A patient of mine who had had a heart attack when she was forty-five called because her menopausal symptoms were driving her crazy. She said she didn't feel like herself at all. She handled her heart problem with more equanimity than her hot flashes.

MENOPAUSE ACROSS CULTURES

There is anthropological research showing that American women experience more symptoms of menopause than women in other cultures and that their symptoms are more severe. It has been suggested that our reverence for youth contributes to this. That seems likely. Postmenopausal women often are depicted as sexless, unproductive, unattractive, and invisible, and so for many American women menopause is accompanied by a sense of endings and loss. It has become a disease that needs to be cured.

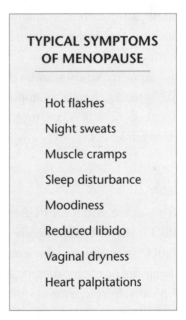

TYPICAL SYMPTOMS OF MENOPAUSE

Hot flashes

Night sweats

Muscle cramps

Sleep disturbance

Moodiness

Reduced libido

Vaginal dryness

Heart palpitations

In many cultures, however, menopause is considered not as the beginning of the end but as a transition from a time of childbearing to one of individualized growth and increased wisdom. Although research is inconclusive, evidence is mounting that cultural diversity and biological differences have an impact on how women experience their menopause, and certainly about how they communicate that experience. In India, many symptoms, such as depression and dizziness, are entirely unknown. Mexican Mayan women report no symptoms at all except absent periods. Women in Botswana report no symptoms other than enjoying sex more without fear of pregnancy. These cross-cultural data indicate that cultural attitudes have an impact on severity of symptoms—or at least on the way those symptoms are interpreted.

WHAT INFLUENCES THE TIMING OF MENOPAUSE?

The average age at which menopause occurs is between forty-seven and fifty-three. Remember that "average" means that many women stop their periods before that age or after; the range can be anywhere from thirty to sixty. The timing of menopause is influenced primarily by genetics, especially the age at which your mother stopped menstruating. Studies show that women who smoke experience menopause three years earlier on average than those who don't, but oral contraceptives, the number of children you have had, and race have no impact on the age of onset.

However, there are some social factors that do make a difference. A study conducted at Harvard's Brigham and Women's Hospital found that women who are living in poverty are 80 percent more likely to begin menopause earlier. Perhaps it is environmental factors, such as stress, poor nourishment, exposure to toxins, and smoking, that lead to earlier symptoms of menopause.[4]

Another study showed that depressed women were 20 percent more likely to experience menopausal symptoms earlier than women without depression. Stress, a symptom of depression, is associated with lowered estrogen levels.[5]

PREMATURE MENOPAUSE

Women are said to be in premature menopause if they have had no periods for three months before age forty. This could be caused by hormone deficiencies, genetic abnormalities, autoimmune disease, viral infections, radiation, or chemotherapy. Women who undergo premature menopause typically have hormones in the menopausal range and experience the same menopausal symptoms as women who go through menopause at a normal age.

SURGICAL MENOPAUSE

Although the majority of women experience menopause naturally, sometimes medications and medical treatments, such as radiation or chemotherapy, can cause the ovaries to stop producing estrogen and trigger menopause. Surgery that removes both ovaries (as in a total hysterectomy) will induce menopause too, and because the change is sudden, as opposed to the gradual change of natural menopause, women may experience more dramatic symptoms.

A patient recently told me that after her hysterectomy she was suddenly depressed, couldn't sleep, gained weight, and was "dry down there." If only someone had explained to her what to expect after her hysterectomy, she would have understood and perhaps prepared herself to relieve these symptoms.

HOT FLASHES

Just recently I was having lunch with a group of friends. One of them, who is in her fifties, starting peeling off her jacket and fanning herself. I hear women asking all the time, "Is it hot in here or am I having a flash?" Hot flashes are very common: between 50 and 85 percent of women experience them, usually during the years leading up to menopause (perimenopause) rather than after menstruation has stopped. These sudden and uncomfortable flashes usually end after a few years, but for 10 to 15 percent of women they may last the rest of their lives. Among the most troubling characteristics of hot flashes is that they can't be anticipated, sometimes coming at inconvenient or embarrassing times. My patients tell me that they get them in the middle of meetings, while they are in waiting rooms, at the gym, and even sometimes while I'm taking their blood pressure. One minute they are fine, and the next they are soaked in sweat.

Here are some practical and natural ways that women I know have handled their hot flashes. It may seem obvious, but try to keep yourself in a cool environment. Turn off the heat. Turn on the AC or fan. Dress lightly or in easy-to-remove layers. Some women find that meditation or yoga helps, others that strenuous exercise provides some relief.

Researchers believe that hot flashes happen as estrogen levels fall. Falling estrogen alters the level of brain chemicals that regulate our temperature center. As this happens, there may be a sense of warmth that may be associated with anxiety, perspiration, and palpitations. Hot flashes are more prevalent in African American women and Latinas compared to white women and are less common in Asian women.

Hot flashes are characterized as mild, moderate, or severe. The more severe the hot flashes, the greater the likelihood of your also experiencing insomnia. One study found that 80 percent of women with severe hot flashes had symptoms of chronic insomnia as well.[6] Chronic insomnia is defined as difficulty falling asleep, staying asleep, or feeling refreshed after sleeping.

How Do You Handle Symptoms of Menopause?

In order to make a decision about how to treat menopausal symptoms, you and your doctor should assess how you feel and how you manage your symptoms. Severity of symptoms is entirely subjective and varies among women. Some women can manage not sleeping; others feel awful all day if their night is disrupted. Some women find that vaginal dryness makes them too uncomfortable during sex to have a normal sex life; others whip out the K-Y jelly and manage just fine. You may want to figure out what you can live with and what is too difficult. Quality of life counts! If you are someone who is finding it very difficult to tolerate the symptoms of menopause, a short-term (less than five years) low dose of hormone, carefully monitored by a physician, might enable you to manage the worst of your symptoms with little adverse health impact.

THE HOT FLASH SCALE

MILD
A sensation of heat that occurs without sweating and does not limit your activities

MODERATE
A sensation of heat accompanied by sweating, although not limiting your activities

SEVERE
A sensation of heat accompanied by sweating that stops your activity

Let's Talk About Hormone Therapy

Unless you have been living on another planet, you probably have heard that hormone therapy (HT), previously extolled as a cure for everything from heart disease to Alzheimer's disease, has fallen out of favor. Most physicians are no longer recommending it with the abandon of previous decades.

Because estrogen is good for you, doctors were prescribing it for postmenopausal women. The thinking was that you don't want to do without something that works to keep you healthy (not to mention young, beautiful, and sexy). Recent research, however, has revealed that this prescription doesn't work and can actually have negative consequences, such as an increased risk of uterine cancer. To try to reduce this risk, progesterone was added to estrogen, but even this combination of hormones has been shown to increase the risk of developing breast cancer in some women. If you have early menopause or surgically induced menopause (that is, a hysterectomy or removal of the ovaries), you will probably be prescribed hormone therapy to mitigate the effects of the sudden onset of symptoms.

A BRIEF HISTORY OF HORMONE THERAPY

Did you ever wonder how hormone therapy got started? It's a pretty weird story and not as scientific as you might have thought. In 1889, a seventy-two-year-old French physiologist, Charles-Edouard Brown-Séquard, in an attempt to introduce new vigor into his virility, injected himself with a combination of mashed testicles of dogs and guinea pigs. No kidding. According to his writings, his "vitality" then returned to a more youthful state.

In 1899, the *Merck Manual for Diagnosis and Therapy* listed Ovariin, a concoction of dried and pulverized cow ovaries, as relief for the symptoms of menopause (which was called the "climacteric" at the time). In the early years of the twentieth century, John Brinkley, an American physician, began using goat testicle transplants to restore men's "vitality." Eventually his medical license was revoked, but not before he performed more than sixteen thousand transplants. And so the notion that hormones could be replaced and would counteract the effects of age was introduced.

Before you get sick to your stomach, remember that the estrogen that most women are prescribed for hormone therapy is Premarin, which comes from the urine of pregnant mares (*pre* = pregnant, *mar* = mare, *in* = urine).

The FDA approved the use of estrogen in 1941 for symptoms of menopause. By the 1950s hormones were big business and drug companies were reaping gigantic profits in sales of estrogens to women hoping to remain forever young. Physicians, responding to the complaints of their patients, were happy to prescribe hormones. Everyone—women, physicians, and the drug companies—was happy until very recently, when objective evidence from research concluded that the hormonal fountain of youth was not all it was promised to be. As more medical information has come to light, it turns out that things are way more complicated than originally thought. Surprise, surprise.

In the 1960s, the medical community thought that we had found the "cure" for aging in estrogen. The concept was promoted by a best-selling popular book written in 1963 by a New York gynecologist, Robert Wilson, called *Feminine Forever*. In this book, Wilson argues that menopause is a disease caused by estrogen deficiency and unless women were treated with estrogen replacement, they would continue to experience inevitable "living decay." It was bad enough that laypeople were swallowing this idea, but I was shocked to learn from a colleague that it was recommended reading for her gynecology rotation in medical school. It's a very good thing indeed that we have come a long way.

IT'S NEVER TOTALLY BLACK OR WHITE

As a cardiologist and a women's health specialist, I think the publicity, both pro and con, surrounding hormone therapy has been extreme, whether it was Wilson's *Feminine Forever* telling us that HT was a perfect solution to horrors of menopause or the results of the widely publicized Women's Health Initiative study, telling us HT will give you a heart attack.

What the recent studies show is that hormone therapy does not reduce the risk of heart disease and stroke, as was previously thought, but it is beneficial for the relief of menopausal symptoms, as was previously thought.

As a physician and a woman, I want to give you a better understanding of how to personalize the almost daily flow of information on HT in the media so that when you are ready to have a conversation with your doctor about menopause and your symptoms, you will be able to make an educated and informed choice about whether you want treatment. In order to more effectively decide whether to take HT or not, let me share a doctor's approach to wading through the information so you understand why different recommendations are made for different women. I hope this will help you feel more comfortable discussing it with your health care provider.

HT 101

Hormone therapy refers to medication that contains one or more of the female hormones. HT can be just estrogen, or a combination of estrogen and progesterone. There are reasons to prescribe one rather than another. If you have a uterus, estrogen will be combined with progesterone, which decreases the risk of uterine cancer. If your uterus has been removed, you are most likely to be prescribed estrogen alone.

It's important to realize that what was thought to be fact a few years ago may no longer be accurate. Most of our current information about hormone therapy comes from a massive study of almost 162,000 women, ranging in age from fifty to seventy-nine, that was conducted by the Women's Health Initiative (WHI). The WHI was established by the National Institutes of Health (NIH) in 1991 with the goal of addressing disease and disability, such as stroke, heart attack, colon cancer, and Alzheimer's disease, in postmenopausal women.

Part of the WHI study involved examining the health risks and benefits of hormone replacement. There were two hormone components to the study: estrogen alone for women with no uterus and estrogen plus progestin (a synthetic progesterone) for women with a uterus. In 2002, after five years, the estrogen and progestin arm of the study was stopped because interim results had shown an increase of 26 percent in the breast cancer rate and an increased risk of heart attack in women taking the hormones. In 2004 the estrogen-only arm of the study was also stopped due to health risks as well, but this risk was an increased rate of stroke. The study also found that estrogen alone increased the risk of blood clots, reduced the risk of hip fractures, and had no impact (as was once believed) on colorectal cancer, and that estrogen and progestin increased the rate of dementia in women over sixty-five.

One of the biggest problems with this study was that the hormone therapy was given to women who were already ten to fifteen years past menopause. These women may have already had asymptomatic heart disease. The study did not address the question of the safety of HT therapy in women in their forties and fifties who were healthy and just entering menopause. In February 2006, the WHI researchers did a further analysis and found that estrogen alone did not offer protection against heart attack for the study participants overall, though the results suggested that it may offer some protection to women between the ages of fifty and fifty-nine.[7] It is clear that the connection between hormones and heart disease needs further evaluation and that you should be very careful to read the fine print of any study before you swallow the results.

The latest news (2006) from the NIH, however, updates the estrogen-only analysis. While researchers found no increased rate of breast cancer, study participants receiving estrogen had 50 percent more abnormal mammograms that required follow-up, including biopsies.[8] Even with this update, the recommendation remains that HT should be used only to treat menopausal symptoms and should be used at the lowest possible dose for the shortest time. Although HT does provide protection against osteoporosis, the problem is that the benefit exists only as long as the hormones are being taken. Therefore, the treatment needs to be for a lifetime.

Because the media hypes results of studies without detailing the important subtleties, it is important not to react too quickly when you see or hear a news item about hormone therapy. Years ago some women insisted on taking HT even though they had no symptoms because they were told it would be good for them. Many women stopped taking HT in 2002 even though they had severe symptoms because they were told it was not good for them. But new information comes in every day, and there should never be complete acceptance or rejection. You and your doctor need to assess the benefits *to you* of having any kind of medication or therapy.

The latest concern about hormone therapy is an increased risk of ovarian cancer. A 2007 research study involving more than nine hundred thousand postmenopausal women, some of whom were using hormone therapy, some who had had HT in the past, and others who had never used HT, found a slightly increased risk of ovarian cancer in women who were currently using HT and had been using it for five years. Previous studies had not shown this association. In the new study, the type of hormone therapy or the method of taking it (patch or pill) didn't matter.[9]

IS HT RIGHT FOR YOU?

Wouldn't life be easier if there were always only a single solution to each problem? Your health status is complicated, and although there are concerns about HT, and especially about taking hormones for more than five years, you also need to be able to live your life. If menopausal symptoms are terribly disruptive and your quality of life is compromised, you should evaluate with your doctor if you are a candidate for HT. Like any decision to take medication, it should be based on your symptoms, your medical history, and your risks for breast and ovarian cancer and heart disease. Your doctor will take your history, determine your menopausal status, and perhaps do some hormonal testing. But be aware that the tests are not 100 percent accurate because hormone levels during perimenopause may be high or low on a given day. The most accurate test is the FSH test, and levels above 40 IU/L (international units per liter) are consistent with menopause.

THERE ARE VARIOUS OPTIONS FOR HORMONAL THERAPY

When hormone therapy is prescribed for relief of menopausal symptoms, therapy is short-term. For osteoporosis, hormones are used as long-term therapy. Long-term therapy, that is, more than five years, is associated with increased risk of breast cancer, stroke, and heart attack. There have been recent studies that indicate that women who started the hormone therapy early in menopause were less likely to have these risks.

In addition to the risks already discusssed, possible side effects of hormone therapy include weight gain, breast tenderness, postmenopausal bleeding, gallstones, and migraine headaches.

Local therapy. Among the unpleasant symptoms of perimenopause and menopause is vaginal dryness. It's a common complaint, affecting between 10 and 40 percent of menopausal women. (Some medications, including ones for cancer treatment, allergies, antidepressants, and high blood pressure, also can cause vaginal dryness.) One completely safe, non-

A GUIDE FOR WHETHER TO TAKE HT

You have to determine whether or not your menopausal symptoms are negatively affecting your quality of life. The following questions can serve as a guide:

• Do you have menopausal symptoms?

• Where are you on the scale of menopausal symptoms? Are they moderate or severe?

• Do your symptoms keep you from you usual activities (sleeping, sex)?

If you are having symptoms that are adversely affecting your life, a low dose of HT should be considered for a short term. However, you should consider the following questions:

Do you have heart disease? If the answer is yes, don't take HT. If women who have a history of heart disease or stroke take HT, they can be at increased risk for a recurrence.

Do you have breast cancer? If yes, don't take HT. Even if you have a family history of breast cancer, it may not be a good idea to take HT, since it puts you at an increased risk for developing breast cancer. If you decide that you want to go on HT, make sure to have a mammogram before you start therapy, and have regular tests.

Do you have osteoporosis? If yes, you may want to take HT. Estrogen improves bone density. But remember it only works for as long as you take it. Once you stop therapy, bone loss begins again. There are other options (see Chapter 9).

Do you have a history of blood clots to the legs or lungs? If so, HT is not the right therapy for you since it increases the risk of recurrent blood clots to the legs, known as deep vein thrombosis (DVT), and clots to the lung, which is a potentially life-threatening condition.

invasive remedy for this problem is using a lubricant. Another low-risk remedy involves applying hormones where they are needed. Local options include:

• Vaginal estrogen cream, which you insert into your vagina several times a week

- Vaginal estrogen ring, a soft plastic ring that is inserted into the upper part of your vagina and releases estrogen for three months
- Vaginal estrogen tablets, which you insert into your vagina regularly

Estrogen skin patches and oral hormone supplements, which also help with vaginal dryness, are generally not prescribed unless you are suffering from other menopausal symptoms.

Skin patches. Skin patches that contain either estrogen plus progestin or estrogen only are applied to the skin either weekly or several times a week (depending on brand) to relieve menopausal symptoms and prevent bone loss. But because they deliver estrogen systemically, they carry the same potential risks associated with other nonlocal forms of HT, such as an increased risk for blood clots. The patch may be better for women with high triglycerides because this method of delivering the medication does not raise triglycerides the way oral HT does. Patch therapy has never been studied specifically on the risk of heart disease, but as with oral HT, it should not be used if you

RISKS AND BENEFITS OF HORMONE THERAPY

BENEFITS OF ESTROGEN

Reduces hip and other fractures

Reduces menopausal symptoms

Increases levels of good or HDL cholesterol

Lowers bad or LDL cholesterol

Does not increase risk for breast cancer

Improves the flexibility of blood vessels

RISKS OF ESTROGEN

Strokes and blood clots

Gallstones

BENEFITS OF ESTROGEN PLUS PROGESTIN

Reduced fractures

Reduces risk of uterine cancer

RISKS OF ESTROGEN PLUS PROGESTIN

Heart attack

Stroke and other blood clots

Hearing loss (attributed to the progestin)

have any history of blood clots, liver disease, cancer, or heart disease. Also, there could be local irritation of the skin.

Oral hormone therapy. If you have no uterus, you would take estrogen alone. If you still have a uterus, combination therapy of estrogen and progestin is given to reduce the risk of developing uterine cancer. Dosages differ depending on your symptoms and on the type of HT you are prescribed. The best idea is to take the lowest effective dose for the least amount of time necessary to manage your symptoms. Usually the hormones are given as tablets. Because estrogen has been associated with potential problems (see page 87), you should be checked by your doctor at least once a year; many doctors will want to monitor your status more often. Since HT may contribute to breast cancer risk, your breasts should be checked frequently and any discharge or lump reported to your doctor immediately.

TESTOSTERONE

A word about testosterone therapy, which is sometimes prescribed to mitigate the symptoms of loss of libido and loss of energy associated with menopause. The treatment is controversial and not recommended to women who are not taking estrogen. Although it may help with the symptoms, the downside—fluid retention, cholesterol abnormalities, and increased hair growth—should be considered as well.

BIOIDENTICAL HORMONE THERAPY

Some women who are reluctant to take commercial synthetic preparations of HT take plant-derived compounds as an alternative to relieve menopausal symptoms. The problem with this is that these compounds have the same chemical structure as the synthetic versions and therefore carry similar risks. But because they are not "drugs," they are not regulated by the FDA.

According to the American College of Obstetrics and Gynecology (ACOG), there is no scientific evidence that bioidentical hormones (as this alternative is called) are safer or more effective than synthetic preparations. ACOG expressed concern that although the structures are the same, these compounds have not been tested and since there are few research trials using them, they may in fact be unsafe. Remember how many women were first thrilled and then disappointed with the conflicting evidence regarding the use of HT? So my advice is that before you jump on the biodentical hormone bandwagon, wait for more research. And if you take these compounds, make sure to alert your doctor.

Nonhormonal Therapy for Menopausal Symptoms

Women who experience mild symptoms of menopause have benefited from lifestyle changes, such as more exercise, dressing in layers, and sleeping in a cool room. Don't smoke. In addition to all the other reasons for not smoking, women who smoke are more likely to have severe hot flashes and earlier menopause (not to mention wrinkles around the mouth).

Because of all the negative publicity surrounding hormone therapy, women have tried to find alternatives to mitigate especially severe symptoms of menopause. These alternative therapies include:

- Antidepressants, especially selective serotonin reuptake inhibitors (SSRIs) such as Paxil, which may improve sleep and reduce anxiety

- Blood pressure medications, such as clonidine, to relieve hot flashes

- Soy products and other dietary supplements, such as vitamin E

- Herbs, such as black cohosh, dong quai, red clover, and ginseng

- Other nonmedical techniques, including massage and stress management

CAUTIONS BEFORE USING NONHORMONAL THERAPIES

The FDA does not regulate complementary and alternative products and treatments, and anecdotal evidence (women telling their friends and physicians) about success is unreliable and unscientific. Recent research suggests that soy products and herbal supplements do not reduce menopausal symptoms.

In the May 3, 2006, edition of the *Journal of the American Medical*

Association, many trials involving these alternative therapies were reviewed. The researchers examined the results of trials of various alternative therapies: antidepressants (such as Paxil), blood pressure medication, antiseizure medication, and others. Isoflavone extracts from red clover and soy were also examined. The goal was to determine if these treatments helped with hot flashes, in terms both of number and intensity. Of the therapies that were tested, antidepressants were the most effective, but not as effective as estrogen.

Most of these studies were found to have serious methodological flaws, the results were inconclusive, and nearly all alternatives had adverse side effects. For example, antidepressants can cause headache, nausea, and insomnia, while clonidine can cause dry mouth and drowsiness. The researchers concluded that estrogen therapy remains the safest and most effective treatment for hot flashes.

LOWERED LIBIDO AFTER MENOPAUSE

Some women experience lowered libido as they approach menopause and after, and this is a problem many of them are reluctant to verbalize. In fact, many women don't define lowered libido as a medical problem at all but assume it is simply a natural part of the aging process, like wrinkles. Of course, it goes without saying that when you are exhausted and doing too much, you may have less urge for sex, regardless of your age. And it is important to rule out anemia, depression, diabetes, and thyroid problems as well, all of which can have an impact on libido. When my patients confide in me that their sex life is not what they would like it to be, I work with a gynecologist, and together with the patient we try to find an effective treatment. There are medications, such as combinations of estrogen and testosterone, that help.

Recently, the steroid DHEA (dehydroepiandrosterone) has been touted as a rejuvenator, restoring the lustiness of youth. Our adrenal glands produce DHEA naturally, and the amount in our bodies drops as we age. Parallel to the way we used to think about estrogen replacement, the theory of the past decade has been that if DHEA worked well in our youth, we should make sure we keep it up to youthful levels with a synthetic version. But, as with all drugs, be very careful. The use of this powerful drug is controversial at best, and experts agree that more clinical studies are needed to understand its impact on the body.

DHEA is what's known as a precursor hormone, involved in setting the stage for the sex hormones, such as estrogen, progesterone, and testosterone. Synthetic versions (usually extracted from yams) can be bought in pharmacies and health food stores without a prescription. Because it is a natural substance, DHEA can't be patented, and therefore there is very little incentive for pharmaceutical companies to support serious clinical trials about its safety and effectiveness.

Although DHEA was once thought to cure everything—obesity, depression, menopausal symptoms, low libido, Parkinson's disease, Alzheimer's—there is very little research to support these claims. Most of the evidence there is so far suggests that not only doesn't DHEA solve all of life's problems, but there are risks associated with taking it, such as increased rates of diabetes. Before you take a quick-fix supplement, talk to your doctor.

SHOULD YOU TAKE CALCIUM AFTER MENOPAUSE?

Whether to take calcium after menopause seems like a simple question, but it's not. It's perfectly reasonable to assume that if your bones are more vulnerable due to lower estrogen after menopause, and calcium helps with bone strength, then you should take extra calcium (see Chapter 9). Perfectly logical? Yes. Medically sound? Well, maybe not.

A 2006 study by the Women's Health Initiative, published in the *New England Journal of Medicine,* showed that calcium supplements did not reduce the risk of fractures from osteoporosis in postmenopausal women, as had been previously thought.[10] In fact, the study found that calcium supplements increased the risk of kidney stones. There was some evidence that a subset of women, those over sixty years old, did benefit by having a small improvement in hip bone density.

This study was carefully done, but as with most studies of this sort, there are questions left unanswered. For example, in this study the women were not pretested for calcium deficiency. There are some who believe that women who adhered to the supplement regime were not typical of the general population. Also, there was no investigation into the eating habits of the women, particularly to see if their diet was high or low in high-calcium foods.

The upshot is that the jury is still out on calcium supplements. Calcium can always be added to your diet naturally through foods, including low-fat dairy products and vegetables such as broccoli, brussels sprouts, and snap peas. I recommend supplementation for women who are not able to get enough calcium in their diet. I also do a blood test to evaluate if my patients have enough vitamin D, since this vitamin plays a major role in calcium absorption.

I feel that it is very important to stress that everything we do has an up-side and a downside. Our bodies are too complex to have an easy black-or-white answer to complicated questions. Everyone ages, and the aging process comes with physical changes. Always weigh the risks and bene-fits of your choices. This is another case in which it's often a good idea to wait and watch.

Your best bet is to see your gynecologist regularly and maintain an active and healthy lifestyle to ward off chronic disease.

SIX

Your OB-GYN

IT USED TO BE THAT THE SPECIALTY OF OBSTETRICS AND GYNECOL-ogy was concerned almost exclusively with women's reproductive health and nothing more. A normal gynecological visit encompassed a physical exam to check your ovaries and uterus, a Pap smear to test for cervical abnormalities, including cervical cancer, and a breast exam to feel for any lumps. Today, however, the role has expanded, and the regular office visit has moved away from the legs-up-head-down position to an examination of the entire body and an evaluation of total health status.

One of the reasons for this change is that for many women their gynecologist is the only doctor they see regularly. Therefore she functions as the primary care physician. Because the total woman is the patient, not just her reproductive organs, now a blood pressure check, cholesterol screening, urinalysis, assessment of bone strength, heart function check, and emotional well-being screening are all normally included as part of the yearly checkup as well. Medical organizations have become aware of how many thousands of women use their gynecologist as their primary care physician, and are trying to educate gynecologists that their speculums are not enough. They are encouraged to examine the whole woman, order necessary blood work, and do other appropriate tests to ensure that their patients are healthy.

As gynecologists increase their scope of care and move from a specialty that dealt with pregnancy, childbirth, and surgery of the reproductive organs to the treatment of menopausal symptoms and other issues common to women at midlife, they often recommend specialists to manage specific medical problems, such as heart disease or diabetes. If you are using your gynecologist as your primary care physician, make sure she functions as the coordinator of all your care and has a record or report from your specialists about medications and test results. If your care is more a team effort than dependent on one individual, it's important that someone be in charge.

WHAT TO EXPECT AT YOUR FIRST VISIT TO AN OB-GYN

As with any initial visit, a new doctor has to get to know you. So a regular checkup should start with a medical history and a complete H and P (see page 13), in addition to a gynecological examination. While you are talking to your doctor about your history, you should take the opportunity to tell her about yourself and any health concerns you may have. Don't be surprised if your doctor asks you personal questions, such as how you feel during sex or if you feel depressed. Believe me, she is not prying, only trying to assess your health condition.

I always start off with the question "What brings you in today?" Once in a while someone responds by saying, "This is the time your secretary gave me for an appointment." Of course, what I am really asking is what is my patient's most pressing medical problem or what medical symptoms is she having. If the reason for the visit is a yearly physical, it's certainly okay to say that. Taking care of yourself is a good thing.

Most women begin seeing a gynecologist when they become sexually active, and they should continue regular yearly screenings through menopause and beyond because you should have a pelvic exam to test for abnormalities of your ovaries, uterus, and cervix. It's very important to tell your doctor about any symptoms you might have, even if you think they are trivial.

For example, irregular menstrual periods, which are common in peri-menopause, can be perfectly normal, or they can be a symptom of uterine abnormalities. If you don't tell your physician that your periods are intermittent or that you have heavy bleeding or if you have had bleeding after menopause (remember, that is defined as no periods for one year), she can't investigate these symptoms. Your doctor should be the one to decide whether further testing is indicated for any of your symptoms.

WHAT TO EXPECT TO ANSWER DURING YOUR INITIAL VISIT

In addition to the questions that are typically asked during an H and P, your OB-GYN might also ask:

- About your menstrual periods
- About your mother's menstrual periods
- About any urinary problems, such as infections, leakage, discharge
- About your alcohol and tobacco use
- About your obstetric history (pregnancies, abortions, births)
- About whether you have ever had an abnormal Pap test
- About your mammograms
- About menopausal symptoms, such as hot flashes
- About your emotional states

The doctor will do a physical exam. If you do not go to an internist for a regular checkup, it will be more thorough and include the entire body. If you do, the checkup may be less elaborate. Your blood pressure, pulse, height, and weight will be recorded. Some of my patients actually refuse to get on the scale, and others don't want to look. Nonetheless, weight is important—it gives the doctor information. The doctor should do a breast exam with you both lying down and sitting up and examine your legs for swelling, varicose veins, and vascular disease.

And then there is the pelvic exam, which most women find uncomfortable, either physically, psychologically, or both. I remember one of my patients telling me about how she "zens" herself out of her body during the pelvic exam because she finds it so difficult. The standard gynecological exam involves placing the women's feet in stirrups and inserting a speculum, which is a plastic or metal instrument, into the vagina in order to see the cervix (the opening to the uterus). The doctor also takes a sample of cervical cells, the Pap smear, to test for abnormalities, and feels (palpates) the uterus and ovaries for size and shape.

Stirrup use began so long ago that no one knows the actual reason why it was started in the first place. A recent study published in the *British Medical Journal,* the first to actually address how a woman feels during this exam, questioned the need for putting women in stirrups.[1] In this study 197 women were divided into two groups; half the group was in stirrups, the other half was not. The doctors found that the women who were examined without stirrups were able to get a Pap smear with less pain than the other group.

My patients frequently ask me to recommend a good gynecologist. Most women prefer a female doctor because they say they feel more at ease with one and better able to communicate. Besides the discomfort of the feet-in-the-stirrups exposure of this most intimate exam, I find that what women want is someone who will spend more than five minutes with them, four and a half of which are spent with the doctor's head between the woman's legs. They want to be heard and have a real conversation and to leave with the sense that someone actually cares about them. That's not really a great deal to ask for!

UNDERSTANDING THE PAP TEST

In the Pap test or Pap smear, the doctor takes a sample of cells from the cervix and sends them to a lab for microscopic analysis. This test provides your first line of defense against cervical cancer (see page 108). Usually it is recommended that women have yearly Pap tests as part of their normal checkups. Even if you have had a hysterectomy, depending on the kind of hysterectomy you have had (see page 109), you may still have a cervix and should be checked yearly. It's a good idea to ask your gynecologist how often you should have regular Pap tests. Everyone has a different health status. For example, women who are HIV-positive should have more frequent Pap tests, every six months.

If your Pap test comes back abnormal, don't panic. It does not necessarily mean you have cervical cancer, but only that your cells show some abnormality, which could be due to an inflammation or an infection. Pap tests, although basically reliable, are not infallible, and there is some incidence of false positives and false negatives. Also, certain medications, including estrogen, can influence the results, as can being a smoker. If you have an abnormal test result, it's a good idea to repeat the test.

Cervical cells go through gradual changes on the way from normal to cancer. Sometimes the results show precancerous cells, which can be treated through various techniques. When abnormal cells are treated early, there is little risk of developing cervical cancer.

If the results of your Pap test are abnormal, further testing may be indicated, such as a colposcopy, which uses an instrument (a colposcope) to shine a light on your cervix. If necessary, a biopsy can be taken of the cervix during a colposcopy as well. Treatment usually involves removing the cells using a laser (a beam of high-energy light that destroys tissue) and can be done in your doctor's office.

YOUR PAP TEST RESULTS

According to the American College of Obstetricians and Gynecologists (ACOG), the professional organization for OB/GYNs, your Pap test will be classified according to the following system:

- *Normal:* no sign of cancer or precancer
- *Atypical squamous cells* (*ASC*): some abnormal cells
- *Squamous intraepithelial lesion* (*SIL*): cells show signs of precancer
- *Atypical glandular cells:* further testing is needed because of an increased risk of precancer or cancer
- *Cancer:* cancer cells pervade the cervix

URINARY INCONTINENCE

The National Institutes of Health (NIH) estimate that more than thirteen million adults suffer from urinary incontinence (UI). Twice as many women as men are affected, perhaps because pregnancy, childbirth, menopause, and the way a woman's urinary tract is structured all have a potential impact on developing UI. Other reasons, such as a stroke, multiple sclerosis, or various neurological and spinal cord injuries, can also lead to UI.

A 2005 study reported in the *Archives of Internal Medicine* found that 45 percent of women age thirty to ninety had urinary incontinence.[2] The older the woman, the more severe the problem. The researchers also found that depression, obesity, and having had a hysterectomy were strongly associated with UI. Nonwhite women and women who had only delivered through caesarian section had less incidence of UI.

Urinary incontinence means that you have problems holding in urine. In other words, you leak. The condition sometimes occurs because of physical changes in the muscles that control the bladder, where urine is stored, and the urethra, the tube from which you eliminate urine. When you urinate, the muscles in the bladder contract and force urine out into the urethra. Problems occur if the muscles involved in the bladder contract suddenly and unexpectedly or the muscles that surround the urethra relax.

Even though this is a common complaint in middle-aged and older women, nobody wants to talk about it. But don't be embarrassed to tell your doctor. It is almost always treatable, and it's certainly not your "fault." Usually urinary incontinence is more about putting a serious dent in the quality of your life than it is about having a serious physical problem. I know women who are afraid to go out or to exercise because of this condition. Some get dehydrated because they are reluctant to drink water. The first thing I tell my patients is that they are not alone.

QUESTIONS THE DOCTOR WILL ASK YOU

If you have urine leakage, it's important for your doctor to ask you a number of questions in order to establish whether you have UI or if there is another reason for the problem. For example, cystitis (a bacterial infection of the bladder) can cause bladder irritation, which may result in leakage. Certain medications (such as diuretics) or medical conditions (such as diabetes or sleep apnea) can also result in frequent urination and leakage. Your doctor's questions will enable her or him to define the problem and decide on the appropriate treatment.

- Does your urine leak before you have the urge to urinate?
- Does urine leak only when you cough, lift, or laugh?

- Is there pain associated with feeling that your bladder is full or with emptying your bladder?
- Do you get up at night to go to the bathroom?
- Do you have blood in your urine?

TYPES OF INCONTINENCE

There are several types of incontinence. Treatment depends on the type you have.

FOODS THAT MIGHT CAUSE YOU TO URINATE FREQUENTLY

Alcohol

Carbonated beverages (especially caffeinated ones)

Coffee

Black or green teas

Citrus fruits

Tomatoes

Spicy foods

Sugar

Honey

Corn syrup

Artificial sweeteners

STRESS INCONTINENCE

Stress incontinence is by far the most common kind. If you leak urine when you laugh or sneeze, you may have stress incontinence, which occurs because the muscles that force the urethra closed become weak. This treatable condition can result from changes that happened during pregnancy, from childbirth, or as a result of lowered estrogen levels related to menopause.

URGE INCONTINENCE

Urge incontinence is caused by bladder contractions that cause you to release urine while feeling a sudden urge to urinate. Urge incontinence can result from overactivity in the nerves that control the bladder; sometimes doctors refer to this as "reflex incontinence." People who suffer from this can release urine simply by hearing water run or drinking even small amounts of water. Various diseases, such as multiple sclerosis or Parkinson's, and injuries to the bladder from surgery can cause nerve damage.

FUNCTIONAL INCONTINENCE

Functional incontinence is usually associated with the elderly and with people who have trouble getting to a toilet for physical reasons, such as being in a wheelchair or suffering from dementia or Alzheimer's disease.

OVERFLOW INCONTINENCE

Relatively rare in women, overflow incontinence occurs, as the name implies, because the bladder is always full to overflowing. This kind of incontinence can result from disease such as diabetes or urinary stones that can block the urethra.

HOW TO DIAGNOSE YOUR UI

Once your doctor knows the cause of the UI, treatment can be targeted effectively. The following tests are recommended so that a diagnosis can be made.

- Urinalysis can determine whether you have an infection or urinary stones.

- Blood tests can reveal some causes of incontinence, such as diabetes.

- Ultrasounds can be used to "see" mechanical problems of the kidneys, bladder, and urethra.

- A stress test, where you cough vigorously to see if urine is released, can be performed.

- A cystoscopy, a procedure in which a tube with a tiny camera is inserted into the urethra, enables the doctor to examine the inside of the urethra and the bladder.

TREATMENTS FOR UI

Once your doctor has determined the underlying cause of your UI, treatment can start. If the reason for the UI is an infection, antibiotics should be prescribed. If you have a mild form of UI, the easiest and most effective treatment is Kegel exercises to strengthen your pelvic muscles. Many women learn about Kegels during and after pregnancy. No equipment is required. You simply clench and unclench your vaginal muscles, thereby strengthening the muscles surrounding the urethra as well. You squeeze the muscles as if you were trying to hold back urine or trying to stop urinating when your bladder is only partly empty. Hold the muscles tight for a few seconds and repeat the exercise often.

There are other treatments for UI, such as electrical stimulation, which can stabilize overactive muscles; biofeedback, to help you learn to get control over your muscles; and various bladder training techniques, which are effective for urge and overflow incontinence. Medications, including estrogen, are also used to treat UI. Injections of Botox (yes, it's used for more than wrinkles) can be administered to paralyze the muscles that control the bladder. Surgery is sometimes recommended to reposition the bladder. Talk to your doctor. UI is treatable.

UTERINE PROLAPSE

One of the more serious underlying causes of UI is uterine prolapse. This unpleasant condition occurs when the ligaments and tissues that support the uterus weaken enough to allow the uterus to fall through the cervix into the vagina. Sad to say, only about 10 percent of women who suffer from this seek help. Other symptoms of uterine prolapse are pressure in the pelvic area and constipation.

There are several risk factors for uterine prolapse: increasing age (the condition is most common in middle-aged women), hormonal changes that occur with pregnancy and menopause, childbirth, chronic coughing, bronchitis, allergies, and physical exertion such as heavy lifting or extreme sports. Young women who have had multiple pregnancies or do extreme physical labor may also experience prolapse.

Sometimes Kegel exercises help with uterine prolapse, but usually other treatment is more successful. A pessary (a removable rubber plastic device inserted in the vagina) can be fitted into the upper portion of your vagina to help prevent the uterus from sagging. (The pessary should be taken out and cleaned regularly in order to minimize the risk of infection.) Sometimes either abdominal or vaginal surgery is required to correct the prolapse so that symptoms are relieved. And in some cases, hysterectomy is recommended.

SEXUALLY TRANSMITTED INFECTIONS

Sexually transmitted infections (STIs; also called sexually transmitted diseases, STDs, or venereal diseases) affect more than nineteen million people in the United States annually, according to the Centers for Disease Control and Prevention.

Here are some statistics:

- More than four million cases of chlamydia occur each year.

- Women are twice as likely not to have symptoms of chlamydia as men (no symptoms may mean no treatment).

- Thirty-one million people in the United States are infected with the genital herpes virus.

- Almost half a million new cases of genital herpes occur every year.

- In couples where one partner is infected with herpes, women have four times the risk of becoming infected as men.

- Twenty-four million people are infected with HPV or genital warts, a condition associated with cervical cancer.

- One million new infections of genital warts occur each year.

- More than eight hundred thousand cases of gonorrhea occur each year.

- Almost 80 percent of women with gonorrhea are asymptomatic, while less than 5 percent of men are asymptomatic (no symptoms may mean no treatment).

I find these statistics staggering. The only good news here is that when diagnosed and treated, most STIs can be managed effectively. But that means the infections need to be recognized. Of course, sexual partners of infected people need to be treated also. If you have any suspicions that you might have an STI, talk to your OB-GYN and get tested.

WOMEN AND STIS

In my opinion, there is not enough public noise being made about women and STIs. According to the World Health Organization, women are more vulnerable to STIs than men for various reasons: biologically, due to greater genital surface area with moist cells, and hormonal changes that may interfere with immunity; culturally, since many women are reluctant to seek treatment because they would be stigmatized; and socioeconomically, since women may have neither the time nor the money to pursue treatment.

In addition, women are at increased risk for complications because they often show no symptoms (some estimates say up to 70 percent of infections in women are asymptomatic) and therefore a serious infection can remain undiagnosed and untreated. Without treatment, problems associated with STIs can become severe. Infection can spread to the uterus and fallopian tubes, which can cause pelvic inflammatory disease (PID), which in turn may lead to ectopic pregnancy (the pregnancy occurs outside the uterus and the baby dies) or infertility. Cervical cancer is also associated with STIs, in particular those caused by the human papillomavirus (HPV); young sexually active women are especially at risk. Women with STIs who are pregnant run the risk of passing the infection along to their baby at birth; the herpes simplex virus, which is extremely common, may cause potentially fatal neonatal infections. This is why it is so important to be screened for STIs, even if you have no symptoms.

The emotional wallop of a diagnosis of STI can be enormous and painful in the extreme. One of my patients, Jessie, whom I treat for high blood pressure, called me because she wanted to come in and discuss "a very personal issue." She said that her blood pressure was fine and it wasn't her heart, but she needed a doctor she could talk to.

When she came in, she told me that she had noticed something on her vagina that eventually was diagnosed as herpes. Her gynecologist said, "Take this medicine, use condoms, and talk to your partner." Jessie was very upset. She couldn't understand how she had become infected. She had been married for seventeen years and her husband had recently died. She wanted to know if her husband had been unfaithful; she needed to understand much more than the gynecologist had told her. Would I help?

The lack of humanity and communication between doctors and patients makes my blood boil. How hard is it to take a few extra minutes to explain something to a person in distress and react to her concerns? I recommended a colleague of mine, a gynecologist who I knew would take the time and trouble to adequately address her questions.

PELVIC INFLAMMATORY DISEASE

Pelvic inflammatory disease (PID) is extremely common, with more than one million women a year in the United States experiencing an episode, according to the CDC. It refers to an infection of the uterus, fallopian tubes, and other reproductive organs and is usually caused by an STI, such as gonorrhea or chlamydia. If not treated, PID can lead to infertility from scarring of the reproductive organs, ectopic pregnancy, abscesses, or chronic pain.

As with other STIs, the more sex partners a woman has, the greater the risk of developing PID, and the more sex partners a woman's partner has, the greater her potential exposure to infections. There is research that suggests that douching may increase the risk of PID. Women who want to use an IUD for birth control should be tested and treated for STIs before the IUD is inserted to reduce the risk of infection.

Symptoms of PID may be nonexistent or very mild. This is not a good thing since serious damage may be done to the reproductive organs without the woman's knowledge. If the PID remains unrecognized, obviously it will remain untreated. If there is any indication, such as lower abdominal pain, pain during intercourse, vaginal discharge, painful urination, irregular menstrual bleeding, or fever, the doctor should order tests for chlamydia and gonorrhea. Sometimes an ultrasound or laparoscope can help to determine whether someone has PID. Antibiotics can help to stop the damage to the reproductive organs, but they can't reverse damage that has already occurred. Therefore, it is important to get treated as quickly as possible. The longer the delay, the greater the risk of becoming infertile.

GONORRHEA

Gonorrhea is a sexually transmitted bacterial infection. Among the estimated one million women infected with gonorrhea, up to 40 percent also have chlamydia. Popular lore to the contrary, gonorrhea cannot be transmitted by toilet seats or doorknobs. In fact, the bacterium that causes gonorrhea can't live outside the body for more than a few minutes. It likes moist places such as the vagina, uterus, urethra, throat, and rectum, which is why condom use is effective against the disease.

More than 50 percent of the women who are infected with gonorrhea and are at an early stage of the infection have no symptoms. Therefore, they may not realize they are infected and so don't get treatment until the infection becomes worse. Symptoms include burning or frequent urination, yellow-colored vaginal discharge, swelling of the genital area, and burning or itching of the vagina. Gonorrhea is treated with antibiotic medicine. Untreated, gonorrhea can lead to PID.

CHLAMYDIA

Like gonorrhea, chlamydia requires a moist place to grow within the body, and can be found in the vagina, cervix, uterus, urethra, throat, and rectum. The bacterium can cause severe pelvic infection, but because so many women have no symptoms and don't realize they have the infection and therefore remain untreated, the pelvic infection can lead to PID and infertility. More than 40 percent of women with chlamydia develop PID. Chlamydia is treated with antibiotics.

Again, because the prevalence of chlamydia is so high and the number of women who are asymptomatic is so high as well, all babies are treated with eye drops at birth because chlamydia can result in serious eye damage to newborns.

GENITAL HERPES

There are eight strains of the herpes virus that affect humans. Genital herpes is caused by the herpes simplex virus, type 2 (HSV-2). Cold sores or fever blisters are caused by another strain of the herpes simplex virus, type 1 (HSV-1). Yet another strain of the herpes virus causes chicken pox and shingles. Although cold sores caused by HSV-1 are not considered a sexually transmitted infection, even HSV-1 can result in genital herpes about 20–40 percent of the time through transmission during oral-genital sex. The blisters from HSV-1 that result in genital herpes are indistinguishable from HSV-2 without further testing.

In genital herpes, the virus enters the body through intimate contact with mucus-covered parts of the body, such as the vagina or the mouth, and through microscopic tears in the skin. Once inside the body, the virus travels to the nerve roots near the spinal cord, where it stays until the infected person has an outbreak of the virus. Then the virus travels down the nerve to the site of the original infection, and redness and blisters, typical signs of herpes, erupt. In women, blisters appear around the vagina or on the cervix; they occur on the penis in men. Usually the blisters are preceded by pain, tenderness, or itching in the genital area. Symptoms can also include pain on urination, vaginal discharge, fever, headaches, and swollen glands in the groin area.

More than half of sexually active adults are thought to carry the herpes virus, which can only be accurately diagnosed through an analysis of the blister during an outbreak or a blood test. Since half of infected women have no symptoms, they may not know if they are infected or not. Sometimes the only symptom of herpes is a mild itching in the genital area. If you have any suspicion that you may have herpes, tell your doctor. This is especially important when you are pregnant because the infection can cross the placenta and affect the baby.

Perhaps because the initial infection so often remains untreated, when women do develop an outbreak, they seem to have more severe symptoms, including inflammation of the urethra, which causes painful urination. Often the symptoms of genital herpes are misdiagnosed as common yeast infections, pimples, or urinary tract infections.

Herpes is related to the immune system, so women who are stressed, sick, or on certain medications may have more frequent and longer-lasting outbreaks. The virus is contagious during the time of the blister outbreak until it is completely healed. (There are also periods of time when the virus is "shed" without symptoms.) Since the herpes virus can spread from one part of the body to another, if you have an outbreak, make sure not to touch your mouth or your eyes without thoroughly washing your hands. Don't share your towel, and be careful with any clothing that comes into contact with the blisters. It is a good idea to avoid all sexual contact during an outbreak. And when there is no outbreak, condom use will lessen the risk of the partner becoming infected. Although herpes has no cure, the symptoms and reduction of contagion can be managed with medication.

GENITAL WARTS

Genital warts, caused by the human papillomavirus (HPV), are thought to be the most common STI in the United States. Much like the herpes virus, the strain of the virus that causes genital warts is related to the strains of HPV that cause the common warts we get on our hands. Most people who are infected with HPV have no symptoms. Genital warts are highly contagious, and often the virus remains dormant and so goes undiagnosed. Symptoms of HPV infection can be chronic itching or genital pain. HPV also can predispose women to cervical cancer (see page 108).

Acquired Immune Deficiency Syndrome (AIDS)

AIDS is caused by the human immunodeficiency virus (HIV), which by compromising the body's immune system makes a person susceptible to various opportunistic infections and disease. HIV is transmitted through bodily fluids (blood, semen, or vaginal secretions). Over the past decade, antiviral therapy has greatly improved the outlook for people infected with HIV, but there is still no cure.

Early in the epidemic of AIDS in this country, the disease was associated primarily with intravenous drug users and gay men. According to the CDC, now 25 percent of all new AIDS diagnoses are in women, with African American women having twenty-seven times the number of diagnoses as white women. Most of these women were infected through heterosexual contact. Very troubling is that the CDC also reports that women are less likely than men to receive prescriptions for the most effective treatment for HIV.[3] HIV in pregnant women can be transmitted to the fetus. Therefore, if you have HIV, it's important to talk to your doctor about treatment before and during pregnancy in order to prevent transmission.

During the first month of my internship, in 1984, nine of the thirteen patients I was following had different infections associated with HIV. Most of them died. I realized what a very long way we have come in the past twenty years when a colleague asked me to speak at a recent conference on HIV and cardiovascular diseases. Individuals with HIV are now living longer because of powerful antiviral medications (some of which raise levels of cholesterol), and because they are living longer they have to be concerned about heart disease and its risk factors.

Hepatitis B

Hepatitis B is considered a sexually transmitted infection because it is spread through semen, saliva, and blood. The disease is caused by the hepatitis B virus (HBV) and can lead to inflammation and scarring of the liver, chronic infection, liver cancer, and liver failure. According to the CDC, 5 percent of people in the United States will get infected with HBV at some time during their lives.

You are at increased risk of contracting hepatitis B if you have sex with someone who is infected, if you inject drugs, or if you have a job that involves contact with blood (as is the case for health care workers). An infected mother can pass the virus along to the baby during birth.

Treatment for hepatitis B involves nonspecific medications to treat symptoms; there is no cure. There is a vaccine available that will prevent HBV, which is recommended for people exposed to blood products and sexually active women of childbearing age. It's a good idea to get a blood test to check if you have the virus before becoming pregnant or early in the pregnancy, so your baby can be treated with the hepatitis B vaccine.

About 70 percent of people exposed to the virus show symptoms, with older people showing more symptoms than younger ones. Sometimes a person infected with hepatitis B has no symptoms at all. A blood test is the only way to confirm the diagnosis. If you do have symptoms, they might include fatigue, yellow skin, loss of appetite, joint pain, or dark urine.

CERVICAL CANCER

Approximately half a million cases of cervical cancer are diagnosed worldwide annually. In the United States, the incidence is much less, due to the success of Pap screening. Cervical cancer is more common in middle-aged and older women (half of the cervical cancer cases occur in women between the ages of thirty-five and fifty), and also in women of lower socioeconomic status. There is a higher incidence of cervical cancer among African American, Hispanic, and Native American women than among white women. Women who smoke are twice as likely to develop cervical cancer; research suggests that there are chemicals associated with cigarettes that may damage cervical cells.

Although the cause of cervical cancer is not known, there are risk factors that are. The primary risk is an infection with the human papillomavirus (HPV). More than 80 percent of cervical cancers are associated with HPV, which is sexually transmitted. Also, HIV, which compromises the immune system, increases the incidence of cancer. Because these risks are associated with sexual activity, risks are lowered by having fewer sexual partners and by avoiding partners who themselves have multiple sexual partners. Condoms don't prevent HPV because the virus can be transmitted from person to person through skin contact.

In June 2006, the FDA approved a vaccine that protects against cervical cancer by preventing HPV infections. The three-shot series is recommended for females nine to twenty-six years old. The vaccine does not replace or obviate the need for Pap tests. The vaccine is already controversial, with women's groups applauding its usefulness and social conservatives fearing that endorsing the vaccine will encourage promiscuous sexuality among young people. Also, it is expensive and so may not be easily accessible to lower-income women. Don't let anyone tell you that medicine isn't political.

Usually the first warning of cervical cancer is an abnormal Pap test result. Other symptoms may include heavy menstrual bleeding, vaginal discharge, low back pain, painful sexual intercourse, bleeding after intercourse or douching, and painful urination.

Treatment options for cervical cancer depend on how invasive the cancer is. At the preinvasive stage, when only the outer layer of the lining of the cervix is involved, a simple surgery to remove the abnormal tissue, called conization, can be done. Laser surgery can also be used to kill precancerous and cancerous cells. There are other surgical techniques available, such as the loop electrosurgical excision procedure (LEEP), where an electrical current, which cuts like a scalpel, is used to remove abnormal cells. Finally, a hysterectomy, which removes the cervix and the uterus, can be done.

Even if the cancer is more advanced and in the invasive stage, most women are treated successfully with hysterectomy, radiation, and chemotherapy.

Hysterectomy

Hysterectomy, the surgical removal of the uterus, is the second most common surgery performed on women in the United States. (The C-section is the most common.) The CDC reports that approximately six hundred thousand hysterectomies are performed every year; one out of nine women will have a hysterectomy, and after sixty years of age, that number increases to one in three.

Interestingly, the rate of hysterectomy varies throughout the United States, according to region. Women in the South and Midwest have a higher rate of hysterectomy than women who live in the Northeast or West.

The most common reasons for undergoing hysterectomy are uterine fibroids and endometriosis (see page 67), conditions that are most prevalent before menopause. Obviously if you want to become pregnant, ask your doctor about options other than hysterectomy, such as drug therapy or myomectomy (removing the fibroid tumors but leaving the uterus intact), that might address your symptoms effectively.

TYPES OF HYSTERECTOMY

If your doctor recommends a hysterectomy, there are alternative types of surgical methods. A total hysterectomy involves removing the uterus and cervix. A radical hysterectomy involves removing the uterus, ovaries, cervix, and fallopian tubes. A partial hysterectomy removes just the uterus. The decision about which kind of procedure you should have is based on the reason for having it, and your physical condition.

ABDOMINAL HYSTERECTOMY

By far the most common method for hysterectomy, especially for women with uterine fibroids, is through the abdomen. The surgeon makes an abdominal incision, sometimes along the "bikini line" or vertically from the navel down, and removes the uterus; the cervix may or may not be removed also (retaining the cervix provides support for the vagina). The procedure requires a hospital stay, and recovery time can range from a few weeks to longer. The advantage of an abdominal procedure over alternatives, such as a vaginal one, is that the doctor has greater visibility and can better see the organs.

VAGINAL HYSTERECTOMY

Removal of the uterus through the vagina is recommended for women who are suffering from uterine prolapse (see page 101) or abnormal bleeding. Vaginal hysterectomy is less invasive than an abdominal procedure and usually does not involve removal of the cervix. If you have this type of procedure, yearly Pap tests are still required for maintaining good health. The surgeon makes a small incision in the pelvic area in order to tie up the fallopian tubes and blood vessels, thereby freeing the uterus from its moorings. It is then possible to remove the uterus through the vagina. This procedure usually requires a hospital stay of one or two days, and recovery time is somewhat faster than with abdominal surgery.

LAPAROSCOPIC-ASSISTED VAGINAL HYSTERECTOMY

Yet another alternative method involves using a laparoscope, which is a tube with a tiny camera that is inserted near the navel. The camera allows the surgeon to see the uterus, and the surgeon makes tiny abdominal incisions to detach the uterus from the fallopian tubes and tie off blood vessels. Once the uterus is detached, it can be removed (if small enough) through a small incision at the top of the vagina or through the vaginal canal. Not everyone is a candidate for this type of hysterectomy; it may not be appropriate for women who have very large fibroids or who have had previous abdominal surgery. Also, not every physician is trained to perform the procedure. For these reasons, it is still relatively rare. The advantages of this procedure are a shorter hospital stay and quicker recovery; on the other hand, there is a higher risk of bladder injury.

AFTER HAVING A HYSTERECTOMY

A hysterectomy has implications for physical function and also for your quality of life. You want relief of distressing physical symptoms, but you have to take into account that this is a major surgery, with hospitalization and recuperation time, which for some women has emotional as well as physical implications. Having a hysterectomy sometimes affects your mental and sexual well-being, either positively or negatively. Some women feel loss, some freedom. Some women report relief and increased sexual interest; others the opposite. A 2000 study about sexual functioning and hysterectomy examined frequency of sexual activity, painful sexual activity, orgasm, vaginal dryness, and libido; the results showed that by and large, sexual functioning improved and frequency of sexual contact increased; problems and discomfort during sex decreased.[4]

Sometimes I feel that I learn more about the patient's experience of medical care from my friends than I ever learned in medical school, perhaps because they are more forthcoming about their fears and feelings. My friend Paula, fifty years old, had very heavy and frequent periods. One day I noticed that she was pale, and she told me she was anemic and constantly tired. Her gynecologist had done a sonogram and discovered a grapefruit-sized fibroid on her uterus. The doctor recommended a hysterectomy, but Paula was reluctant. Like most of my patients, she searched the Web for information and went for second, third, and fourth opinions.

A hysterectomy was a reasonable and responsible recommendation, not only for medical and health reasons but to restore her quality of life. And when she asked for my opinion (the fifth), I told her as much. But fear is a terrible thing, and she was scared—scared of the surgery, scared of being changed and becoming unfeminine, scared even of becoming fat from not being able to exercise for weeks after the surgery. Therefore she delayed the surgery and continued to be weak and anemic.

Ultimately she had the hysterectomy; her symptoms improved and she feels better. But living through this experience with her showed me how important it is to focus on the entire patient, the psychosocial issues as well as the physical ones. And I coach my patients that if they go to multiple doctors, they should be very clear about what they are hoping for from the consultation, be it confirmation of a diagnosis, reassurance about the correct treatment, other options, and so on. Unless the patient is clear, it is possible that the doctor won't respond to her need.

Ovarian Cancer

Ovarian cancer is diagnosed in more than twenty-two thousand women every year in the United States, and the American Cancer Society estimates that there will be about fifteen thousand deaths from ovarian cancer this year. If diagnosed early and treated while the cancer is in its early stages and contained in the ovary, the survival rate is good, around 95 percent. The problem is that very few ovarian cancers (only 19 percent) are diagnosed early because they are often without symptoms. Usually symptoms show up only in the later stages, and even then they are easily confused with other problems.

Symptoms

Typical symptoms are abdominal discomfort like that associated with gas or indigestion, nausea, diarrhea, feeling bloated, and weight fluctuations. Usually women who exhibit these symptoms are treated for gastrointestinal problems. If the symptoms remain unexplained and don't go away, it's important to get to the root of the problem. Don't just chew antacids and hope for the best.

Tests

Some of the tests that might help to diagnose ovarian cancer include:

- A pelvic exam to determine whether there are any abnormalities of size or shape to the ovaries

- An ultrasound to distinguish between healthy tissue, fluid-filled cysts, and tumors
- A blood test that measures CA-125, a tumor marker that if high may be an indication of ovarian cancer
- If cancer is suspected, a biopsy may be indicated; if so, the entire ovary should be removed to avoid any risk of cancer cells escaping

RISK FACTORS

No one knows what causes ovarian cancer, but there are some risk factors that increase your chance of getting the disease.

- A family history (mother, sister, daughter) of ovarian cancer or breast and colon cancer
- Having had breast or colon cancer
- Age (most ovarian cancers occur in women over fifty)
- Never having been pregnant
- Being overweight
- Race (white women have a higher risk of developing and dying from ovarian cancer than black women)

There are also some studies that suggest that using talc in the genital areas for many years might increase the risk of ovarian cancer. And there is some evidence that hormone therapy after menopause might increase the risk as well.

What might lower your risk for ovarian cancer often seems to be related to decreasing the number of times you ovulate. Therefore, the following may lower your risk:

- Multiple pregnancies
- Breast-feeding
- Birth control pills
- Surgical removal of the ovaries

There is also evidence that reducing fat in your diet can lower your risk of ovarian cancer.

If you understand the risk factors, you can make more informed decisions—always a good idea.

SEVEN

Breast Health

U NTIL RECENTLY BREAST HEALTH AND GYNECOLOGIC DISORDERS were the only women's health concerns discussed in medical school. I was pleased when I was invited to be the keynote speaker at a luncheon to raise breast cancer awareness at the Pierre Hotel in New York City in 2003. I began my talk by commending these women for successfully raising awareness and for helping to raise funds for research on treatment for breast cancer. Because of the efforts of the American Cancer Society, Susan G. Komen for the Cure, and the National Cancer Institute, women with breast cancer are diagnosed earlier and living longer. Happily they now need information to help them take care of their whole body, and I was pleased to have the opportunity to educate them about their risks for heart attack and stroke.

UNDERSTANDING YOUR BREAST

From puberty we are aware of our breasts, and of changes that occur in how they feel. Most of us have experienced swollen and tender breasts as part of the normal fluctuations of our menstrual cycle. The breasts, which are supported by our chest muscles, are composed of fat and different types of glandular tissue that are responsive to hormones. It is this combination of elements that can make normal breasts feel lumpy and uneven, especially in premenopausal women who have normal hormone fluctuations. Hormones are responsible for enlarging breast tissue during pregnancy to prepare the mother for breast-feeding (lactation). And oral contraceptives or hormone therapy can cause breasts to be enlarged and uncomfortable. One of my patients complained that she had to buy a bigger bra after she started hormone therapy.

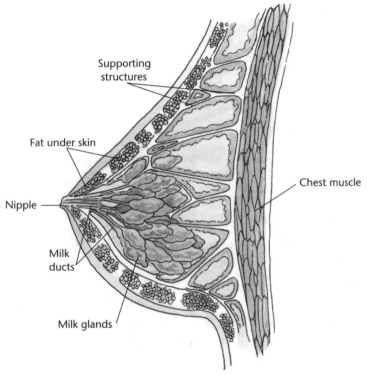

Supporting structures

Fat under skin

Chest muscle

Nipple

Milk ducts

Milk glands

THE BREAST AND SUPPORTING STRUCTURES

GOOD BREAST HEALTH

Some women develop breast lumps right before their periods, which go away during their periods. Because of this, you should schedule a clinical breast examination (that means that a doctor does the exam) during the week after your period. After menopause, because of the reduction of hormones, the breasts are easier to examine. Don't get nuts if you feel something abnormal. There are various reasons other than cancer why your breasts might feel odd. For example, an infection such as mastitis, which is an inflammation of the mammary glands that occurs commonly in women who are breast-feeding, may make your breasts feel unusual.

Or you may get a bruise, which might make your breast sore. Or there might be a blood deposit under the skin from an injury that may feel like a lump and appear black and blue. A breast examination is the best way to find out. You need to transfer your anxiety into action because early evaluation will lead to a quicker diagnosis, relief of anxiety, and prompt treatment if necessary.

NONCANCEROUS CAUSES OF BREAST LUMPS

- An injury or trauma to the breast that produces a bruise or a lump
- Infection, such as an abscess or mastitis, that causes the breast to be hot, tender, swollen, and red. Infection is usually accompanied by fever
- Fibroadenoma, a common, painless benign breast tumor, characterized by well-defined borders

---

I practice what I preach. One morning my mother called to say she felt something in her breast. After I asked her a lot of questions about it, she told me that she had banged into the wall the night before. I told her to relax and explained that she probably had a bruise under her skin. But I made sure that she made an appointment to see her doctor for a clinical examination. It's always a good idea to check out any abnormality. A clinical breast examination can be performed by your primary care physician, your gynecologist, or a breast specialist.

Lumps are not the only reason to go for an examination. Some women experience breast pain, which should also be investigated. When my friend Margie, who is forty-five, called me on a Sunday morning frightened because she had an uncomfortable pain in her breasts, I asked her the same questions I ask my patients. I asked her whether the pain was new or she had had it before. I asked if she was premenstrual, because hormonal stimulation of the breast, related to the menstrual cycle, can be accompanied by breast pain. I asked if she had had any injury to her chest or if her bra was too tight—trauma to the breast or pressure from your bra can result in breast pain. Some women with very large breasts find that they strain their chest muscles, which causes pain. I asked her if she had a breast cyst, because sometimes enlargement of a breast cyst can also cause pain. I tried to reassure her that the causes of breast pain are usually benign, but I sent her for a mammogram to be sure.

EXAMINING THE BREASTS

There are several options for examining breasts. These include self-examination, examination by a physician, and radiological tests such as mammography, ultrasound, and such emerging modalities as MRI. If you read the morning paper or watch the news, you have probably heard that these techniques are less than perfect. That's true; nonetheless, they are what we have. It is important for you to know how to make the best use of what's available for your own breast health.

If this book had been written ten years ago, it would say that the standard of care for examining your breasts would be a monthly self-examination. This has fallen out of favor because of a long-term recent study of women working in a Shanghai factory. Half the women were given instruction on self-examination of the breast; the other half received no instruction. After ten years, the researchers found that there was no reduction in the death rate from breast cancer in the women who performed self-examination.[1] Therefore many concluded that self-examination is a waste of time.

There have been other criticisms of self-examination as well. Some doctors find that women get so anxious that they are afraid to touch their breasts at all. Others feel that since breasts are constantly changing, many women get unnecessarily frightened and undergo unnecessary biopsies. The American Cancer Society no longer recommends self-examination.

I agree that self-examination is not perfect, but you know your own body and you are most familiar with what is normal for you. It's my feeling that you need to be able to recognize changes in your breasts so that you know when to call the doctor. In addition to lumps, you should call the doctor if you see discoloration, discharge, or dimpling of your nipples, or if you have any pain or swelling of the lymph nodes in your armpit.

To ensure good breast health, you should have a yearly breast examination done by your physician even if you do not have any symptoms. During the examination your doctor will do what you should also do: examine your breasts for symmetry, for any discharge or discoloration or dimpling of the nipple, or for any palpable nodules (lumps that can be felt). Masses that require further testing are usually hard, irregular in contour, and attached (fixed in one place); your doctor will also feel the lymph nodes under your armpit for any enlargement. If a nodule is detected, you may be referred for a mammogram and/or a biopsy. In general, benign nodules do not have irregular borders, are firm, and move freely. But no one wants to confuse a malignant tumor with a benign one, so most women are sent for further testing, even if the doctor thinks all is well.

According to recent guidelines (2006) published by the American Cancer Society, good breast health and strategies to reduce your risk of breast cancer include having a clinical breast exam after the age of twenty and regular mammography after age forty.

MAMMOGRAPHY: WHO, WHY, HOW OFTEN

Regular mammograms are recommended for women over the age of forty and are especially important for women over sixty-five, because women over sixty-five have the largest number of diagnosed breast cancers and the highest rate of mortality of any age group. In addition to the standard film mammography that most women have, there is another technique, called digital subtraction, that is particularly useful for women under fifty with dense breasts. It is just common sense that if you have regular mammography screening and you develop a problem, that problem will be caught earlier than if you don't have the screening.

With regular mammograms cancers can be diagnosed at an earlier stage; those women whose cancers are caught early and treated are more likely to outlive the disease.[2] Mammograms are particularly useful in the early diagnosis of cancer of the mammary duct, called ductal carcinoma in situ (DCIS). The mammogram can pick up a particular pattern of calcifications that might indicate DCIS before a lump appears.

No test is perfect, and a mammogram is simply a radiological test. It can't tell us if a specific mass is absolutely benign or malignant. That is why if a mammogram reveals a suspicious mass, it is followed up with a biopsy to determine whether or not the mass is cancerous. Mammograms have a certain percentage of false positives, which means that the test suggests a problem when in fact there is none. Although false positives can make you crazy and may lead to an unnecessary biopsy, the mammogram is still the best test there is for routinely detecting breast abnormalities.

WHAT INCREASES YOUR RISK FOR BREAST CANCER?

Certain factors increase your risk for developing the disease:

- Family history of breast cancer
- Family history of ovarian cancer
- Never having had children
- Having had HT, particularly the combination of estrogen and progesterone, for longer than five years
- Increasing age (over sixty-five)
- Nonwhite race (African Americans have the highest risk)
- The age you were when you first began menstruating (younger than twelve puts you at higher risk)
- The age you were when you had your first baby (the older, the greater the risk)
- The age you were when you had menopause (the older, the higher the risk)
- Obesity
- Drinking more than two alcoholic drinks a day

The fewer risk factors you have, the better. If you have several of these factors, you are at increased risk. For example, an African American woman over sixty-five whose mother had breast cancer and who has been taking HT for fifteen years has a higher risk than an African American woman without a family history and not taking hormone therapy. All women should have regular checkups.

WHAT TO DO IF YOU FIND A LUMP

Don't panic. Be proactive. Most breast masses are benign and harmless. However, you can't diagnose yourself, and only a doctor will be able to rule out malignancy.

No doubt your doctor will recommend that you go for a mammogram. If your mammogram looks fine, which means not suspicious, many doctors will recommend follow-up mammograms after six months to ensure that everything remains normal. Occasionally an ultrasound may be recommended to help determine if a mass is a liquid-filled cyst or made up of solid tissue, or to locate the lump before a biopsy.

Most of the lumps that women find are cysts, which are benign. Cysts occur most frequently in women in their forties. Generally women younger than forty or postmenopausal women who are not on HT don't get cysts. The best way to ensure that your mass is a cyst is to have an ultrasound, which can detect differences between solid and cystic masses. It may be recommended that you have a needle aspiration to drain the cyst of liquid.

Generally if you find a lump, there is a kind of natural progression to diagnosis. First you see your doctor, who may recommend a mammogram. If the mammogram is suspicious or inconclusive, you usually will be sent for another kind of imaging test, an ultrasound or an MRI. Finally, if the suspicions have not been cleared, a biopsy is usually recommended. If you or your doctor find something suspicious (that is, a lump that is not a cyst) or something abnormal is seen on a mammogram, try to leapfrog over other tests and go right for a biopsy.

When my friend Cathy found a lump, she had a series of imaging tests: two mammograms, a sonogram, and an MRI. Nothing conclusive could be established until she finally had a biopsy, which proved negative for cancer. But by the time all the tests were completed and she had the reports back from her doctor, she was a wreck. She had been terrified; no one moved quickly enough for her; she felt that her life was put on hold for weeks and weeks. Her health really suffered from the emotional toll of waiting.

Cathy's experience has happened to many women, so many that the Agency for Healthcare Research and Quality did a research study in order to assess whether or not noninvasive imaging tests, such as sonograms and MRIs, are accurate enough to effectively test for cancer in women whose mammogram or physical exam reveals a potential problem. They concluded that biopsies were the most reliable technique for confirming a diagnosis and that the imaging tests missed too many cancers.

SHOULD YOU GET A BREAST MRI?

The value of getting an MRI is, like so much in medicine, dependent on the circumstances. There has been a great deal of professional discussion about what is the best imaging test for breast cancer, and people were asking whether it was a good idea to skip mammograms and go right to an MRI for diagnosis. Just recently the *New York Times* published an article on the accuracy of using MRI to diagnose breast cancer. The article reported on a study published in the *New England Journal of Medicine* (March 2007) on women who had breast cancer and were using MRI to look for cancer in the noncancerous breast. They found that MRIs were superior to mammography in picking up these cancers. Mammography misses these cancers 10 percent of the time. Other studies have shown MRI to be a beneficial technique for detecting early cancer in women who are at high risk for breast cancer, those who have had previous breast cancer, and those who have received chemotherapy for Hodgkin's disease. In other words, the value of MRI depends on your specific medical history.

WHAT YOUR DOCTOR WILL DO

If you find a lump, your doctor will do a careful history and physical and ask you about the lump, especially when you noticed it and if it has changed (grown larger or smaller), if it is tender, and how its presence is related to your menstrual cycle. The doctor might also ask about your periods, whether you have ever been on hormones (either oral contraceptives or hormone therapy), and whether there is any history of breast cancer on either side of your family. Unfortunately if your mother or sister (first-degree relative) has had breast cancer before the age of fifty, you have three to four times the risk of women without this family history. The doctor will also ask about your children, if you have any, and how many. The reason for these questions is that there is an association between breast cancer and estrogen, and it is thought that the more exposure (in years) you have had to estrogen, the more at risk you might be.

It's important that your doctor ask you to indicate what area is of concern to you to ensure that everyone is on the same page. Your doctor may be feeling a lump that you are not aware of, and you might have felt something that the doctor isn't aware of. Always talk to your doctor.

The doctor will examine the lump to see first if it is a normal glandular node or not. You should be examined in two positions, lying down and upright. Your arms should be over your head.

Facts About Breast Cancer

- Breast cancer is the most common cancer among women in the United States, accounting for nearly one of every three cancers diagnosed.

- One out of seven women in the United States has breast cancer.

- About 75 percent of breast cancers in the United States are diagnosed in women over fifty years old.

- Every year, more than 210,000 women in the United States are diagnosed with breast cancer.

Although the statistics sound grim, there is good news too. Breast cancer rates are continuing to decline, especially for those tumors that are estrogen-receptor-positive, which represent 70 percent of all breast cancers. Doctors attribute the decline to the fact that fewer women are taking HT since the Women's Health Initiative results linking HT with cancer were published.

My philosophy in practicing medicine is always to use common sense and the latest research in making decisions and to individualize the best care for my patients. When I was doing my medical training, my mother called to ask my advice because her gynecologist had given her a prescription for hormone therapy. She was confused about why she needed it and whether or not I thought it would be good for her. She had to ask me because the doctor had not explained anything to her. My mom did not have menopausal symptoms, and I was concerned about the relationship between hormones and the stimulation of breast tissue. I had a theoretical concern that it could lead to breast cancer. Now my mother thinks I was a genius.

SOME STRATEGIES TO LOWER YOUR RISK FOR DEVELOPING CANCER

It would be wonderful if there were a way to prevent getting cancer. Unfortunately, there isn't. Women who have a family history of breast cancer have a greater risk than others of developing the disease themselves. Women who have been on HT for many years have an increased risk as well.

Many of your risks you can't control, such as your genetic history. However, since you can control some things in your life, such as diet and exercise, it seems smart to adopt some lifestyle strategies to help lower your risk.

- Do regular exercise (thirty minutes at least three times a week; five times a week is even better).

- Keep yourself at a healthy weight because excess fatty tissue promotes estrogen and estrogen is linked to breast cancer.

- Avoid long-term hormone therapy (longer than five years).

- If you have a family history of breast cancer and are interested, you can have genetic testing to see if you have the breast cancer gene (see page 124) and then make decisions accordingly.

- Some women who are at high risk decide to have prophylactic mastectomies.

- Avoid having more than one alcoholic drink a day.

- Have yearly mammograms after age forty.

QUESTIONS WOMEN ASK ABOUT BREAST CANCER

DO DRUGS REDUCE THE RISK OF DEVELOPING BREAST CANCER?

The Breast Cancer Prevention Trial was designed to see whether taking the drug tamoxifen could prevent breast cancer in women who were at increased risk of developing the disease. Researchers concluded with a definite "it depends"—on age and race, as well as on the woman's individual risk factors.[3]

In another large breast cancer prevention study, postmenopausal white women were given either the drug tamoxifen or another drug, raloxifene, which is used to prevent osteoporosis. Both drugs were equally effective in reducing invasive breast cancer by around 50 percent, but raloxifene did not reduce noninvasive breast cancer as well as tamoxifen. Both drugs were associated with serious side effects, such as blood clots to the legs and lungs. Tamoxifen increased the risk of uterine cancer, while raloxifene did not.[4] Always read the fine print and talk to your doctor.

SHOULD YOU GET GENETIC TESTING FOR BREAST CANCER?

Cancer genes are passed along in families just like other genes. If you inherited genes called BRCA1 and BRCA2, it can increase your risk for developing breast cancer. However, we are talking about risk, nothing more. Not every woman who inherits a BRCA1 or BRCA2 gene will get breast cancer. Only about one of ten breast cancer cases can be explained by inherited genes.

A simple blood test can check for these genes. If no gene is found, that doesn't mean you won't develop cancer, only that you are not at increased genetic risk. (You can be at risk due to other factors.) Deciding whether or not to take the test is entirely a matter of individual choice.

The pros: if you have the test, it might provide you with information that will help you to make better medical choices, or you might choose to be monitored more often for signs of cancer. You might consider taking preventative medication, such as tamoxifen. Some women decide to have surgery to remove their breasts prophylactically.

My friend Judy had both breasts removed when she was in her early forties. She had the test and found out she had the gene that predisposed her to breast cancer. She told me that all she did all day was worry about getting cancer and dying from it, as both her mother and aunt had done at an early age. She said that reducing her anxiety about getting cancer was worth the surgery, and afterward she felt she could move on with her life. However, you have to know yourself. Some women who decide to get prophylactic mastectomy have difficulty adjusting to it emotionally. Breast reconstruction after surgery is an option that has been shown to relieve some of the psychological stress.

The cons: if you have the test, you might suffer from increased anxiety and worry. There may be other disadvantages to you as well, such as having problems with various kinds of insurance if your test results do not remain private.

Only you and your doctor can determine whether knowing your genetic predilection for cancer would be useful information to you.

WHAT IS THE EFFECT OF WEIGHT AND EXERCISE ON BREAST CANCER RISK?

We all gain weight as we get older. That's just the way it is. Not only do the pounds appear seemingly of their own accord, but once they're on, it is harder and harder to take them off. Not only do I have to eat less than I used to, but I have to exercise more simply to maintain my weight. But keeping your weight under control is not a matter of mere vanity (although feeling good about the way you look never hurt anyone); rather, it's a matter of good health.

Weight gain has been associated with breast cancer especially in postmenopausal women who had not taken HT. For this group, women who gained about forty pounds from the time they were eighteen years old (it sounds like a lot but it is very easy to do) had a 16 percent increased rate of breast cancer.[5]

And again, I can't stress enough how important it is to exercise. A study published in 2006 found that women who had breast cancer and who were obese or overweight had less risk of dying from the cancer if they had been physically fit and active before their diagnosis than women who were not fit. Not only did they have a lower mortality rate, but women who exercised, especially those who did cardiorespiratory exercise (see page 40), expressed an improved sense of well-being.[6] Therefore, if you have had breast cancer, it might be well worth it to engage in an exercise program, especially one that works on heart rate and breathing.

WHAT IS THE EFFECT OF CALCIUM ON BREAST CANCER?

Many of my patients are confused about calcium, and I don't blame them. As I said earlier, it seems obvious that if you are postmenopausal and thus losing the benefit of estrogen on the bones, you should take calcium supplements. However, there is increasing evidence that not all forms of calcium have the same value.

Researchers who want to understand the role of diet in disease studied the relationship between calcium intake and breast cancer. The Cancer Prevention Study, which tracked almost seventy thousand post-menopausal women, found that taking more than 1,250 mg of dietary calcium a day was associated with a lower risk of developing breast cancer. But notice that it is *dietary* calcium that makes a difference—that is, calcium you eat in food (two or more servings of dairy products daily)—and not calcium in the form of supplements.[7] (Read more about calcium in Chapter 9.) The foods that contain calcium also have other antioxidants and vitamins that are good for you.

CAN A SOY-RICH DIET LOWER YOUR RISK FOR BREAST CANCER?

The role of soy products is also confusing to many women. Here's how the reasoning works: because Asian women eat a diet that is rich in soy, and because Asian women have a lower rate of breast cancer than American women, many people infer that there is a relationship between eating soy and reduced incidence of breast cancer. Some doctors believe that soy may indeed lower breast cancer risk because soy foods contain a plant-based estrogen. However, other doctors believe that these plant-based estrogens may actually *increase* the recurrence of breast cancer in women who have already had the disease. In other words, research into the correlation between breast cancer and a soy diet is highly controversial and inconclusive. And remember that this research has been done primarily on dietary soy and not on soy supplements.

For example, a 2002 study reported in *Carcinogenesis* compared Asian American women who ate soy to non–Asian American women who did not.[8] They found that if the Asian American women had been eating soy foods all their lives, they had a reduced rate of breast cancer, but if they began eating soy (about four times a week) only in adulthood, they had no significant reduction in breast cancer rates. The study suggests various questions: Were there other lifestyle issues that had an impact? Was the absence of meat in the diet the reason for the improved rates rather than the presence of soy products? Did these women exercise more? There is no strong evidence either way that adults who eat soy-based products have a lower risk than those who don't.

CAN REDUCING FAT IN THE DIET LOWER THE RISK OF BREAST CANCER?

Once again, how fat in the diet might affect breast cancer risk is inconclusive. We just have to wait and see. Many of the studies that have researched the connection between dietary fat and breast cancer risk have serious flaws, making their conclusions invalid. My opinion is that it probably couldn't hurt to reduce the amount of fat you eat—always a healthy choice. And if research supports the idea that in addition to cardiovascular benefits, such a diet has breast cancer benefits, those of us who have been careful with fats will be at an advantage.

UNDERSTANDING BREAST CANCER

If you have had a diagnosis of breast cancer, your doctor will do tests to ascertain the stage of the cancer, which means how far from the breast, if at all, the cancer has spread. This makes a difference, because treatment is dependent in large part on the stage of the cancer. The chart below defines what the stages mean and what the usual treatment is for each stage. It goes without saying (or it should by now) that all decisions you make regarding treatment have to be thoroughly discussed with your doctor.

Cancer Stage	Standard Treatment
Carcinoma in situ (the cancer is localized at the site where it started)	Local surgery (lumpectomy) with radiation or mastectomy
Stage I: no larger than 2 centimeters and not spread beyond the breast	Surgery to remove cancer and surrounding tissue; removal of some of the lymph nodes under the arm Mastectomy Chemotherapy
Stage II: cancer is smaller than 2 centimeters but has spread to lymph nodes or the cancer is larger than 5 centimeters and has not spread to lymph nodes	Surgery to remove cancer and surrounding tissue; removal of some of the lymph nodes under the arm Mastectomy Chemotherapy

Cancer Stage	Standard Treatment
Stage IIIA: cancer is smaller than 5 centimeters and has spread to lymph nodes or the cancer is larger than 5 centimeters and has not spread to lymph nodes	Chemotherapy prior to surgery followed by radiation Mastectomy and removal of the lymph nodes under the arm Radiation therapy Chemotherapy
Stage IIIB: cancer has spread to tissue near the breast or cancer has spread to lymph nodes inside the chest	Chemotherapy, surgery, radiation
Stage IV: cancer has spread to other organs	Chemotherapy, radiation
Recurrent: cancer that has come back after treatment and can occur anywhere in the body	Surgery, radiation, or both Chemotherapy

In addition to the size and spread of the breast cancer, identifying the cell type helps to determine the chemotherapy medication that will be most effective. For example, breast cancer cells that are estrogen-receptor-positive, which means that the cancer cells need estrogen to grow, will be treated with antiestrogen drugs such as tamoxifen and amastrozole.

Herceptin is a drug that is used in women with an aggressive form of cancer, called HER2-positive, either alone or in combination with other kinds of chemotherapy. It has been found to reduce the recurrence of breast cancer by as much as 50 percent. The combination of chemotherapy and Herceptin in women with HER2-positive tumors showed 87 percent of women to be free of cancer at three years compared to 75 percent in the women who received chemo in addition to mastectomy or lumpectomy.

LUMPECTOMY OR MASTECTOMY?

In many cases there is an option to surgically remove either a portion of the breast where the cancer is located (called a lumpectomy) or the whole breast (called mastectomy). Doctors recommend one or the other treatment depending on the size of the tumor and its location. Generally both procedures have the same survival rates. Lumpectomy when used with chemotherapy decreases the chance of recurrence better than lumpectomy alone.

A good friend of mine who had a lumpectomy and chemotherapy fifteen years ago was recently diagnosed with recurrent breast cancer. She started beating herself up because she had opted for a lumpectomy and chemotherapy and now thought that if she had had a mastectomy, the recurrence might not have happened. She spoke to many doctors, and all agreed that in her case it made no difference. Sometimes, even after following all the best medical advice, recurrence happens. Unfortunately there is no therapy that totally eliminates the risk.

HOW MUCH INFORMATION DO YOU REALLY WANT?

Many women who are confronted with a serious diagnosis feel that their lives are suddenly totally out of their control. One of the ways some women gain a sense of control is by acquiring information, the more the better. Of course, that is their right. Modern medicine no longer shields a patient from unpleasant news, as was done not so long ago, and families no longer have the right to censor the information that the doctor gives the patient. Many women with a diagnosis of breast cancer want to be informed and want the opportunity to make decisions in partnership with their doctors. But there are always people who prefer not to know too much and instead to be told what to do.

TAKING CARE OF YOURSELF IF YOU HAVE HAD BREAST CANCER

According to guidelines published by the American Society of Surgical Oncology, if you have had breast cancer, you should be sure to have:

- A clinical breast physical exam
  - Every three to six months during the first three years of treatment
  - Every six to twelve months during the fourth and fifth years
  - Annually after five years
- Annual mammography
- Annual pelvic exam
- Monthly self-examinations

Not everyone is comfortable with the same amount of information or the same levels of choices in decision-making. How much is right for you? It's a very personal consideration, but one well worth making before you engage in a conversation with your doctor. Maybe certain kinds of information are more important to you than others. Maybe you should consider the level of detail and specificity you want. In a study about the level of involvement women recently diagnosed with breast cancer wanted to have in their treatment, a wide discrepancy was found: 22 percent wanted to select their own treatment, 44 percent wanted to select treatment in collaboration with their doctor, and 34 percent wanted the doctor to make all decisions about treatment. Although the women had diverse positions about treatment decisions, they all wanted the same information: what were the chances of a cure and what was the risk of the disease spreading.[9]

BREAST RECONSTRUCTION

Many women who undergo mastectomy consider breast reconstruction, which can be done at the same time as the mastectomy or at some future time. The new breast can be made from the patient's own tissue from another part of the body or by using implants (see Chapter 14).

The combination of increased awareness, regular medical care, and mammograms have saved women's lives. The best way to maintain good breast health is by being your own advocate, maintaining a healthy lifestyle (see Chapters 16 and 18), and making sure you follow up on any symptoms.

EIGHT

Know Your Own Heart

UNTIL VERY RECENTLY, HEART DISEASE WAS THOUGHT TO BE A man's problem. Medical research was conducted almost exclusively on men, and medication was calculated according to what men needed, as were rehabilitation therapies. Women, it was thought, simply didn't have heart disease. It has been a long, hard road to convince the medical establishment that women are indeed *not* small men who have similar, if weaker, symptoms and presentations of illness.

In the past few years, doctors have begun to recognize that the "classic" heart attack, with the red-faced man clutching his chest and sweating, is not the only way a person—that is, a woman—can suffer a heart attack. Unless someone is looking, women can have easily missed symptoms, such as seeming indigestion, back pain, or just feeling lousy. Breathlessness or fatigue can be other easily misdiagnosed warnings. Because women's symptoms of heart disease don't look like men's, doctors often don't diagnose the problem until there is a full-blown crisis.

My friend Ali told me about a visit she made to a cardiologist with her husband. The doctor spent a lot of time explaining to her husband why he had some risk factors (he had diabetes and high blood pressure) and why it was so important for him to be on medication and monitored. When Ali asked if she should make an appointment to see him also, he blew her off, saying she was too young to worry. She is fifty-nine. He never thought to ask about her history or her risk factors. In fact, her father had died of heart disease when he was in his fifties, and she certainly should have been evaluated. But she was a woman and so somehow not considered to be at risk. He was completely wrong, because heart disease is definitely a women's health issue, killing more women than all cancers combined.

Doctors are not the only ones who need to be informed about the risks of heart disease to women. According to the American Heart Association, nearly 60 percent of women realize that heart disease is women's greatest health threat—which is a good thing because they can take steps to ensure good care. But as aware as most women are about their vulnerability to heart disease, only 26 percent believe they are at risk. Maybe that number reflects a kind of it-can't-happen-to-me denial or a residue of the belief that heart attacks are for men, but believe me, it can happen to any of us.

It has now been several years since the publication of my first book, *Women Are Not Small Men* (recently republished as *The Women's Healthy Heart Program*), in which I sought to raise awareness about the risks of heart disease in women and detailed the symptoms that are unique to women and are often overlooked. Gender differences in diagnoses, treatment, and clinical trials are just beginning to be recognized and addressed. But it's still in its early days and there is a great deal to correct.

WHAT IS HEART DISEASE?

It's important to realize that heart disease involves a great deal more than heart attacks. It also involves structural issues such as valve problems, heart muscle problems such as heart failure, plumbing problems such as clogged arteries that supply the heart, and problems of the electrical system such as arrhythmias.

You may have heard the term cardiovascular disease, which refers not only to heart disease (the *cardio-* part) but also to diseases of the

THE FACTS ABOUT WOMEN AND HEART DISEASE

- Heart disease is the number one killer of women.

- In the United States, 7.2 million women have heart disease.

- In the United States, nearly half a million women die of heart disease each year.

- Heart disease is the leading cause of death in women over thirty-five.

- Heart ailments disable and kill more women than cancer.

- One in 2.6 women will die of heart attack, stroke, or other heart problems.

- Women under fifty who get heart attacks die at twice the rate as men.

- Half of all heart attacks occur in people who do not have elevated cholesterol.

- After menopause, the risk of heart attack increases.

- Death rates due to cardiovascular disease are 50 percent higher in African American women and 30 percent higher in Hispanic women than for other groups.

blood vessels (the -*vascular* part) throughout the body, such as those involved with heart attack, stroke, high blood pressure, and peripheral vascular disease. A third of all women from forty-five to fifty-four years old have cardiovascular disease, according to the American Heart Association, and many of them don't know it.

In this chapter, I want to introduce you to the cardiovascular system, share information about common cardiovascular conditions, outline the symptoms to watch out for, and tell you the steps you need to take to prevent problems. My goal is also to help you get better care in the doctor's office.

UNDERSTANDING YOUR HEART

Let's start with some basic information. If you are familiar with the terms when your doctor says something, you'll be better able to understand it. The heart is divided into four chambers: the right atrium and left atrium (the plural is *atria*) and the right ventricle and left ventricle. The atria are the upper chambers of the heart and receive the blood coming in from your body, while the ventricles, the lower chambers, pump the blood out of the heart to other parts of the body. Electrical impulses cause the heart to "beat"—that is, the chambers to expand and contract—in an organized way, a kind of natural pacemaker. Blood is prevented from flowing from one side to another by the septum, which is a thin wall of muscle that divides the heart. The right side accepts blood that is returning from other parts of the body and sends it to the lungs for oxygen. The left ventricle delivers blood to the aorta from which it goes to vital organs.

Heart valves—there are four: tricuspid, mitral, pulmonic, and aortic—are small flaps of tissue that open or close depending on changes in the pressure in the atria, ventricles, or vessels. These valves are like doors designed to ensure that blood flows only one way. The tricuspid and mitral valves regulate blood flow from the atria to the ventricles by opening when the heart fills with blood and closing when the heart contracts. The pulmonary and aortic valves guard the openings from the ventricles to the aortic and pulmonary arteries.

The heart muscle is enclosed in a small sac known as the pericardium; this is the heart's shock absorber. On top of the heart muscle are the coronary arteries, which supply blood to the heart muscle.

CORONARY ARTERY DISEASE

When the coronary arteries are damaged by atherosclerosis, it is called coronary artery disease (CAD). Atherosclerosis refers to the narrowing of the arteries caused by the buildup of plaque (plaque is clusters of cholesterol; it has nothing to do with dental plaque) on the lining of the artery walls, called the endothelium. Narrowed arteries have difficulty delivering sufficient blood to the parts of the body they supply.

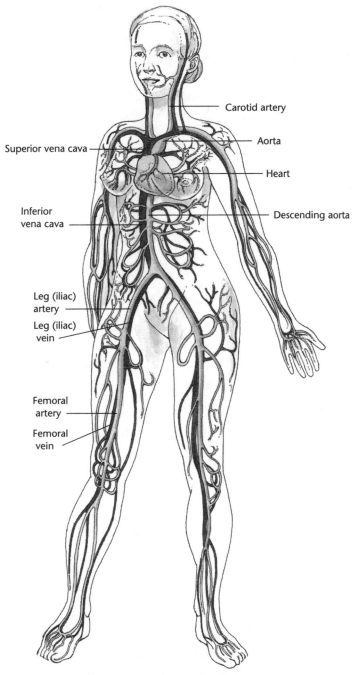

Carotid artery

Aorta

Superior vena cava

Heart

Inferior
vena cava

Descending aorta

Leg (iliac)
artery

Leg (iliac)
vein

Femoral
artery

Femoral
vein

ARTERIES, VEINS, AND THEIR BRANCHES

Woman's body with just the heart and blood vessels. The analogy is that of a tree and its branches. The aorta originates in the heart; it is the trunk of the tree and delivers oxygenated blood through its branches to the heart, brain, arms and legs, and abdomen.

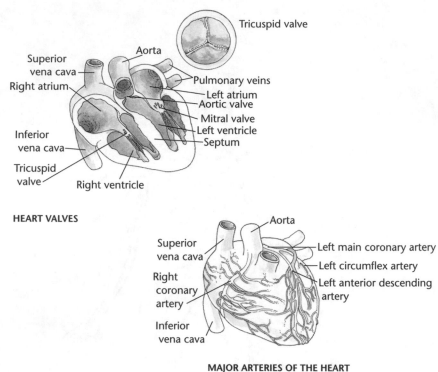

HEART VALVES

MAJOR ARTERIES OF THE HEART

Atherosclerosis is the primary cause of heart attack in post-menopausal women. The damage to the arteries can be accelerated by smoking, high blood pressure, high cholesterol and triglycerides, and diabetes. Smoking is a serious risk factor because it excites the platelets (blood-clotting cells), increasing their tendency to form clots. Although younger women generally have less plaque than older women, younger women who smoke can get heart attacks from a sudden clot.

HEART ATTACK

A heart attack (also called a myocardial infarction or MI) occurs when there is an obstruction of blood flow and oxygen to the heart muscle. The obstruction is usually caused by a blood clot that has broken away from the cholesterol plaque in a coronary artery. Once blood flow is cut off, the section of heart muscle that the blood was supplying can become damaged, and if blood flow is not restored within about 30 minutes, the damage can become permanent. Another mechanism that causes heart attack is an arterial spasm. This is a temporary and abrupt contraction of the artery that causes restricted blood flow to the heart.

Women's symptoms of heart attack can be easily overlooked or misdiagnosed. Some women have shortness of breath and seem unreasonably tired. There might be pressure in the upper abdomen, which could be mistaken for a stomachache, or upper back pressure, which could be interpreted as muscle aches. Few women jump to call their doctors or rush themselves to the hospital if they feel excessively tired or somewhat achy, which is what makes education about women's symptoms of heart attack vitally important for women and their doctors. Some people experience no symptoms at all with a heart attack; this is called a silent MI and can happen to anyone, but is more common in women who have diabetes.

WOMEN'S HEART ATTACK SYMPTOMS

If your doctor calls any of these symptoms "atypical," he (it's usually a he) has not studied the symptoms of heart attack in women.

- Unusual fatigue
- Shortness of breath, especially during low levels of activity or even at rest
- Nausea
- Dizziness
- Lower chest pain
- Back pain
- Upper abdominal discomfort

The following symptoms are typical of men's heart attack, but of course women can have them too.

- Pressure or pain in the center of the chest
- Chest pain that spreads to the neck, shoulder, or jaw
- Chest pain with a feeling of faintness, sweating, nausea, shortness of breath

TIME IS OF THE ESSENCE

If you have any symptoms of a heart attack, don't wait. Don't start cleaning up the house before calling 911, as one of my patients did. Don't ignore the symptoms and say it is probably stress and indigestion, as another of my patients did. Yet another of my patients didn't want to inconvenience the doctor on the weekend and thought she should wait until normal office hours to call. If you think you have heart symptoms, what you want to do is to get medical attention immediately. What's the worst thing that can happen? You'll be wrong and sent home.

Heart attacks have a 50 percent death rate if they happen outside of a hospital, with death usually occurring within the first twelve to twenty-four hours, but two-thirds of women never make it to the hospital. Even more disturbing, 90 percent of women who have heart attacks have at least one risk factor (high blood pressure, diabetes) that if diagnosed could have been treated, possibly preventing the heart attack. That is why women need to learn the symptoms and not be afraid to call 911. Once on your way to or in the hospital, you can get medications that may greatly improve your chances of survival.

HOW IS A HEART ATTACK DIAGNOSED?

It is important to diagnose a heart attack as quickly as possible and treat it so that the heart damage is kept to a minimum. Usually, a heart attack can be diagnosed by:

- An electrocardiogram (also called an ECG or EKG), a simple, non-invasive procedure that records the electrical activity of the heart and can detect whether your heart muscle is being deprived of oxygen.

- Blood tests to measure cardiac enzymes and proteins that are released from the heart muscle during a heart attack.

- An echocardiogram, which uses sound waves to "see" the heart and can assess what areas of the heart that have been damaged.

- Cardiac catheterization, which uses dye and X-ray pictures to image the arteries. This procedure may be lifesaving, because once the blockage causing a heart attack is identified, the doctor can open it up with a balloon and place a stent in the artery to keep it open (see page 165).

TREATMENT FOR HEART ATTACK

Medications are used help to relieve pain, thin the blood to reduce the work the heart has to do, and treat underlying conditions, such as high blood pressure and high cholesterol. The first medication that is given is a full dose of uncoated aspirin; this should be done while you are still at home or in the ambulance.

Once on the way to the hospital you should be given oxygen as well as nitroglycerin to relax and widen the blood vessels. Beta-blockers are given to reduce the work of the heart. After the blood tests and the ECG are done, the focus is on opening up the clogged artery causing the heart attack. This can be done with either clot-busting medications or an angioplasty (see page 165). It's best to get to the hospital within six hours of the beginning of symptoms. Within that time, there is a better success rate in opening the artery. So don't waste time.

You'll find a full discussion of heart medications at the end of this chapter.

WHAT TO DO AFTER HAVING A HEART ATTACK

Before you are discharged from the hospital, your doctor should recommend that you make changes for a healthy heart: eat a heart-healthy diet (see Chapter 16), get regular exercise (see Chapter 18), stop smoking, and lose excess weight. I refer all my patients to cardiac rehabilitation and an organized program of exercise, nutritional counseling, and stress management that should begin three weeks after a heart attack. These programs are covered by many insurance plans. Studies show that women are less likely than men to be referred, however. If you are a woman and have had a heart attack and your doctor doesn't recommend it, ask for it. Don't become another statistic of a woman who doesn't get referred to cardiac rehabilitation.

ANGINA

Angina, or in full, angina pectoris (literally "chest pain" in Latin), is a form of coronary artery disease characterized by decreased blood circulation to the heart. Although it is usually considered a man's disease, it affects more women than men, especially African American and Hispanic women. Symptoms differ for men and women. Usually, decreased circulation triggers chest pressure in men, but women often display other symptoms, such as shortness of breath or fatigue on exertion. Unlike a heart attack, angina usually does not result in permanent heart damage. There are different forms of angina, which I will explain below.

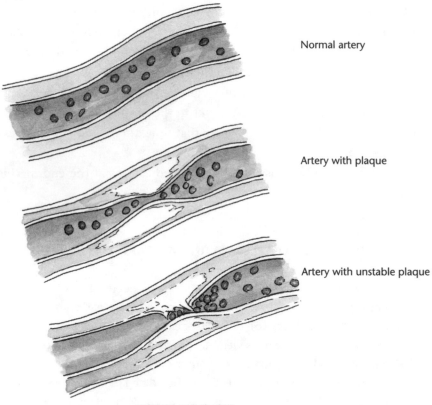

Normal artery

Artery with plaque

Artery with unstable plaque

ARTERIES AND PLAQUE

Atherosclerosis is the culprit for angina as well as for heart attack. The reduced blood flow causes less oxygen to get to your heart. As your body tries to compensate, you can become short of breath. This is especially true when you experience strong emotions or engage in certain physically stressful activities. At these times your heart rate and blood pressure increase, and if you have coronary artery disease, blood flow cannot increase appropriately, putting extra stress on your heart. Some typical stressors include:

- Anger

- Emotional distress

- Excitement

- Exertion of the arms and upper body

- Walking uphill or up steps

- Walking after a heavy meal

- Exercising in the cold

I know some women with angina who refuse to acknowledge that they can't catch their breath and who make various excuses about why they are so tired. It is as if they feel inadequate in some way because they are having trouble breathing. It's important to know that if you have a heart problem, this is not a personal failure. You may not be ready to think you have heart disease, but delaying an evaluation or not sharing your symptoms can be dangerous. If you experience shortness of breath, extreme fatigue, or any of the other symptoms of angina or heart attack, call your doctor.

> ### WHEN TO WORRY ABOUT CHEST PAINS
>
> People get chest pains for all kinds of reasons, and they are not always indicative of heart disease. For example, if your pain lasts only for a few seconds and disappears when you move to the side or drink something, most likely it is not angina. However, if you have any of the symptoms for heart attack that last more than a few minutes and don't go away, you should get medical attention quickly.

STABLE ANGINA

Stable angina occurs when there is what I call a predictable supply-and-demand problem. When your heart needs increased blood flow to accommodate exertion or other stresses, you can't get it because one (or more) of the arteries is narrowed. The increased demand and lack of supply causes pain or shortness of breath. The pattern is predictable because when the exertion stops, there is no need for increased blood flow, and the pain stops. The cause of the angina is a fixed—that is, stable—obstruction of the arteries. That means it's there all the time. Stable angina usually does not progress to a heart attack.

The first step in any diagnosis is to have a real conversation with your physician. She will ask questions about your medical history and physical condition and ask you about your symptoms, which you should describe in detail. Be prepared for the following questions:

- When did the symptoms first start?
- What provoked the symptoms?
- How long did they last? How frequent are the symptoms?
- What made them go away? Did you rest or take medication?

Remember, just state the facts. Don't say "I thought I had a gallbladder attack." It is your doctor's job to make an objective assessment of the symptoms. Your job is to describe how you feel.

Unstable Angina

Unstable angina differs from stable angina because it is not predictable. Symptoms can be longer-lasting or more frequent, or they may occur when at rest. They can even wake you from sleep. These are 911 symptoms, and you need to get to the hospital! Unstable angina is a more dangerous condition than stable angina and is associated with a higher risk of heart attack. It is a pre-heart-attack condition. Symptoms of unstable angina can also occur after a heart attack if you have been diagnosed with coronary artery disease.

> **DON'T DIAGNOSE YOURSELF**
>
> If you experience any of the warning signs of a heart problem or any chest discomfort that lasts longer than a few minutes, call 911 and go to an emergency room. You could have unstable angina or a heart attack.

Unfortunately, even if you have done everything required to keep your angina stable, sometimes the situation becomes unstable for no apparent reason. Plaque in the arteries may break off and start a series of reactions leading to the formation of a clot that blocks the flow of blood to the heart; this may cause a heart attack if you wait too long to get medical help. This problem can occur in people without angina as well.

VARIANT ANGINA

Variant angina refers to chest pain that occurs randomly and without explicit cause (such as exertion). The pain is caused by spasms of the artery, which narrows the artery and blocks the flow of blood to the heart. About 25 percent of women with variant angina have a history of migraine headaches or Raynaud's phenomenon. Raynaud's is a condition in which sporadic blood vessel spasms interrupt the flow of blood to the fingers, toes, ears, and nose.

MICROVASCULAR ANGINA

Microvascular angina is hidden heart disease. It is caused by impaired flexibility of the blood vessels that supply the heart. Women who have this condition have symptoms of chest pain and shortness of breath. Unfortunately there is no single test available at this time that will clinch the diagnosis. When I went to medical school, I was taught that this form of heart disease was benign. However, recent research shows that 30 percent of women who have microvascular disease have heart attacks. But when these same women go for an angiography (a radiological test to examine the arteries), they are often told that their angiograms are normal. In fact, they aren't. The angiograms look normal because the disease is in smaller blood vessels not seen by the angiogram or the cholesterol buildup is so evenly distributed in the larger blood vessels that the obstruction is not obvious.

Esther, a fifty-six-year-old retired schoolteacher, came to me complaining of chest pain. I performed an exercise echocardiogram (see page 164) on her, which revealed that she had reduced blood flow to the heart muscle. I referred her for an angiogram, and the doctor performing the angiogram told her her arteries were all clear. But she still had symptoms. I told her that I thought they were due to a more subtle artery problem and recommended medication. She said she wasn't about to take medication for something that no one could see, and decided not to continue her care with me. A year later her primary care physician told me she had had a heart attack.

Microvascular angina is difficult to diagnose, but a doctor who listens to you and pays attention to all your test results, such as a positive stress test, can save your life.

Diagnosing Angina

After assessing your symptoms, your doctor might recommend the following tests to see whether you have angina:

- ECG, to determine whether there is damage to the heart
- Chest X-ray, to see if the pain could be caused by lung disease
- Exercise stress test, which uses an ECG to record your heart function during exercise, such as riding a stationary bicycle or walking on a treadmill
- Cardiac catheterization to locate any blockages after an abnormal stress test
- Blood tests to measure cholesterol and other fatty substances (called lipids) that increase the risk for angina

Treatment for Angina

Your doctor will recommend lifestyle changes, just as for a heart attack. Angina can be treated with medications, angioplasty, and bypass surgery (see page 168). Recent studies show that stable patients do as well with medication as with stents. Medications used to treat angina as well as other heart problems because they improve blood flow to the heart are aspirin, beta blockers, calcium channel blockers, statins, and nitrates.

Risk Factors for Coronary Artery Disease

Coronary artery disease is not only for the old, nor is it a natural or inevitable part of the aging process. One of the biggest challenges I face in my practice is to convince women under forty that they are at risk for CAD. CAD, like other medical conditions, is associated with certain risk factors. For women in particular, high triglycerides, low HDL cholesterol, obesity, and diabetes are stronger risk factors than in men. If you can eliminate some of these risks, you have a better chance of staying healthy.

Risk factors include:

- Family history of heart disease
- Smoking
- Elevated LDL (bad) cholesterol
- Low HDL (good) cholesterol
- High triglycerides
- Diabetes
- High blood pressure
- Sedentary lifestyle
- Obesity

You can't do much about your family history of heart disease. It is what it is. But you can do something about a lifestyle that puts you at risk. If you don't exercise and you eat a high-fat diet or smoke, your chances of developing heart disease are much greater than if you take reasonably good care of your physical well-being. Being overweight and not getting regular exercise increase your chances of developing heart disease. These are risk factors you can do something about.

CHOLESTEROL AND HEART DISEASE

Cholesterol, which people talk about as if it is a dirty word, is actually necessary for our bodies to function properly. Some cholesterol is produced by our bodies; we also take cholesterol in from foods. You might be surprised to learn that cholesterol is an important part of the chemical structure of estrogen. But where cholesterol is concerned, you can have too much of a good thing.

Cholesterol is carried around the body on lipoproteins. The cholesterol that is attached to low-density lipoproteins, LDL, is "bad," and the cholesterol attached to high-density lipoproteins, HDL, is "good." Very-low-density lipoprotein (VLDL) cholesterol is made up of triglycerides, which are broken down by the body into free radicals, which are products of our bodies' energy use that promote atherosclerosis and are thus very bad. High cholesterol increases your risk for heart disease from arteriosclerosis. When total cholesterol is low, the risk decreases.

LDL Cholesterol

If the LDL cholesterol is high, plaque can form in the walls of the arteries. All plaque is not the same. Stable plaque is less likely to rupture and cause a heart attack than unstable plaque. Unstable plaque can break off from the artery walls and cause a clot that could lead to a heart attack. If a clot blocks the flow of blood to the brain, it could cause a stroke. Therefore, you don't want to do anything to increase your LDL level, and you want to do whatever you can to reduce it. One thing you can do is to reduce the amount of fat in your diet.

HDL Cholesterol

The reason HDL cholesterol is referred to as the "good" cholesterol is because HDL cholesterol travels away from the heart, helping to remove LDL cholesterol as it goes (think vacuuming) and thereby reducing your risk of heart attack. Premenopausal women generally have higher levels of HDL cholesterol because estrogen helps to keep the levels high. After menopause, the HDL levels may decrease, which means that the LDL cholesterol isn't being removed as effectively. Low HDL cholesterol is a more powerful risk factor for women than for men.

Having high HDL cholesterol doesn't take away the risk of also having high LDL cholesterol. My patient Jenny learned that the hard way. Her primary care doctor kept telling her that her HDL cholesterol was the best he'd ever seen and that he wished all his patients had her HDL level. Unfortunately, although Jenny's HDL was high, it was not enough to protect her from high LDL cholesterol, and she had a heart attack. It is important that all components of your lipid panel (an analysis of the cholesterol in your blood) be evaluated and assessed together.

Triglycerides

Triglycerides, another type of blood fat, have been shown to increase the risk of heart disease in women. Women with elevated triglycerides often have high LDL cholesterol and low HDL cholesterol. Even if your cholesterol level is normal, if you have elevated triglycerides, your risk of heart attack increases. High triglycerides can be due to diabetes, oral contraceptives, or excessive consumption of alcohol. You can lower your triglyceride level by losing weight, lowering your intake of dietary fats and sugars, decreasing alcohol consumption, and exercising regularly. Sometimes medication is required to lower triglyceride levels.

What You Can Do About High Cholesterol

I recommend that women over twenty have a fasting lipoprotein profile, which will measure total cholesterol, LDL, and HDL cholesterol levels and triglycerides. The recommended first line of treatment for elevated cholesterol is an improved diet (low in fats), regular exercise, and medication if your doctor recommends it. Not so very long ago, the treatment for high cholesterol was HT; now we know it is not the best option.

UNDERSTANDING CHOLESTEROL LEVELS

Ideal cholesterol levels are dependent on your personal risk for heart disease, but basically, the chart below offers some general guidelines. (All figures are in mg/dl.)

LDL (Bad) Cholesterol

Equal to or less than 70	Where you want to be if you have diabetes or heart disease
Equal to or less than 100	Good
100–129	A little elevated
130–159	Borderline high
160–189	High
equal to or more than 190	Very high

HDL (Good) Cholesterol

Less than 50	Low
Equal to or greater than 60	Good; it reduces the risk for heart disease

Total Cholesterol	
Less than 200	Where you want to be
200–239	Borderline high
More than 240	High

Triglycerides	
Less than or equal to 150	Good

OTHER RISK FACTORS

Diabetes and Excess Weight

If you have diabetes, you have a fivefold greater risk for heart disease, atherosclerosis, and coronary artery disease. Being overweight also puts you at greater risk, especially if you carry your fat around your waist— the so-called spare-tire or apple body type. Extra weight can put a strain on the heart, raise blood pressure, increase LDL cholesterol, triglycerides, and increase your chance of developing diabetes.

BLOOD PRESSURE AND HEART DISEASE

Women who have high blood pressure, or hypertension, increase their risk of developing heart disease by 25 percent and also increase their risk for stroke.

Your blood pressure reveals the amount of pressure put on the walls of the blood vessels as blood moves around your body. You want enough pressure to reach all the cells, but not too much that it strains the vessels. Blood pressure is easily and painlessly measured. You can even do it yourself. The blood pressure cuff is a medical instrument that assesses the pressure in your arteries when the arteries are contracting (systolic) and relaxing (diastolic). The pressure is given in millimeters of mercury (mm Hg), with the systolic pressure given over the diastolic pressure. For good heart health, you want a reading of 120/80 or less. This is especially important if you have diabetes.

It is normal for your blood pressure to go up when you're excited or nervous (such as when you are going to a doctor for the first time, a phe-nomenon called white-coat syndrome). But if either number is consistently high, it is called high blood pressure or hypertension.

Hypertension is dangerous because there is constant pressure exerted on the blood vessels, which can damage them and cause them to become stiff and inflexible. This makes your heart work harder than it should, and in order to compensate, the muscle (remember, the heart is a muscle) gets thicker. A thickened heart muscle can predispose you to irregular heartbeats (arrhythmias). Hypertension also stimulates athero-sclerosis, which increases the risk of heart attack. If you have hypertension, you also have an increased risk of stroke, heart failure, kidney disease, and blindness. You want to monitor your blood pressure and treat it if it gets high.

> **UNDERSTANDING YOUR BLOOD PRESSURE READINGS**
>
> ---
>
> Optimal blood pressure: under 120/80
>
> Prehypertension: between 120/80 and 139/89
>
> Hypertension: over 140/90

Prehypertension means that although your blood pressure is not high enough to be called hypertension, you are at increased risk of developing it. Women who are fifty-five years old and older and have prehypertension have a 90 percent risk of developing high blood pressure later in their lives. Therefore it pays to do everything possible to lower your blood pressure while you can. Exercise helps to reduce blood pressure, as does a low-salt diet. You can take steps to lower your stress levels also, doing whatever works for you as long as it is healthy, such as walking, yoga, meditation, or gardening. Sometimes medications are necessary.

Symptoms of Hypertension

Most people have no idea they have high blood pressure, and so they remain untreated. But if you find yourself feeling dizzy, having vision problems, or having frequent headaches, get yourself tested.

WHO GETS HIGH BLOOD PRESSURE?

Anyone can develop high blood pressure, and many women have it without realizing it. One of my patients kept going to doctors for their opinion about her blood pressure because she was told it was high enough to require medication. She couldn't believe it and didn't want to take the medicine. Another one thought it was a personal failing if she wasn't perfect physically. She also thought that high blood pressure was for old people and she was young. She was sixty-two. I told her that half of women over age forty-five have high blood pressure.

Typically women at midlife have many of the risk factors for hypertension, including:

- Overweight
- Diabetes
- Sedentary lifestyle
- Stress
- Excessive alcohol consumption
- A diet high in salt

The risk of hypertension increases with age, and African American and Hispanic women have an even greater risk than other groups. In fact, African American women living in the United States have the highest prevalence of high blood pressure in the world.

If you have high blood pressure, don't feel like it's a personal failing. Consider yourself lucky to know about it and to be able to treat it before you have serious health consequences.

When you go for a medical visit, questions the doctor might ask include:

- Do you have a history of high blood pressure?
- Do you have headaches or dizziness or shortness of breath?
- Have you been taking any new medications?
- Do you take medication for pain, particularly nonsteroidal anti-inflammatory drugs such as ibuprofen?
- Are you physically active?
- Do you have any history of diabetes or heart attack?

- Do you have high cholesterol?
- Do your legs and ankles swell?

TESTS FOR HYPERTENSION

Other than taking your blood pressure with a blood pressure instrument, your doctor may order tests of other major organs. The doctor should examine your eyes to see if there is damage from high blood pressure. A urinalysis can check for protein in the urine, which may indicate kidney damage from high blood pressure and diabetes. Blood tests are also done to evaluate for kidney damage. If your doctor thinks that the hypertension comes from a kidney problem, a sonogram will be ordered. An echocardiogram (ultrasound of the heart) may be recommended because hypertension increases the thickness of the heart muscle and can predispose you to arrhythmias and heart failure. I see many young women in my practice who have high blood pressure without any family history and who look perfectly healthy. I do blood tests to check for kidney problems, and urine tests that may indicate secretion of hormones from a tumor in the adrenal gland, possible causes of hypertension.

HOW TO TREAT HYPERTENSION

The best way to treat hypertension is to avoid getting it in the first place. Keep your weight down, exercise regularly, follow a low-salt diet (no more than 2 grams of sodium a day), don't smoke, and try to reduce stress. Medications commonly prescribed to control blood pressure are diuretics, ACE inhibitors, and beta-blockers. Remember to let the doctor know if you are pregnant or planning to be pregnant so she can choose medications that would not harm the fetus.

STROKE

A stroke occurs when the brain is deprived of blood flow and oxygen, usually due to a blockage (a blood clot or a plaque rupture) in an artery in the brain. A stroke can also occur if there is a sudden burst at a weak point in an artery, called an aneurysm, causing a hemorrhage. When brain tissue is deprived of oxygen, it stops working and the area of the body its nerves control stop working too. Although more men than women have strokes, women are twice as likely to die from stroke as men.

No one really understands why this should be so. As far as I am concerned, the first step is to actually notice the gender difference; only then can it be analyzed.

As with heart attacks, the symptoms of stroke in women can be more subtle than in men. Women can experience tingling in the face or a slight headache, and they often don't reach out quickly to get early medical attention. Gina, fifty years old, was referred to me by her doctor because she was overweight and needed to start an exercise program. When I took her medical hisory, I found out that two weeks before she came in to see me she had had a half hour of tingling and numbness in the face. The symptoms went away, but she was left with a headache. I suspected that she was having stroke symptoms and sent her to the emergency department. The CT scan of her head showed that she indeed had had a stroke, probably the very day she had the tingling and numbness in the face. She is now on blood thinners and cholesterol medication and doing fine. But I remind every woman I see to pay attention to their bodies and not to ignore symptoms. They could be warnings of heart attack or stroke.

A friend of my parents found herself unable to speak, just for a minute or so. She said she felt funny, as if her head went blank, but since

---

TYPES OF STROKE

- *Ischemic strokes* are caused by a ruptured plaque, similar to a heart attack. Almost 80 percent of strokes are ischemic.
- *Embolic strokes* are caused by a clot (called an embolism) that travels through the bloodstream into a blood vessel in the brain.
- *Hemorrhagic strokes* occur when an aneurysm, a blood-filled pouch in a weakened area of the artery, bursts, leaking blood into the brain.
- A *transient ischemic attack* (TIA or ministroke) should be taken seriously as a warning that you are at higher risk of stroke. The difference between a TIA and a stroke is that symptoms of TIA are temporary and last only minutes or hours. Don't ignore this. If you have a TIA, you should get medical help right away.

she returned to normal so quickly she never did anything about it, or informed her doctor. When my parents told me about it, I told them that this had probably been a TIA, and I carried on about the importance of getting checked out. I don't want you or anyone you care about to ignore a TIA.

Signs and symptoms of stroke

- Sudden numbness or weakness of face, arm, or leg, localized to one side
- Trouble speaking (aphasia)
- Confusion
- Sudden difficulty in seeing
- Sudden difficulty in walking, balance, coordination
- Sudden dizziness
- Sudden severe headache
- Difficulty swallowing

As with other types of cardiovascular disease, women can have nontraditional (that is, male) signs of stroke. One of my patients, fifty-two years old, who had high blood pressure and was obese, came to me complaining that she had been having headaches. An imaging test showed that she had had a small stroke. She was astounded because she had no history of stroke in her family. It had never occurred to her that she was at risk. In a way, the headache and subsequent diagnosis served as a warning to her. A good thing too because after her condition was diagnosed she got so scared that she started to exercise and lose weight. She is also working to stop smoking.

Risk factors for stroke

- Hypertension
- Smoking (especially in combination with oral contraceptives)
- Elevated cholesterol
- Diabetes
- Family history
- Atrial fibrillation (see page 175)

- Arteriosclerosis
- Sedentary lifestyle

How Is a Stroke Diagnosed?

There are very sophisticated tests and technology available to diagnose strokes.

- A CT (computed tomography) scan, also called a CAT scan, is a special imaging test that shows soft tissues and blood vessels very clearly and can be used to assess what area of the brain was affected by the stroke. It can also locate a hemorrhage.

- Another type of scan, called a carotid Doppler, which is an ultrasound of the arteries in the neck, can identify where a plaque rupture might have occurred.

- A magnetic resonance angiography (MRA) uses magnets to provide images of the blood vessels in the brain.

- Magnetic resonance imaging (MRI) uses magnets to provide images of the brain.

- An ECG can evaluate atrial fibrillation and the presence of clots in the heart.

- An echocardiogram can visualize blood clots in the heart.

Treating Stroke

The first thing to do is to get medical attention immediately. If the stroke is caused by a blood clot, sometimes a clot-busting drug, called tPA (tissue plasminogen activator), can restore blood flow if you get it within three hours of the onset of symptoms. Call 911, since every minute counts. The paramedics who come are trained to give you this drug, saving precious time. There are other medications for stroke as well, including cholesterol-lowering drugs, blood thinners, and blood pressure medications.

Not long ago, I gave a lecture and during the question-and-answer period a woman stood up to thank me. It seems that she had had a headache and her vision became blurred. She had just finished reading my book about women and heart disease. When she checked the book, she realized she could have symptoms of a stroke, and she took herself to the emergency department. The doctors there told her how lucky she was to have gotten to the hospital in time to get the clot-busting drugs. Because of her speed and their attention, she recovered fully.

EMERGING RISK FACTORS FOR HEART DISEASE

Some women have heart disease although they have none of the traditional risk factors associated with it. They don't smoke, their cholesterol levels are normal, they exercise, they are not overweight, they do everything right. Yet they have heart disease. If you are among this group of women, it is a good idea to be screened for nontraditional risk factors that are just being identified. In most instances, there is little to be done about having them. But if your doctor knows you are at increased risk, you can be monitored more often or treated more aggressively than otherwise.

RISK FACTORS AND RISK MARKERS

What's the difference between a risk factor and a risk marker? With a risk factor, there is research to support that the factor increases risk for a certain disease; there is also research showing that once an intervention is made (such as inspiring a couch potato to exercise), the risk is reduced. Risk markers, on the other hand, show an association with a disease, but there are no studies yet showing that lowering the risk marker reduces risk for a disease.

HOMOCYSTEINE

One of the recognized risk markers for heart disease is an elevated homocysteine measurement. Homocysteine is a protein that is found in blood, and normally it has no impact on the arteries. However, some people's bodies don't efficiently clear out homocysteine, which can damage the artery walls, causing cholesterol buildup. High levels of homocysteine have been associated with heart attack and stroke.

Studies have shown that one of the reasons for high levels of homocysteine is a lack of B vitamins, especially folic acid, that are needed to remove homocysteine from the blood. For this reason, many doctors recommend eating foods rich in these vitamins, and that can't hurt. However, a recent study reported in the *New England Journal of Medicine* showed that taking B vitamins to lower homocysteine levels did not reduce heart disease risk, as was previously believed.[1] In my practice, I do not recommend B vitamin supplements or routine screening for homocysteine levels. The women who I think should be screened are those who have heart disease or a family history of heart disease and who do not have traditional risk factors.

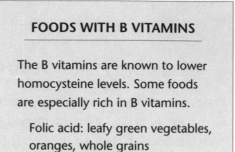

FOODS WITH B VITAMINS

The B vitamins are known to lower homocysteine levels. Some foods are especially rich in B vitamins.

Folic acid: leafy green vegetables, oranges, whole grains

Vitamin B_6: baked potato with skin, bananas, whole grains

Vitamin B_{12}: meat, fish, eggs

LIPOPROTEIN (A)

Another emerging risk factor for heart disease is lipoprotein (a) or Lp(a). It is similar to LDL (bad) cholesterol and a blood clotting protein (thrombin), which are risk factors for atherosclerosis in women. We know that levels of Lp(a) increase at menopause. If you don't have the traditional risk factors for heart disease, yet have heart disease or a family history of heart disease, your doctor may screen for Lp(a) levels. Several studies have shown that estrogen and niacin can help lower Lp(a) levels, but no studies have shown that a lower level reduces the risk of heart disease. So even if you have high levels of Lp(a), you don't need to start HT therapy or niacin supplements.

HIGH-SENSITIVITY C-REACTIVE PROTEIN

High-sensitivity C-reactive protein (hs-CRP) is a marker of inflammation, and elevated levels have been found in people with heart disease, so CRP level serves as a predictor of future heart disease. Elevated levels of high-sensitivity C-reactive protein (hs-CRP) in women have been associated with a 21 percent higher risk of heart attack, even when LDL cholesterol is low. In fact, the Cholesterol Recurrent Events (CARE) study found that CRP levels were more accurate than cholesterol measures in predicting heart problems.[2]

Aspirin and statin medication have been shown to lower levels of C-reactive protein in women without heart disease. For women with heart disease, statin therapy has been shown to reduce the progression of disease, lowering CRP even after the cholesterol was adequately lowered. Therefore, women with heart disease should be treated with statin medication and aspirin.

However, I don't recommend medication to lower CRP in healthy women with elevated levels. A sensible diet and regular exercise for improved heart health is my most effective prescription for women to remain healthy.

If you have blood drawn for a CRP blood test while you have an active infection or a flareup of arthritis, the CRP level may be elevated. Don't be concerned. Simply repeat the test after the infection has cleared up.

Fibrinogen

Fibrinogen is a blood-clotting protein that the body needs to help with healing. However, elevated levels can be dangerous because blood clots can form more frequently and can obstruct the arteries, leading to heart disease and stroke. Women who have a family history of heart disease often show elevated levels of fibrinogen, as do women with high blood pressure and smokers. Levels of fibrinogen can also become elevated in response to inflammation. Cholesterol levels are associated with fibrinogen as well. People who have high LDL (bad) cholesterol and triglycerides and low levels of HDL (good) cholesterol also have elevated fibrinogen levels.

As with the other emerging risk factors, if you have heart disease and none of the traditional risk factors or early family history of heart disease, you should have your fibrinogen levels checked. Losing weight and stopping smoking help lower the fibrinogen levels. Estrogen replacement in postmenopausal women also reduces these levels. Discuss possibilities for treatment for high fibrinogen with your doctor.

WHITE BLOOD CELL COUNT

The white blood cell count is another way to assess women's risk for heart disease. White blood cells fight off infection, such as pneumonia or the common cold, and increase in number in response to inflammation. However, in a study of postmenopausal women, those women with persistently elevated white blood cell counts had a 40 percent greater risk of heart attack and 46 percent greater risk of stroke.[3] Again, if you don't have any of the traditional risk factors but have symptoms of heart disease, it's a good idea to have your doctor evaluate your white blood cell levels. Unfortunately, there are no studies that show that treatment with antibiotics to lower your white count lowers your risk for heart disease.

LUPUS

Lupus, an autoimmune disease that primarily affects women (90 percent of those with the disease are women), is also associated with a higher risk of heart attack, stroke, and blood clots. Women age thirty-five to forty-four with lupus have a fiftyfold increased risk for heart attack. Traditional cardiac risk factors, such as diabetes and high blood pressure, are more common in women who have lupus than in the general population. Other factors, such as increased homocysteine levels (see page 155) and early menopause, might play a role. Some researchers think that the chronic inflammation typical of lupus and the long-term use of steroids to treat it may also influence the rate of heart problems.

Another cause of heart attacks in women with lupus is the presence of antiphospholipid syndrome. This is an autoimmune condition that can occur with or without lupus, but a third of women with lupus have antiphospholipid syndrome. If you have it, there is an increased risk of vascular clotting, leading to an increased risk of heart attacks, strokes, and deep vein thrombosis. Such women also frequently have miscarriages due to a clot in the blood supply to the placenta.

The risk of heart disease is so high in women with lupus that many doctors feel it should be considered one of the risk factors for CAD. If you have lupus, your blood pressure and cholesterol levels should be carefully monitored. I test my patients for lupus and antiphospholipid syndrome if they have a heart attack or stroke and none of the common risk factors.

PSYCHOSOCIAL FACTORS AND HEART DISEASE

The medical field is increasingly recognizing the importance of managing psychological factors such as anxiety and stress in maintaining good health, including heart health. Finally!

STRESS

Stress increases the risk of heart attack. And which of us are not stressed? We care for our kids and our parents, work at our jobs, deal with our family and friends, and try to keep ahead of the chaos in our lives. All this stress can cause adrenaline and cortisol to pump excessively through your body. The excess adrenaline and cortisol can lead to hypertension and affect the flexibility of the arteries, which in turn makes them more susceptible to plaque buildup.

Women's hearts are more vulnerable than men's to stressful events, such as the death of a loved one. This recognized condition has been termed "broken heart syndrome." Women experience the symptoms of a heart attack, and it is not until weeks later, when it is obvious that the heart isn't damaged, that it becomes clear that the symptoms were the result of stress. Highly emotional experiences, even an argument or a surprise party, can cause stress hormones to be released that can have a negative impact on the heart.

PERSONALITY

Your risk of heart disease is related to your personality. If you are what is called a type A—racing around, driven to excel, impatient—your risk for heart disease, including hypertension and heart attack, is greater than if you move more slowly and take time to smell the roses. On the other hand, if you are type D—negative, depressed, distant, and insecure— you have an increased risk of heart disease as well. It's really related to anger. Type A personalities are generally angry or easily angered, while type D's suppress their anger, leaving them depressed. Both types are correlated with greater risk. Anger and hostility increase the production of stress hormones, so try and put something in place in your life to reduce stress. Exercise is good. Alcohol and overeating are not. Best to be type B and roll with the punches.

PANIC ATTACKS

Panic attacks can have symptoms that are very similar to those of heart attacks, so much so that it is often hard for a doctor to distinguish between them until tests are conducted. If the doctor can't, you can't either. Don't assume that sweating, dizziness, or difficulty catching your breath are simply symptoms of a panic attack. It could in fact be a heart attack. If you know you are susceptible to panic attacks, make sure you talk to your doctor about how to evaluate whether or not your symptoms are panic- or heart-related.

SOCIAL SUPPORT

Research on heart disease has shown a clear connection between living a long life and having adequate social support. A study conducted by the NIH showed that women who have a family history of heart disease are at increased risk of having it themselves if they are isolated. This risk is even greater than for high-risk men. Especially in today's world, where family members and friends are often living far apart, it can be difficult to provide yourself with emotional support. But this emotional nourishment is important, so reach out and touch someone.

RISK FACTORS FOR WOMEN ONLY

HORMONES

Our natural estrogen provides us with some protection against heart disease. After menopause, women's risk for heart attack increases by a factor of two or three. This observation is what led doctors to recommend estrogen replacement for postmenopausal women. However, as we now know from recently conducted research, HT does not help to keep your heart healthy.

When you are young and have normal levels of estrogen, you have higher levels of "good" HDL cholesterol and lower levels of "bad" LDL cholesterol and triglycerides. Estrogen also helps to prevent plaque from breaking off and causing a heart attack. Of course, there are younger women who get heart disease and have heart attacks; doctors speculate that those women may be less responsive than normal to the estrogen their bodies produce.

As you get closer to menopause, LDL cholesterol and triglyceride levels go up, increasing your risk of heart disease. As estrogen levels decrease with menopause, blood vessels become less flexible and blood pressure levels rise. Arteries become susceptible to the buildup and rupture of plaque. The role of hormones shows up in the big difference between women and men in heart attack timing: women are usually ten years older than men (and about ten years after menopause) when they have heart attacks.

Research shows that to ensure a healthy heart after menopause, you have to begin controlling whatever risk factors you can *before* menopause. The cardiovascular problems that may surface during menopause have been developing for decades. Prevention, including a healthy diet and regular exercise, can make a huge difference in your heart health.

ORAL CONTRACEPTIVES

Oral contraceptives are hormones (see Chapter 5), and if you are young and in good health and don't smoke, they may be a good form of birth control. However, if you are over thirty-five or have risk factors, such as high blood pressure, or you smoke, you should probably not take oral contraceptives because your risk of heart attack increases. Oral contraceptives also increase the risk of blood clots developing in the legs and lungs. If you have a history of clots or if you develop them while on oral contraceptives, talk to your gynecologist about alternative methods of birth control.

POLYCYSTIC OVARY SYNDROME (PCOS)

Polycystic ovary syndrome (PCOS), which is a common endocrine disorder (see Chapter 11), also increases the risk for heart disease. Research shows that women with PCOS, especially premenopausal women, have significantly increased risk factors, such as higher cholesterol and triglycerides, diabetes, hypertension, and atherosclerosis. If you have PCOS, you should be monitored for early detection of heart disease.[4]

PREGNANCY-RELATED PROBLEMS AND HEART HEALTH

Pregnancy is a time of hormonal changes, and some of the conditions associated with pregnancy can have an impact on your heart health long after the baby is delivered. For example, preeclampsia, a condition of high blood pressure, protein in the urine, and edema (swelling) that occurs during pregnancy (see Chapter 5), has been associated with an increased risk of a midlife heart attack and stroke. If you have had preeclampsia, it is important to have regular checkups with your health care provider to monitor your heart disease risk factors, such as blood pressure, weight, and blood sugar.

Gestational diabetes, a form of diabetes that also occurs during pregnancy (see Chapter 5), may lead to type 2 diabetes in later life. One of my patients recently told me that her blood sugar was elevated in pregnancy and never got better, even though her gynecologist had told her it would. If you had gestational diabetes, it is important to have regular checkups to follow your blood sugar levels.

There are some researchers who hypothesize that preeclampsia and gestational diabetes are linked to heart disease risk through the mechanism of insulin resistance, a prediabetic condition. In a recent study of almost five thousand women conducted by researchers at the Mayo Clinic and reported at the 2006 meeting of the American Heart Association, there was double the risk of stroke and one and a half times the risk for high blood pressure and heart attack in women who had these pregnancy-related conditions. Some of these women had protein in their urine, which is an early sign of kidney damage due to high blood pressure.

Remember that what happens in pregnancy is an important part of your medical history. Make sure you share this information with your doctor. As always, you should exercise regularly and follow a healthy eating plan (see Chapters 16 and 18) to continue to reduce your heart disease risk throughout your life cycle.

TESTS AND PROCEDURES FOR CORONARY ARTERY DISEASE

There are various tests and procedures that help locate and fix problems that relate to heart disease. However, it is vitally important to remember that fixing the problem is not the same thing as curing the disease that caused it. In other words, you still have to do whatever you can to reduce your risk for heart disease. If you have symptoms, your doctor will usually recommend one or more of these procedures in order to assess how your heart is working.

EXERCISE STRESS TEST OR ECG STRESS TEST

The exercise stress test shows how the heart muscle responds to a need for extra oxygen. It is used to evaluate the causes of chest pain or other symptoms and to determine whether there are blocked arteries or heart rhythm irregularities. During a stress test, a machine records the heart's electrical activity and blood pressure is taken during gradually increased physical stress, such as during exercise. This test is sometimes called an exercise tolerance test.

This noninvasive procedure can be done in a physician's office or as an outpatient at a hospital. After checking your blood pressure, a technician performs an ECG to see your heart rhythm at rest. Then you begin to exercise, either on a treadmill or on a stationary bicycle, and the doctor monitors your heart rhythm throughout exercise for changes that indicate blocked arteries. After you exercise, your blood pressure and ECG are monitored until you return to your baseline heart rate and blood pressure. In addition to testing for blocked arteries, how long you can exercise before becoming fatigued and your recovery time to your baseline heart rate are important indicators of your heart health. I always tell my patients that the longer they stay on the treadmill, the longer they will live.

For many years the ECG stress test was considered useless for women. This was because the stress test was often abnormal and when the woman had further testing, she was found not to have heart disease. This is called a false positive test. Sometimes false positives occur because the woman is unable to stay on the treadmill long enough for the test to be accurate. If you feel that you might not be able to do the treadmill, ask for another option. There are exercise imaging studies that can be done without the treadmill in conjunction with the electrocardiogram to determine if there are blocked arteries.

NUCLEAR STRESS TEST

Sometimes, in addition to an exercise stress test, your doctor may want to see how your blood flows through the arteries to the heart and will suggest a nuclear stress test. For this test, a small amount of radioactive material is injected into a vein while you are at rest, and during the peak of exercise on the treadmill your heart is scanned to see the blood flow to the heart. Pictures are then taken to help identify which areas of the heart are receiving oxygen. This test is more accurate in women than a treadmill stress test; however, there may be false positives here because of the breast getting in the way of the image. Also, this test uses radiation.

STRESS ECHOCARDIOGRAM

A stress echocardiogram is a stress test that is done with an ultrasound of the heart both at rest and during exercise. The patient has a resting ultrasound test, then walks on the treadmill; another image is taken as soon as you finish exercising. The rest and exercise images are compared. If you have a blocked artery, after you exercise the heart won't contract as strongly as at rest. The advantage of this test is that it does not use radiation and gives information about heart muscle function, valve function, and heart muscle damage from high blood pressure. I like to use this test for

---

TIPS FOR GOING FOR YOUR STRESS TEST

- Wear comfortable clothing and sneakers. (I sometimes have to lend a patient my sneakers when she shows up for the stress test with high-heeled mules.)
- Ask whether or not to take your medications before the test.
- Don't waste time putting on body lotion. The sticky pads that we use to monitor the ECG will slide right off.
- Ask about instructions for eating and drinking before the test.
- Make sure the stress test environment is safe. Emergency medications and equipment such as a defibrillator must be available.
- Make sure the doctor is in the room when you have the stress test.

women because it helps to distinguish whether their symptoms of short-ness of breath are due to a blocked artery or hypertension. But for women with chronic lung disease a nuclear stress test would be a better option because the ultrasound pictures are more accurate.

My patient Glenda called me, very upset. She was scheduled for hip surgery and her surgeon wanted to make sure that her heart was strong enough to get through the stress of the surgery. So he recommended that she come for a stress test. She told me in frustration when she came in, "I can't walk because my hip hurts. That's why I am having the surgery—so I can exercise. If I could get on a treadmill, I wouldn't need it." It was clear to me that she was right and shouldn't have an exercise stress test. But there are alternatives. I scheduled her for a pharmacologic stress test, where medications are given to simulate the stress of exercise. This test can be done with ultrasound (stress echo) or nuclear imaging.

CARDIAC CATHETERIZATION

Coronary catheterization or angiography is a medical procedure used to locate arteries that have become narrow or blocked by plaque, causing di-minished blood flow to the heart. During the procedure a catheter (a thin tube) is inserted into the artery, usually in the groin. A specialist called an interventional cardiologist uses X-ray images to guide the catheter through the arteries until it arrives at the heart, and then dye is injected to locate the artery that is blocked.

ANGIOPLASTY

Once the problem area is located, another, thinner catheter with a de-flated balloon on its tip is inserted through the first one. When it reaches the blockage, the balloon is inflated to widen the opening of the artery and improve the blood flow. Once the blood flow has improved, the bal-loon is deflated and the catheter removed. Sometimes a stent (a tube made of mesh or metal) is placed in the blocked artery to keep it open.

STENTS

In medicine, although we would all like to have everything crystal clear, very often we are left with mostly shades of gray. The controversy re-garding stents is a good example of how advances in technology and medicine have to be carefully studied and understood. Bare metal stents have been used for years to prop open blocked arteries and to avoid restenosis, a repeat narrowing of the artery. Although with the use of stents the rate of restenosis was reduced, it remained unacceptably high—about 25 percent within the first six months after the procedure. The development of stents coated with medication to prevent reblocking, the drug-eluting stents, greatly reduced the problem. But studies have shown that one year after placement of the drug-eluting stent there is an increase in the risk of developing a sudden blood clot (thrombosis) that would obstruct the artery. Therefore, both types of stents were associated with problems.

TIPS ON STENTS

- Be informed. Before the procedure ask your doctor what type of stent is being used and why that type is right for you.

- Tell your doctor if you are prone to blood clots or if you think you might have to have surgery or biopsies within a year of having the procedure. This is important because both the aspirin and clopidogrel medications cannot be stopped for one year after the procedure. Even if your dentist tells you to stop the blood thinners, don't do it unless you speak to your cardiologist.

- Medications are expensive, especially clopidogrel. Some drug plans offer mail-order options that lower the price. Pharmaceutical companies also offer assistance plans to help those who can demonstrate financial need.

However, these problems may not only be about the stents. People who have stents need to be treated with two types of antiplatelet medication, aspirin and clopidogrel (Plavix) for a year or longer, then aspirin alone, according to the latest recommendations from the American Heart Association, American College of Cardiology, and the Society for Coronary Angiography Intervention. The medical therapy cannot be stopped safely. Sometimes patients do not take their medications reliably, and those patients who don't are more likely to have another heart attack and die. Some people stop taking clopidogrel because it is expensive;

some are concerned about their (completely non-life-threatening) black-and-blue marks. Another problem is that sometimes dentists and surgeons, concerned about bleeding, tell their patients—without communicating with the cardiologist—to stop these necessary medications for nonemergency procedures.

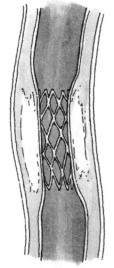

ARTERY WITH STENT IN PLACE

Drug-eluting stents are used for small arteries. They are not appropriate for individuals who need frequent surgical procedures, who are prone to blood clots, or who will have difficulty taking the blood thinners or remembering to take them. Never stop your blood thinners unless you have discussed it with your cardiologist. If you need a stent, don't be scared off by negative publicity. Discuss with your doctor which stent is right for you—and make sure to take your medication afterward, without interruption.

CT ANGIOGRAPHY (CTA)

The CTA uses X-rays and computer analysis to assess the condition of the blood vessels and therefore is a much less invasive test than a traditional angiogram. The test is best used for women who come to the emergency room with symptoms of shortness of breath or chest discomfort yet have normal electrocardiograms and blood tests. If the CTA is normal, it may save you from being admitted to the hospital unnecessarily.

This technique may also be useful for women who do not have a clearly positive or negative stress test. However, it's not a substitute for a traditional angiogram, which must be done before placing a stent or prior to coronary artery bypass surgery. Like an angiogram this test uses dye and radiation.

There are a few downsides to this test. Since the radiation dose is calibrated for men and not adjusted for a woman's size, women often get a higher dose. Also, the test is usually not covered by insurance. The CT angiogram is not accurate if you are obese, or have heavily calcified blood vessels, or have had a stent.

Make sure you let your doctor know if you think you may be allergic to the dye with either type of angiogram. If so, you should be given premedication to prevent the allergic reaction.

CARDIAC MRI

A cardiac MRI (magnetic resonance imaging) uses radio waves and magnetic fields to "see" inside the body. It is different from a traditional X-ray because it shows clearer pictures of internal organs and tissue and can give doctors information about the size and thickness of the chambers of the heart, the buildup of plaque, the condition of the arteries, and if there are any blockages. It can also identify small amounts of plaque that are potentially responsible for future heart attacks. It is also used to check the extent of heart damage after a heart attack.

CORONARY ARTERY BYPASS SURGERY

Coronary artery bypass surgery (CABG, often referred to as "cabbage") is the most common cardiac surgery performed in the United States. The procedure reroutes the blood flow around the blocked arteries so that the heart muscle gets the oxygen and other nourishment it needs. Before surgery, an angiogram identifies where the blockages are located. To bypass these blocked areas, the surgeon takes veins from the legs or arteries from the chest wall, wrist, or stomach and grafts one end to the aorta and the other to a place just past the obstruction. Women have a higher rate of complications after CABG compared to men, which might be due to the fact that women are generally older than men when they have the procedure and are more likely to have complicating risk factors such as diabetes, high blood pressure, and high cholesterol. Evaluate with your doctor if you are a good candidate for this procedure.

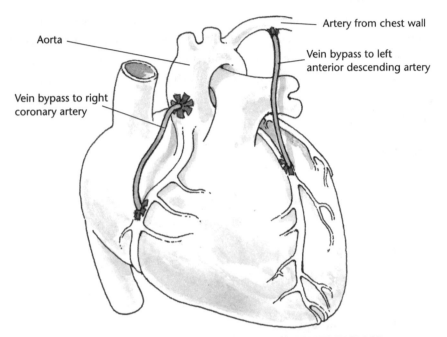

OBSTRUCTED ARTERIES WITH BYPASS GRAFTS IN PLACE

OTHER CAUSES OF CHEST PAIN

When people have serious chest pain, the first thing they assume is that they are having a heart attack. But there are other, quite serious medical reasons for chest pain, such as pulmonary embolism and pericarditis. Another reason for chest pain that is not related to heart disease is acid reflux disease (see page 217). I want you to know about these problems too.

PULMONARY EMBOLISM

A pulmonary embolism (PE) can occur if a blood clot originating in the legs, pelvis, or elsewhere travels to the lung, where it obstructs the flow of blood, depriving the lungs and other organs of oxygen. It is a very serious condition and can be fatal if not treated. Anticlotting medication, if given in a timely way, can resolve the problem. Unfortunately, however, many times PE is not diagnosed correctly and therefore not treated.

The signs of PE are very similar to that of a heart attack: chest pain, shortness of breath, sweating, feeling faint, racing heartbeat. One of the useful distinctions between pulmonary embolism and a heart attack is that with pulmonary embolism the chest pain is sharp and can increase when you take deep breaths (because the condition involves the lungs), whereas with a heart attack, the chest pain or sensation of chest pressure is unrelated to types of breathing. But this is not a distinction that you can make without a doctor, and they are both life-threatening conditions. If you have symptoms of a pulmonary embolism, get emergency medical care immediately.

Risk factors for pulmonary embolism

- Genetic predisposition to blood clots
- Immobilization (such as bed-ridden, long plane or car rides)
- Obesity
- High blood pressure
- Pregnancy
- Oral contraceptives
- Hormone therapy
- Cancer

If you have symptoms of PE, you need to see a doctor. Some typical questions the doctor may ask are:

- Have you recently had surgery?
- Have you recently been bedridden?
- Have you been on a long plane ride?
- Do you smoke?
- What is your blood pressure?
- Are you taking HT or oral contraceptives?
- Is there a family history of blood clots?
- Have you had a history of blood clots?

TESTS FOR PULMONARY EMBOLISM

Because symptoms can be similar to those of a heart attack, usually the first test is an ECG. If the ECG is normal, then your blood oxygen level is measured. If lower than normal, a lung scan or a CT pulmonary angiogram (CTA) scan can show if a blood clot has traveled to the lung. A sonogram of the leg veins may also be done to see if the clot originated there. Sometimes the clot is the result of a deep vein thrombosis (DVT), which is a clot that has formed in the legs, resulting in swelling. If you have painful or swollen legs, have your doctor check it out. You don't want a clot traveling to your lungs.

TREATMENT

Once diagnosed, treatment is intravenous blood thinners. In severe cases, clot-busting drugs may be used. After a few days, when you are stabilized, you will be put on an oral medication called warfarin (Coumadin), which is a blood-thinning medication that has to be carefully and continuously monitored for correct dosage.

PERICARDITIS

Pericarditis refers to an inflammation of the sac that surrounds the heart. This condition can be a complication of open-heart surgery, such as CABG or a valve replacement, or it may occur a few days after a heart attack. Another possible cause for pericarditis is infection.

With pericarditis, you may feel a sharp pain when you lie down that gets better when you sit up. You may also feel pain when you inhale. The condition is diagnosed through an ECG, and the treatment is usually medication, such as aspirin or ibuprofen. Sometimes steroids are prescribed.

PERIPHERAL ARTERY DISEASE

Peripheral artery disease (PAD) is a condition similar to coronary artery disease. In PAD, fatty deposits build up in the inner linings of the artery walls and restrict blood circulation, mainly in arteries leading to the kidneys, stomach, arms, legs, and feet. In its early stages a common symptom is cramping or fatigue in the legs and buttocks when you are doing some activity. The cramping usually subsides when you stop the activity. For some people who have severe PAD, the pain occurs even at rest. Tests used to diagnose PAD are ultrasound and MRA of the arteries to the legs.

People with PAD also have fatty buildup in the arteries of the heart and brain, making them at higher risk of death from heart attack and stroke. If you have diabetes and you smoke, it increases your risk for PAD. Treatment for PAD is directed at risk factors such as high cholesterol, smoking, and high blood pressure; medications are also used to help prevent blood clots. Sometimes angioplasty or bypasses are performed. If you are diagnosed with PAD, your doctor should check you for coronary artery disease, as these conditions commonly coexist.

ARRHYTHMIA

Heart Rhythm Disorders

Robin, a fifty-four-year-old woman who is a smoker, came to see me because she had palpitations and thought she was going to die. To help me assess what was going on, I asked her about how much coffee she drank, and if she ever felt dizzy or faint. I examined her, especially her thyroid, and asked about her family history. When I gave her a stress test, her baseline heart function was normal; however, I did see that she had skipped heartbeats when she began the test and that they went away when she was doing more vigorous exercise. I was able to reassure Robin that this pattern indicates a benign problem and she didn't need to worry—though I did point out that she was putting herself at greater risk of a heart attack by smoking. The most common reason women come to see me is for an irregular heartbeat, so it's important to understand the heart's electrical system in order to get a sense of what's normal and what's not.

Blood and nutrients are supplied to the body through the regular beating of the heart. The heartbeat is controlled by regular electrical impulses. Normally, the heart beats 60 to 100 times a minute. When something goes wrong with the electrical impulses and the heart does not beat regularly, the result is a rhythm disorder, or an arrhythmia.

If the heart rhythm is too fast, it is called tachycardia. At any age, you can experience a sinus tachycardia, a rapid heartbeat that is caused by the sinus node (specialized cells that pace the heartbeat) sending out electrical signals faster than normal. This can occur as a response to:

- Fear or stress

- Infection

- Caffeine (from coffee, tea, chocolate)

- Medication (such as epinephrine and digoxin)

- Thyroid disease

- Lung disease

- Reduced heart function

If the heart rhythm is too slow, it is called bradycardia. Sinus bradycardia is defined as a heart rate of less than 60 beats a minute. For some very fit people, this rate could be normal. For others, it might be caused by medications or indicate a sluggish thyroid.

Generally an occasional skipped beat is not a cause for concern, but it is important to identify why it is occurring. My patients describe the sensation of arrhythmia as palpitations, pounding heartbeats, or fluttering heartbeats. Usually when whatever is causing the disturbance is removed, the arrhythmia resolves. However, sometimes the altered heartbeat is due to an underlying abnormality of the heart muscle, perhaps from a heart attack or a valve problem. High blood pressure can also cause arrhythmias. Your doctor has to determine the source of the arrhythmia.

Types of Arrhythmias

Arrhythmias are classified by the location of the problem: the atria or the ventricles. Arrhythmias that do not begin in the ventricles are generally called supraventricular arrhythmias.

PREMATURE SUPRAVENTRICULAR OR PREMATURE ATRIAL CONTRACTIONS

In this condition, the heart beats early (that is, before the next beat normally would be expected) and the beat originates in one of the the upper chambers of the heart (the atria). This condition occurs in people of all ages but becomes more common as you get older. When it happens occasionally in women with normal heart function, this condition is usually not serious. But if it occurs frequently and is associated with dizziness, light-headedness, or fainting, you should consult your doctor.

SUPRAVENTRICULAR TACHYCARDIA AND PAROXYSMAL SUPRAVENTRICULAR TACHYCARDIA

This is a series of rapid heartbeats that can begin and end suddenly. They originate in the upper chambers of the heart, the atria. This condition is common in women in their twenties and thirties and may be precipitated by caffeine or stress or caused by certain medications. If the symptoms are severe or continue, you should have an ECG. Treatment is designed to slow the heart rate. This can be accomplished through medication and by eliminating caffeine and other stimulants. If medications do not clear up the problem, a procedure known as radiofrequency ablation is performed to correct the electrical impulse causing the arrhythmia.

RADIOFREQUENCY ABLATION

Radiofrequency ablation is a procedure that is used most often to treat supraventricular tachycardia. During this procedure, a physician inserts a catheter through a vein in the groin and with the help of imaging guides it to the spot inside the heart where the electrical signals causing the abnormal rhythm are generated. Using an electrode attached to the catheter, radiofrequency energy, a low-voltage high-frequency form of electrical energy, is applied to the cells that are causing the rapid heartbeats, destroying them. The procedure has a very high success rate and a very low complication rate.

WOLFF-PARKINSON-WHITE SYNDROME

This syndrome causes very fast heart rates due to an abnormality in the accessory pathways between the atria and ventricles. The electrical signal bypasses its normal route and ricochets back and forth between the atria and the ventricles. The resulting fast heartbeat can cause you to faint or collapse and should be evaluated. Radiofrequency ablation can be used effectively, especially for those people who do not want to take medication for prolonged periods.

SICK SINUS SYNDROME

The sinus node is thought to be the heart's natural pacemaker, but sometimes abnormal heartbeats, either very slow or very fast, can be caused by a malfunction of this node. Occasionally there are no symptoms and no treatment is needed. But if you become dizzy and tired or experience other symptoms, a pacemaker may be required.

ATRIAL FIBRILLATION

In atrial fibrillation, an irregular heart rate is caused by electrical signals in the atria firing rapidly, irregularly, and ineffectively. Atrial fibrillation usually occurs in women over fifty who have a history of hypertension, coronary artery disease, congestive heart failure, or thyroid disease. For some unexplained reason, women who are treated for atrial fibrillation generally don't do as well as men treated for the same condition.

Because there is a risk of stroke in people who have atrial fibrillation, treatment usually involves blood-thinning medication. Rate control medications such as beta-blockers and calcium channel blockers are used to slow the heart rate. Sometimes an electrical shock to the heart is used to restore normal rhythm. A specialized form of radiofrequency ablation, known as pulmonary vein ablation, is also used in cases where the atrial fibrillation is difficult to control, but it is only 65 percent successful. Studies show that patients who are treated with a combination of rate control medication and blood thinners have fewer strokes.

VENTRICULAR TACHYCARDIA

A fast heartbeat can be caused by electrical signals from the ventricles. This type of arrhythmia is common in women with heart disease and requires immediate treatment, as it can be life-threatening. Treatment depends on what is causing the problem. Sometimes cardioversion (electric shock to the heart) is required to restore the heart's natural rhythm. Some patients have an automatic implantable defibrillator inserted.

VENTRICULAR FIBRILLATION

In this life-threatening arrhythmia, electrical signals in the ventricles fire in a fast, uncontrolled manner, causing the heart to quiver rather than pulse. This arrhythmia requires quick action with electrical shock to recover a normal heartbeat.

DIAGNOSING ARRHYTHMIAS

If you have an arrhythmia, some of the questions the doctor might ask are:

- How often do you have palpitations?
- Are you dizzy or light-headed?
- Did you ever faint when you were having palpitations?
- Do the symptoms occur with exertion or exercise?
- Have you had a heart attack?
- Do you have a heart murmur?
- Are you taking any cold medications?
- How much caffeine, in coffee or tea or chocolate, do you consume?
- How would you describe your level of stress?
- Are the palpitations related to your period?
- Are the palpitations associated with your hot flashes?

Tests that your doctor may order include:

- *ECG.* An ECG can provide baseline information about your heart rhythm. If you have it done during the time of an arrhythmia, the

> **AUTOMATIC IMPLANTABLE CARDIO DEFIBRILLATOR**
>
> An automatic implantable cardio defibrillator is a small device implanted in the chest with a special wire that is inserted into the heart. It is used to control sudden fainting episodes that are caused by arrhythmias; it works by automatically shocking the heart when necessary so that normal rhythm is restored.

doctor should be able to locate the place in the heart (atrial or ventricular) that is abnormal.

- *Holter monitor.* If the ECG does not reveal information about the problem, a Holter monitor may be recommended. This device is worn for twenty-four to forty-eight hours (electrodes are attached to your chest and the small recording device can be kept in your pocket) and constantly records your heart rhythm. Usually you are asked to keep a diary of your activities that the doctor can match to the heart rhythms.

- *Event monitor.* Because some arrhythmias occur less frequently than once a day, another monitor, called an event recorder, can be worn for a longer time, usually a month. It works like the Holter monitor but records heart rhythm when a button is pushed. The idea is to record the "event" of the arrhythmia.

- *Echocardiogram.* An echocardiogram may be recommended to evaluate if there are structural abnormalities of the heart muscle or valve that is the cause of the arrhythmia. An instrument called a transducer is placed on your chest near your heart, picks up the echoes of sound waves, and translates them into electrical impulses that can be read by your doctor.

- *Stress test.* A stress test can be done to see whether exercise is the cause of the arrhythmia. (See page 163 for a full description.)

A few years ago I saw a sixty-year-old patient who was complaining of severe shoulder pain. Because of her financial and social situation she had never been examined fully. Instead when she complained of pain, she had been sent for X-rays. She told me that no one had ever asked her to take her clothes off. I needed to get to the root of her pain, which meant I needed to examine her shoulder. What it showed shocked me. She had had a pacemaker implanted—but in the wrong place, near her armpit. No wonder she had pain. The other doctors only needed to examine her and not blindly send her for testing. Of course, I arranged for an electrophysiologist (a cardiologist who specializes in pacemakers) and an arrhythmia surgeon to fix the problem, and she was fine.

VALVULAR HEART DISEASE

The four heart valves (pulmonic, aortic, tricuspid, and mitral) control the flow of blood between the chambers of the heart. When the valves don't open or close properly, you have valve problems. Valve problems can be very mild and without symptoms or life-threatening.

The valves can have two basic kinds of problems: stenosis, when the opening of the valve is narrow, which causes the heart to work harder, and insufficiency, which refers to leaking because the valve isn't closing properly. (Many women are told that they have a murmur. This means that the doctor hears abnormal closing sounds.) Symptoms of valve disease are usually chest pain, shortness of breath, or feeling light-headed or faint during exertion. Treatment of valve disease depends on the severity of the problem. Many people have no symptoms and require no treatment. Others, with more serious conditions, may require medication, such as diuretics or anticoagulants, to improve blood flow. In extreme cases, surgery may be required to repair the valve.

If your doctor suspects you have valve problems, she probably will suggest an echocardiogram to visualize how the blood is pumped through the heart. Sometimes, due to obesity or body shape, an "echo" is not effective and another similar ultrasound test, called a trans-esophageal echocardiogram (TEE), can be used to evaluate valve problems. This test works by passing a tube into the esophagus so that the sound waves of the heart can be heard and recorded. Transesophageal echo is also done to look for blood clots in the heart.

MITRAL VALVE DISEASE

A normal mitral valve allows the blood to flow freely from the left atrium to the left ventricle and closes to prevent regurgitation (backup). There are three main kinds of mitral valve problems: mitral valve prolapse, mitral valve stenosis, and mitral valve regurgitation. These are quite common in middle-aged women, and I want you to understand the difference.

MITRAL VALVE PROLAPSE

In mitral valve prolapse small amounts of blood may leak backward into the upper chamber of the heart because the valve does not close properly. This causes a heart murmur. One of my male professors in medical school referred to this condition, which affects more women than men, as the "click-chick phenomenon" because the doctor hears a clicking sound with the stethoscope. In fact, this condition has often been seriously overdiagnosed in women. When strict criteria for diagnosis are applied (the Freed criteria), only 2 percent of the population have it. Women who really do have mitral valve prolapse have fewer complications than men and lead perfectly normal lives. So don't be frightened unnecessarily if you are told you have a heart murmur.

If you have mitral valve prolapse, antibiotics used to be recommended routinely before certain procedures, such as dental work, colonoscopy, and some gynecological procedures, in order to prevent endocarditis. Now antibiotics are recommended only for individuals who have had valve replacement or repair, certain types of congenital heart disease, or a history of endocarditis. Endocarditis is an infection of the heart valve that leads to heart valve damage.

MITRAL VALVE STENOSIS

Mitral stenosis refers to a narrowing of the valve into the left ventricle that prevents proper opening and therefore limits the blood flow to the heart. Mitral stenosis is two to three times more common in women than in men. The most common cause of mitral stenosis is rheumatic fever. Other causes are congenital abnormalities, lupus, and rheumatoid arthritis.

MITRAL REGURGITATION

In patients who have mitral regurgitation, blood leaks out of the left ventricle into the left atrium, which causes the heart to pump extra hard so that normal blood flow can be maintained. Sometimes this condition is called mitral valve insufficiency. Mitral valve regurgitation occurs in about 2 percent of the population. The underlying causes of mitral valve regurgitation are mitral valve prolapse, an enlarged heart, heart attack, and endocarditis.

AORTIC STENOSIS

Aortic valve stenosis, or aortic stenosis, happens when the aortic valve becomes narrow, preventing the valve from opening fully. The narrowing causes the blood flow from your aorta to become obstructed. Because there is an obstruction, the heart has to work harder to pump, especially when called upon to deliver more blood, as with increased exertion. When the heart works harder than normal, the muscle walls become thick. If you have aortic valve stenosis, the doctor can usually hear an abnormal heart sound or heart murmur. If you suffer from aortic stenosis, in addition to fatigue and shortness of breath, you may experience angina and heart failure. Severe aortic valve stenosis requires surgery to replace the valve. The surgery has a 95 percent success rate in patients who have no coronary heart disease and who have normal heart function.

AORTIC REGURGITATION

Aortic regurgitation is the backing up of blood from the aorta into the left ventricle because the aortic valve does not close properly. Some people have no symptoms at all; others can feel fatigue, shortness of breath, and arrhythmias, and have swelling of the ankles and feet. The most common cause of chronic aortic regurgitation is infection such as rheumatic heart disease, hypertension, and endocarditis. It could also be congenital, meaning that's the way you were born.

HEART FAILURE

Heart failure means that the heart is unable to do its job—it fails to pump blood effectively. It can occur for a variety of reasons: structural heart defects such as heart valve problems, a virus that has damaged the heart muscle, high blood pressure, or coronary artery disease. It is a progressive disease, and as you get older, the likelihood of getting it doubles with each decade. There are two types of heart failure: systolic failure, which is poor pump function due to weakened heart muscle function, and diastolic heart failure, where the heart function is normal but the pressure within the heart is high. Symptoms may be the same for both types.

Medical conditions, such as diabetes, anemia, or thyroid disease, can increase the risk for heart failure by putting extra strain on the heart. You are also at increased risk if you are overweight, smoke, or abuse alcohol.

The causes of heart failure in women are different than for men. Women are more likely to have high blood pressure, valve disease, or diabetes as their underlying cause. Men are more likely to have heart failure due to previous heart attacks. Another cause is peripartum cardiomyopathy, a condition that develops within the last month of pregnancy or soon after delivery and so is the one form of heart failure truly unique to women. Peripartum cardiomyopathy occurs in one out of ten thousand pregnancies. The risk is greater in women over thirty, African American women, and women pregnant with twins or other multiples. The symptoms improve in 50–60 percent of women, but the problem can reoccur with subsequent pregnancies.

Symptoms of Heart Failure

Although the heart is "failing," it keeps working, only not as efficiently as it should. If you have heart failure, you might become short of breath and tired, especially when you exercise. You might also retain water and notice that your ankles and legs are swollen and that you have gained weight.

Diagnosing Heart Failure

Questions the doctor might ask include:

- Are you short of breath?
- Can you sleep flat on your back?
- Are your ankles and legs swollen?
- Do you have thyroid disease?
- Do you have diabetes?
- Do you have palpitations?
- Have you fainted recently?
- Do you have a persistent cough?
- Lack of appetite?

It is important to discover the underlying cause of the heart failure in order to treat it properly. Usually the doctor will recommend an echocardiogram, an ECG, or cardiac catheterization to discover the cause.

TREATMENT FOR HEART FAILURE

Most often, medications are used to treat heart failure. ACE inhibitors expand blood vessels in order to enable the blood to flow more easily and take some pressure off the heart. Beta-blockers, another type of medication, improve how the left ventricle pumps. Diuretics help the body eliminate the water that has built up. Other drugs may be used as well. If the heart failure is due to high blood pressure, that should be treated. If it is due to an abnormal valve, surgery might be necessary.

CARDIOVASCULAR MEDICATIONS

Medications for heart problems are used to reduce the risk of heart attacks and strokes. Like many medications, heart medicine treats the symptoms rather than cures the disease. Cardiovascular disease is such a serious problem for women, and so many women are treated for various problems associated with heart disease, that I want to familiarize you with at least some of the medications commonly prescribed.

CORONARY ARTERY DISEASE

ASPIRIN

Aspirin has been around for more than a hundred years. In fact, Hippocrates in 400 B.C. used the bark of the willow tree, which contains the active ingredient in aspirin, to treat fever and pain. Its value in treating heart disease was discovered accidentally. In the late 1940s a California physician realized that of the four hundred men in his practice that he had treated with aspirin for pain, not one had suffered a heart attack. A clinical study in the 1980s showed that when men took aspirin every other day their risk of a first heart attack was reduced by 32 percent.

And what about the women? In 2005 one of the largest aspirin studies involving women was published. Nearly forty thousand healthy women forty-five years and older took 100 mg of aspirin every other day.

The study showed that aspirin reduced a first heart attack and stroke in healthy women over the age of 65. The researchers also found that taking aspirin reduced the risk of a first stroke caused by a blood clot (ischemic stroke) by 24 percent. This study did not evaluate women who had previously had a heart attack, nor did it include many women at high risk for heart attack.[5]

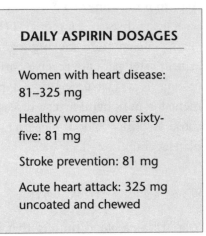

DAILY ASPIRIN DOSAGES

Women with heart disease: 81–325 mg

Healthy women over sixty-five: 81 mg

Stroke prevention: 81 mg

Acute heart attack: 325 mg uncoated and chewed

There are many studies that show that women who have suffered a previous heart attack do benefit from daily aspirin to prevent a recurrent heart attack. Aspirin reduces the risk of death from a second heart attack by 25 percent and the chance of having a second heart attack by 49 percent. Still, despite its proven benefits, aspirin therapy, like other heart medications, is underprescribed to women.

Aspirin is effective for reducing heart attacks and stroke because it is an antiplatelet medication, that is, a medication that prevents blood clots from forming. However, there are side effects and risks you should watch out for if you take daily aspirin. These include stomach upset and bleeding. Your blood pressure should be carefully controlled as well to prevent a stroke caused by bleeding in the brain.

Aspirin is recommended for:

- Women of any age with previous heart attack or ischemic stroke, TIA, stents, or angina

- Healthy women over sixty-five

- Women at high risk: those who have diabetes, vascular disease, or multiple risk factors for heart disease

- Healthy women over forty-five, who may reduce their risk of stroke with aspirin therapy

CLOPIDOGREL

Aspirin is only one of a number of medications recommended to women with heart disease. Clopidogrel (Plavix) is another medication that prevents platelets from sticking together. It is primarily used in addition to aspirin after patients receive coronary artery stents, particularly drug-eluting stents (see page 165). Clopidogrel also has some benefit for treatment for peripheral artery disease. The side effects of clopidogrel are those of "thin" blood: bleeding, black-and-blue marks, and a reduced platelet count.

WARFARIN (COUMADIN)

Warfarin is a blood thinner that inhibits blood-clotting proteins in the liver. It is used to prevent stroke if you have atrial fibrillation and to treat DVTs and pulmonary embolism. It reduces the risk of clots to mechanical heart valves. It also reduces the growth of blood clots that form in the left ventricle after a heart attack.

Coumadin has interactions with many medications, including hormone therapy and oral contraceptives. It also can be affected by foods. Your blood has to be tested regularly to see if your Coumadin dose is accurate. It is an important calibration because if your blood is not thinned enough, there is risk for blood clots; if it's too thin, there is a risk for bleeding.

Coumadin should not be taken during pregnancy because it is associated with birth defects.

> **WARNING IF YOU ARE ON BLOOD THINNERS**
>
> Avoid taking additional blood thinners or supplements with blood-thinning properties, such as vitamin E or garlic capsules.

> **FOODS THAT INTERACT WITH COUMADIN**
>
> Dark leafy vegetables contain vitamin K, which makes Coumadin less potent. If you eat a lot of salads, let your doctor know and she will dose the medication accordingly.

HEPARIN

Heparin is an intravenous medication that enhances the activity of your natural blood-thinning proteins. It is used in the hospital for patients who have had an acute heart attack, pulmonary embolism, or DVTs, until Coumadin can be taken as an outpatient.

Low-molecular-weight heparin, enoxiparin (Lovenox), is administered by injection under the skin and can be used on an outpatient basis. Recent studies show that it may be more protective against stroke than regular heparin.

NITROGLYCERIN

Nitroglycerin can be given intravenously in the hospital when someone is having a heart attack, or by pill, patch, or spray. If taken under the tongue for symptoms of chest discomfort or shortness of breath due to coronary artery disease, relief is quick. I recommend to all my patients with coronary artery disease that they carry a bottle in their purse for an emergency. The bottle has to be in a dark place, and once opened, the medication is good for only three months. Long-acting forms are prescribed for daily therapy. Side effects include headache, dizziness, and low blood pressure, especially when added to other blood-pressure-lowering medications such as beta-blockers and calcium channel blockers.

CHOLESTEROL-LOWERING MEDICATIONS

Diet and exercise can lower cholesterol levels 12–15 mg/dl. This may be enough for women who have only mild elevations of cholesterol, but severe elevations of cholesterol, and even mildly elevated to normal values in women who have heart disease or diabetes, might require medication such as statins.

STATINS

Statins reduce the production of cholesterol in the liver. They lower the risk of heart attack by 36 percent in women and risk of death due to heart attack by 21 percent. A 2005 study published in *Circulation* showed that only one in five women on cholesterol medication and at high risk for heart disease actually had their cholesterol lowered.[6] Although the women were on cholesterol medication, their doctors were not following their cholesterol levels carefully. All they needed to get the benefit of the medicine was a dose adjustment.

Like all medications, statins have side effects. You need to have your liver function checked regularly if you take statins. If you have muscle aches and weakness or feel unusually tired and headachy, tell your doctor. Constipation is also a common side effect. Women, especially those who have a petite frame, are over sixty years old, take multiple medications, and use erythromycin or calcium channel blockers while on statins, have more side effects.

Some statins can be affected by grapefruit juice (see page 47), calcium channel blockers, and the antibiotic erythromycin. Don't worry if you need to take antibiotics; your doctor will probably tell you to temporarily discontinue the statins.

The most commonly prescribed statins are atorvastatin (Lipitor), simvastatin (Zocor), pravastatin (Pravachol), and rosuvasatin (Crestor). Pravachol and Crestor are not affected by grapefruit.

EZETIMIBE

Ezetimibe (Zetia) lowers cholesterol by interfering with the absorption of cholesterol from the intestine. It lowers LDL ("bad") cholesterol by 18 percent when used alone and by 12 to 20 percent when used in combination with a statin. If you can't take statins, Zetia is a good alternative, but many patients take both Zetia and statins. I like to add Zetia to statin therapy because it allows me to keep my patients on a lower dose of statins, and the lower the dose, the fewer the side effects.

People on Zetia sometimes complain of gastrointestinal upset and muscle aches and may have abnormal liver tests. Your doctor will monitor your liver function, and you should be sure to tell the doctor about any side effects you experience.

FIBRIC ACID DERIVATIVES

Fibric acid derivatives, such as fenofibrate (Tricor) and gemfibrozil (Lopid) lower triglycerides, and for my patients whose triglycerides are

300 or more, I start with one of these drugs. In addition to lowering triglycerides these medications also raise HDL (good) cholesterol and lower LDL (bad) cholesterol.

As with many of these drugs, liver function needs to be measured regularly because one of the side effects is elevated liver enzymes. As with statins, muscle aches and weakness are other potential side effects, although these side effects are more likely in patients with kidney disease. For patients without kidney disease who are on a combination of statin and fibric acid derivative, to minimize side effects I use lower dosages of each medication and make sure my patients do not miss their appointment for the follow-up laboratory tests. Gastrointestinal side effects include bloating, diarrhea, and constipation.

If you take Coumadin and fibric acid derivatives, you need to have your blood monitored more closely because the latter tend to increase the blood-thinning effects of Coumadin. Often your doctor will make an adjustment to your dosage of Coumadin.

OMEGA-3 FISH OIL

Omega-3 fish oil lowers triglycerides and is recommended for people with high triglycerides. Although omega-3 fish oil is available in health food stores, prescription formulations (Lovaza is the brand name) are purified and have a specific known quantity of fish oil in each capsule. The dose to lower triglycerides is 3 to 4 g daily. If you have had a heart attack, 1 g daily is recommended. In addition to a fishy taste, potential side effects may include a rash or gastrointestinal problems such as bloating and gas.

Although there is a potential for increased risk of bleeding when omega-3 fish oil is added to other blood thinners, most patients do fine. But it is important to be monitored for bleeding.

NIACIN

At first glance, niacin looks like the perfect solution to high cholesterol because it raises HDL (good) cholesterol and lowers LDL (bad) cholesterol. Niacin is generally prescribed to lower triglycerides. It is also used to raise HDL cholesterol in women with low HDL cholesterol and at high risk of heart disease. The American Heart Association recommends niacin for women at high risk for heart disease in their 2007 guidelines. The reason that only high-risk women are targeted for niacin is because we know HDL is an important risk factor for heart disease.

The problem with niacin is some of the side effects. My patient Madge started to take some niacin that she bought in a health food store because she read an article in the *New York Times* extolling how fabulous niacin was in raising HDL cholesterol. Soon she thought that she was getting her hot flashes back. She didn't realize that one of the most common side effects of niacin is flushing. It is interesting that in one study of prescription niacin, women were more likely than men to stop the medication because of side effects. Even if the niacin you take is over-the-counter, you should tell your physician because of the possibility of abnormal liver function, hyperglycemia, and increased uric acid. Taking niacin along with other cholesterol medications may increase the risk of muscle pain and liver test abnormalities. I often use combination therapy to treat cholesterol, but I explain to my patients that they must follow up regularly for their blood tests. There could be increased side effects if taken along with supplements (see Chapter 13) such as kava and red yeast rice.

High Blood Pressure

Diuretics, which promote the excretion of water from the body, are the first-line medication to reduce blood pressure and are now thought to be superior to beta-blockers. Diuretics can be used alone or in combination with other types of blood pressure medications. They are also prescribed for heart failure patients to relieve the body of excess fluid.

Some diuretics cause a loss of potassium and magnesium. This problem can be monitored by blood tests that measure for these electrolytes. To avoid this problem, potassium replacement is commonly prescribed along with diuretics. Low potassium levels are associated with muscle cramps and arrhythmias. There are diuretics, such as triamterene, that prevent

> **IF YOU ARE ALLERGIC TO SULFA**
>
> Let your doctor know if you are allergic to sulfa medications because diuretics contain sulfa.

potassium loss. But triamterene should not be taken with an ACE inhibitor because there is a risk of overly high potassium. If an ACE inhibitor is added to the diuretic, potassium replacement may not be necessary.

Dehydration is another potential side effect of diuretic therapy. Some people don't realize that you can and should drink water if you are on these medications. Even though diuretics are effective blood pressure medications, if you have urinary frequency or incontinence the diuretic may make it worse. Ask your doctor for alternative blood pressure therapy.

ANGIOTENSIN CONVERTING ENZYME (ACE) INHIBITORS

ACE inhibitors, or ACEIs, promote a chemical reaction to relax the blood vessels. These medications also reduce the onset of heart failure in people who have had a heart attack and improve survival in people who have heart failure.[7] ACE inhibitors reduce the risk of heart muscle thickening in individuals who have high blood pressure. They are prescribed to diabetic patients to protect the kidneys from the damaging effects of diabetes. Many ACE inhibitors are available as a combination pill with a diuretic.

The most common side effects are rash and a dry cough. The dry cough is dose-related and more common in women. If you are on ACE inhibitors, and are taking potassium, you may need to discontinue it to prevent overly high potassium levels. A less common but more serious side effect is swelling and tingling around the mouth and tongue. If this occurs, you need to stop the medication immediately because you may be having a serious allergic reaction. Talk to your doctor.

> **FOR PREGNANT WOMEN**
>
> ACE inhibitors should not be taken if you are pregnant or trying to become pregnant.

ANGIOTENSIN II RECEPTOR BLOCKERS (ARBs)

ARBs work like ACE inhibitors, relaxing the blood vessels to lower blood pressure. They also protect the kidneys from damage in people who have diabetes, and are used as treatment for heart failure. The side effects are also similar to those of ACE inhibitors, with the exception of the cough, which is uncommon with ARBs. Therefore patients who get a cough on an ACE inhibitor are usually prescribed an ARB. As with ACE inhibitors, there is a risk for overly high potassium.

> **FOR PREGNANT WOMEN**
>
> ARBs should not be used if you are pregnant or thinking of becoming pregnant.

You should not take nonsteroidal anti-inflammatory drugs (NSAIDs) such as ibuprofen (Motrin) if you are taking ARBs or ACE inhibitors because they will interfere with the blood-pressure-lowering effect. Using ACE inhibitors and ARBs together increases the risk of excessively low blood pressure.

CALCIUM CHANNEL BLOCKERS

Calcium channel blockers lower blood pressure by relaxing or widening blood vessels. There are two types of calcium channel blockers: those that slow the heart rate in addition to relaxing blood vessels and others that primarily relax blood vessels, such as amlodipine (Norvasc), which may increase the heart rate slightly. Another calcium channel blocker, nifedipine, particularly the short-acting form, has caused low blood pressure and angina symptoms in patients with coronary artery disease.

The side effects of calcium channel blockers can be constipation, acid reflux, swelling of the ankles, dizziness caused by low blood pressure, and headaches. Another side effect, overgrowth of the gums, requires discontinuation of the medication.

BETA-BLOCKERS

Beta-blockers (such as metoprolol and propranolol) have been available for nearly forty years and are used to treat angina and arrhythmias; they also are given prophylactically after a heart attack to reduce the risk of a second heart attack. Beta-blockers are also used in pregnancy for arrhythmias and high blood pressure. When they are prescribed for blood pressure, they are usually added to another medication, such as a diuretic, ACE inhibitor, or ARB. I generally use beta-blockers to reduce high blood pressure in patients who have an arrhythmia or coronary artery disease.

Beta-blockers have side effects, like all medication. They can cause fatigue and sleep problems. They can precipitate asthma attacks in people who suffer from asthma. They also exacerbate Raynaud's syndrome where your fingers and toes turn color when exposed to a cold environment—outdoors in winter, in air-conditioning, or the freezer. This is not life-threatening but can be annoying. Also, it is difficult to lose weight on beta-blockers because the medication slows metabolism by 10 percent.

If they are combined with other medications that lower blood pressure, beta-blockers can increase the risk of lower-than-expected blood pressure. That is why when I prescribe combination therapy, I use low dosages to start and increase slowly as needed. If combined with certain calcium channel blockers, there is a potential for very slow heart rates, and therefore you should be closely monitored by your doctor.

> ## STOPPING BETA-BLOCKERS
>
> When beta-blockers are discontinued, they should be tapered, not stopped abruptly, because stopping too suddenly can precipitate chest pain in people with coronary artery disease and cause a sudden rise in heart rate in people with normal hearts.

CLONIDINE

Clonidine, available by pill or patch, is used after other agents have been tried but blood pressure has not been adequately lowered. The patch is applied weekly and the pill is taken two or three times per day. It can cause dizziness and fatigue and slow your pulse rate. The light-headedness or dizziness is more marked when you change position, so when you first start the medication avoid abrupt changes in position. If the medication is stopped abruptly, you will get a sudden rise in blood pressure. The side effects are less common with the patch, but the patch has a 20 percent chance of producing a rash.

FOR PREGNANT WOMEN

Hypertension in pregnancy is treated with a few different medications. Methyldopa has been used the longest, and in terms of safety it is the first choice. Beta-blockers, calcium channel blockers, and labetalol are also used.

LABETALOL

This blood pressure medication has properties similar to the beta blockers. It is used if the other medications are not effective in controlling blood pressure. It is more commonly used in the emergency room for patients who come in with severe hypertension, in which case it can be given intravenously and it can also be prescribed by pill as a long-term medication. Side effects include nausea, vomiting, sweating, dizziness, and headaches.

NONSTEROIDAL ANTI-INFLAMMATORY DRUGS (NSAIDS)

One day three patients came to the office who were all taking their blood pressure medication, yet they all had high blood pressure. After the third patient, Colleen, my nurse, came to me and said something was wrong. She thought that all of the blood presssure machines in the office might be broken. I went in to see one of the patients. This woman had had a blood pressure of 110/70 for the last five visits, but now it was reading 140/90, without any weight gain or change in diet. I asked her the magic question: had she been taking any pain medicine recently? I knew that the other two patients had. She said yes, she had been taking high-dose ibuprofen for a knee injury for the last three months. When I asked her if she had followed up with the orthopedic surgeon, she said she couldn't get a convenient appointment, and besides, her knee was feeling better. I stopped the ibuprofen and made sure she got an appointment with the orthopedic surgeon.

All the interest in anti-inflammatory pain medication started in 2004, when data were released showing that rofecoxib (Vioxx), an anti-inflammatory pain medication (a type known as a COX-2 inhibitor), increased heart attack and stroke risk. The drug company that made the drug, Merck, voluntarily took it off the market. Celecoxib (Celebrex), another COX-2 inhibitor, is still prescribed, although the FDA mandated a warning that it too is associated with heart attack risk, but to a lesser extent than Vioxx (the dosage is weaker). I never prescribe COX-2 inhibitors because when I reviewed the pharmacology of the drug, I was concerned that it could increase my patients' blood pressure and potentially cause heart attacks.

Because of the information about COX-2 inhibitors, researchers began investigating the heart attack risk associated with other pain medications, such as the NSAIDs ibuprofen (Advil) and naproxen (Aleve), as well as the non-NSAID pain reliever acetaminophen (Tylenol). In a study of more than seventy thousand women it was found that high doses of these medications, defined as more than fifteen tablets per week, increased the risk for cardiovascular disease by 86 percent with the NSAIDs and 68 percent with acetaminophen (Tylenol). Aspirin is an NSAID but does not increase heart attack risk; in fact, it prevents heart attacks and strokes.

So what's a woman to do if she is trying to exercise to prevent heart disease and has arthritis?

- Make sure you tell all of your doctors your medical history and which medications you take or have recently taken.

- Ask the doctor who is taking care of your arthritis how long you need to take these meds.

- Be confident that small amounts of NSAIDs for short-term use are safe.

- Don't stop taking aspirin if you are on it to prevent a first or second heart attack or stroke.

- Ibuprofen may interfere with the protective effects of aspirin, so take the ibuprofen several hours after you take your aspirin.

- Ask about nonpharmaceutical ways to manage pain, such as physical therapy, heat, or cold.

- If medication is necessary, start with acetaminophen, narcotic pain relievers, or non–COX-2 inhibitors short term at the lowest dose.

- Start an exercise program (see Chapter 18) for exercises that are low-impact and won't exacerbate joint pain.

NINE

Taking Care of Your Bones and Muscles

TAKING CARE OF YOUR BONES

It's easy to take your bones for granted—that is, until one breaks. Then it becomes clear that it is really important to take care of them. Think of your bones as the support structure for the house you live in. If you thought you had termites eating away at the beams, you would certainly do something about it. You wouldn't wait around for the house to start falling down around you. As with your house, without good maintenance for your bones, you are asking for trouble.

WHAT ARE BONES?

Bones are living tissue, made up of cells, nerves, blood vessels, and minerals. Bone cells have various functions: making new bone, carrying nutrients to and from blood vessels in the bone, and breaking down and reforming bone. These processes continue throughout your life. Not only do your bones support your physical structure and protect your internal organs (for example, the skull protects the brain), they also enable you to move (along with muscles and joints) and play a role in cell formation as well as the storage and metabolism of calcium and other minerals.

Bones consist of calcium and other minerals that cause them to be hard; strong, hard bones are necessary to support your weight. Dietary calcium—that is, the amount of calcium that you take in via your diet—and vitamin D affect how much calcium is stored in the bones. Calcium is stored in the bones, providing bone density and bone strength, and when the body needs it, is released into the bloodstream.

> ### EXERCISE FOR BONE HEALTH
>
> Many of my patients are confused about what weight-bearing exercise is. Weight-bearing exercise does not mean that you need to lift weights. It means that you should exercise upright, so your bones and muscles carry your weight. Walking, jogging, dancing, and playing tennis are all weight-bearing exercises and should be done several times a week. Swimming, on the other hand, although very good exercise for your heart, is not weight-bearing and so not especially useful for developing bone strength.

Normal bone metabolism involves a balance between bone building and bone breakdown. We are at our peak of bone mass from late childhood until the age of thirty. After the age of thirty, bone mass begins to decline, which means that the building part does not keep pace with the breakdown part. After forty, as estrogen decreases in the body, bone loss speeds up. As you approach and go through menopause, bone loss increases still more.

This normal aging of the bones depends on many factors. Among them are:

- The amount of calcium in your diet
- Your activity level
- The types of exercise you do
- What medications you take

- Whether you smoke or drink

- The timing of menopause

- Whether you are on hormone therapy

Although hormone therapy prevents bone loss, it is effective only for the time you are on it. Once you stop, the benefit to your bones stops as well. Smoking accelerates bone loss. (There is nothing good about smoking!) The earlier you have menopause, the greater the risk of osteoporosis because of lowered estrogen. If you have premature or surgical menopause, it is wise to talk to your doctor about doing something to protect your bones.

KEEPING YOUR BONES STRONG

Bone loss can lead to trouble. If your bones get to the point where they are brittle, they can be susceptible to fractures and break easily. Also, you can develop deformities of the spine, such as kyphosis, a condition where your upper spine is so curved that you appear bent over. Finally, bone loss can cause osteopenia (below-normal levels of bone mass) and osteoporosis (porous, brittle bones), conditions that are very common in middle-aged and older women.

> Foods that are high in calcium include:
> - Dairy foods, such as low-fat milk, cheese, yogurt
> - Canned salmon with bones, sardines
> - Dark green leafy vegetables
> - Calcium-fortified foods, such as orange juice and cereal

Since bone mass decreases dramatically at menopause, women at midlife, especially those who are not taking HT, should take whatever steps available to protect against bone loss. I recommend that my patients do what I do—get weight-bearing exercise and eat foods rich in calcium and vitamin D. Weight-bearing exercise not only is good for strengthening the bones but also improves balance and coordination, thereby reducing the risk of falling and breaking a bone. It also helps to develop muscles that help to support your bones, making them less vulnerable to fracture. If for some reason you don't eat a diet rich in calcium, which is found primarily in dairy foods, supplements may be advisable. Discuss the use of calcium supplements with your doctor. If necessary, and if recommended by your doctor, take prescription medication that prevents bone loss (see page 201).

Diagnosing Bone Loss

Don't wait to break a bone. Take a bone density test, called a DEXA (dual-energy X-ray absorptometry) scan, which shows your bone density. "Density" refers to the amount of calcium in the bone; the higher the density, the stronger the bone and the less likely you are to have a bone fracture. This outpatient and painless radiological test can show if you have bone loss, osteopenia, or even osteoporosis. Postmenopausal women should take a bone density test every few years.

The bone density score is a comparison between your score and that of a young healthy adult:

- 1: normal
- -1.5 to -2.5: osteopenia
- <-2.5: osteoporosis

How Much Calcium is Necessary to Protect Bones?

The amount of calcium that you need for bone health varies according to your age. According to the National Academy of Sciences, women between the ages of nineteen and fifty require 1,200 mg a day, with 400 units of vitamin D to help with absorption. Postmenopausal women (over the age of fifty) have the highest calcium requirement of any age or gender group and should aim for a daily calcium intake of 1,200 to 1,500 mg.

CALCIUM REQUIREMENTS		
Age of Woman	Calcium (mg daily)	Vitamin D (IU)
19–50	1,200	400
50+	1,200–1,500	400
70+	1,500	600

CALCIUM SUPPLEMENTS

Calcium supplements come in two forms: calcium carbonate and calcium citrate. Calcium carbonate has a higher concentration, but it needs to be taken with meals. The calcium in calcium citrate is more efficiently absorbed. You should not get more than 2,500 mg of calcium total a day, from all sources, so be careful if you take calcium supplements and have a diet rich in calcium. Side effects of calcium supplements can be constipation, flatulence (gas), upset stomach, and kidney stones.

TO TAKE SOY OR NOT?

There is no evidence that eating soy foods (the active ingredient is isoflavones) has any impact on bone density in women. Isoflavone supplements are not recommended because they contain varying levels of the substance and have not been researched sufficiently.

Having enough vitamin D to properly absorb calcium may also present a problem. If you are among the lucky few who can actually find twenty minutes a day to be outside in the sun each day, which is what is recommended to have sufficient vitamin D, that's great. But for many of us who have to be in an office early and leave after dark, this might not be easy to do. So we have to get our vitamin D from other sources, either foods or supplements. Foods rich in vitamin D are eggs, fatty fish, cereal, and fortified milk. I recommend 400 IU of vitamin D daily. Be careful—more than 2,000 IU of vitamin D can be harmful, causing nausea, vomiting, weakness, and mental confusion.

THE CALCIUM CONTROVERSY

Although there have been many studies about the benefit of calcium supplements and vitamin D on bone density and risk of fractures, the results have been inconsistent and unclear. The study done by the Women's Health Initiative found that women who take calcium may still be at risk for osteoporosis if they have other factors that compromise their bone health. Women over sixty and those with low dietary calcium may benefit from calcium supplements but also may have an increased risk of kidney stones. If you take calcium supplements, you need to remember to drink a lot of water!

A recent study of the effects of calcium supplements with vitamin D (1,200 mg calcium) on fractures for women over seventy showed that they were effective in preventing hip fractures—but only if taken consistently.[1] You don't really need to spend money on research and clinical trials to know that if you don't take a medication or supplement consistently, it won't work.

OSTEOPENIA

Osteopenia is not a disease. It is a term that means you have below-normal bone density and are at greater risk for fractures and for developing osteoporosis, which is considered a disease. Think of it as a preosteoporosis condition. It is estimated that over thirty-four million American women have osteopenia. If you have a bone density test and are diagnosed with osteopenia, you should begin bone strengthening measures and be monitored by your doctor.

A friend of mine who is extremely fit and who works as a dance instructor complained to me about having a chronic stomachache and diarrhea. She asked me whether it could be from the medication her doctor had prescribed for osteopenia after her bone density test came back low. However, since she was so fit and should not have been a candidate for osteopenia or osteoporosis, and since she complained of a stomachache, I thought it was possible that stomach problems were preventing her from absorbing calcium properly. I suggested this possibility, and she went back to her doctor to ask about it. It turned out I was right. But I applaud her for questioning what was going on and investigating her problems, even though her doctor thought he had handled them. It is always a good idea to discover the underlying cause of a condition, rather than simply throw medication at it.

OSTEOPOROSIS

Osteoporosis, which means "porous bones," is a disease characterized by the significant loss of bone mass, which can lead to a risk of fractures. According to the National Osteoporosis Foundation, more than 80 percent of people who have osteoporosis are women, making this a serious women's health issue. Unfortunately, many women have no idea that they are at risk for developing osteoporosis because there are no symptoms until a bone breaks. It's a silent disease. That is why prevention is key. The bones that are affected most commonly are of the spine, hip, and wrist.

WHAT CAUSES OSTEOPOROSIS?

Bones, like other tissues in the body, are constantly breaking down and being replenished. After about age thirty, more bone is broken down (about 0.4 percent a year) than can be replaced. This is normal. With proper nutrition, losing bone mass at a normal rate should not cause osteoporosis.

Osteoporosis can occur if there is not enough bone mass established by the age of thirty or if the bone loss that occurs after thirty happens very quickly. Bone loss accelerates after menopause, when women lose bone mass at the rate of about 3 percent a year.

RISK FACTORS FOR OSTEOPOROSIS

White, postmenopausal women have the highest risk for developing osteoporosis. If you have a family history of osteoporosis, it also increases your risk. Certain chronic medical conditions, such as kidney disease, or endocrine problems, such as hyperthyroidism, can also increase bone loss. Drugs such as steroids, blood thinners, seizure medications, and thyroid replacement medication can increase the risk for osteoporosis.

Bone health is one of the things in life for which "too thin" is not an advantage. Women who weigh less than 127 pounds for most of their adult life have a greater risk of developing osteoporosis than heavier women. Lifestyle issues, such as lack of exercise, smoking, or drinking to excess, can also increase the risk of developing serious bone loss. Anorexia affects the bones as well.

Some facts about osteoporosis:

- Osteoporosis affects eight million women in the United States.
- Four times as many women as men develop osteoporosis.
- Women over fifty have a 40 percent risk of developing a fracture due to osteoporosis sometime in their lives.

- Twenty-five percent of postmenopausal women will develop spine deformity.

- Caucasian and Asian women are more likely than others to develop osteoporosis.

- Smoking increases bone loss.

TREATMENT FOR OSTEOPOROSIS

The first lines of defense are diet and exercise. But if you have lost bone mass, there are medications that will slow bone loss and others that help rebuild bones. For these medications to work, they have to be taken consistently and as directed.

MEDICATIONS FOR BONE LOSS		
Type of Medication	**What It Does**	**Side Effects**
Bisphosphonates (alendronate, risedronate, ibandronate)	Slow bone breakdown; decrease chance of fractures	Nausea, heartburn, digestive problems, ulcers
Selective estrogen receptor modulators (SERMs) (raloxifene)	Increase bone density and decrease vertebral fractures and hip fractures	Hot flashes, increased risk of blood clots
Calcitonin (shot or nasal spray)	Increases bone mass in spine	Nausea, diarrhea, flushing
Parathyroid hormone (teriparatide)	Improves bone density in spine and hip	Nausea, dizziness, leg cramps

Bisphosphonates. Bisphosphonates, such as alendronate (Fosamax), risedronate (Actonel), and ibandronate (Boniva), reduce fracture rate by 45 to 55 percent. Their unpleasant side effects can be minimized if you follow the directions: take with a glass of water thirty minutes before you eat any food. Stay in an upright position for thirty minutes after taking the pill to prevent irritation to the esophagus. Although this may be inconvenient, it is less inconvenient than breaking a bone. You can pay your bills, water your plants, or stare out the window. If you take antacids, calcium supplements, or multivitamins, it's best to wait two hours after you take the bisphosphonate to take them.

As with all drugs, especially those taken over the long term, there are certain people for whom the drug may not be appropriate. Recent studies have shown that bisphosphonates may increase the risk of osteonecrosis of the jaw (ONJ), especially in cancer patients who have taken chemotherapy. ONJ is a serious disease; the bones begin to die through infection. Sometimes the jaw doesn't heal after dental trauma, such as a tooth extraction. Physicians recommend that patients on Fosamax and other bisphosphonates try to avoid major dental work while taking these medications. It's always a good idea to talk over the risks and benefits of a medication with your doctor.

SERMs. A selective estrogen receptor moderator (SERM) such as raloxifene (Evista) has the beneficial effects on the bone of estrogen but without the increased risk of breast and uterine cancer. Compared to the bisphosphates, when the medication is discontinued, the bone density drops immediately. If you are going to be on bed rest for a prolonged period of time, talk to your doctor about stopping it because there is a risk of blood clots, particularly when you are immobilized. It's also a good idea to discuss these medications with your doctor if you are taking thyroid replacement medication or Coumadin (see page 184).

Calcitonin. A hormone released by the thyroid gland in response to elevated calcium, calcitonin (Miacalcin) decreases bone breakdown. It is not first-line therapy and is prescribed to women with osteoporosis who are five years postmenopause and cannot tolerate the bisphosphonates. The preparation is taken by nasal spray; you should avoid other nasal sprays when using calcitonin.

Teriparatide. This medication contains proteins similar to those in parathyroid hormone and prevents osteoporosis. Short-term use of teriparatide (Forteo) increases bone density and decreases risk of fracture, reducing vertebral fractures by 60 percent and nonvertebral fractures by 53 percent. You are taught to give yourself injections under the skin. But be careful: low blood pressure and dizziness can be side effects.

UNDERSTANDING ARTHRITIS

There are many different types of arthritis. All types of arthritis cause pain, sometimes result in deformity in the joints, and have a negative impact on quality of life. The two most common forms of arthritis are osteoarthritis and rheumatoid arthritis.

A little anatomy lesson may be helpful in understanding the disease. Bones connect at the joints. Cartilage covers the ends of the bones and keeps them from rubbing against each other when we move. Osteoarthritis involves deterioration and damage of the cartilage.

Facts about arthritis:

- Women have higher rates of arthritis than men in every age group.

- Arthritis is the most frequent and disabling chronic condition among women.

- More than forty-three million people in the United States suffer from arthritis.

- Women with arthritis have more severe activity limitations than men in every age group.

- More than 60 percent of people over sixty-five are affected.

DIAGNOSING ARTHRITIS

Your doctor should give you a complete medical history and exam if you complain of joint pain. Sometimes analysis of the fluid around the joints can determine the type of arthritis you have. Radiological tests, X-rays, CT scans, and MRIs can reveal the condition of the joints. Blood tests can reveal antibodies that signal the presence of rheumatoid arthritis.

OSTEOARTHRITIS

Osteoarthritis is very common, affecting more than twenty million people in the United States. Increasing age is a risk factor because the disease is caused by normal wear and tear of the body—what orthopedists like to call repetitive use. It is this repeated use of the joints that leads to wear and tear of the cartilage. Before the age of forty-five, osteoarthritis affects more men than women, but after age fifty-five, women are more frequently affected. The joints that are most commonly affected by osteoarthritis are in the hands, wrist, feet, spine, hips, and knees. Obesity makes osteoarthritis worse because the excess weight puts more stress on the joints. Being middle-aged and overweight makes you a good candidate for developing osteoarthritis.

In advanced cases of osteoarthritis, the cartilage between the bones can be seriously damaged or totally lost. If that happens, then there is no cushion between the bones, which leads to pain, swelling, and limited mobility. When the joints get inflamed, spurs, which are bone outgrowths, can develop. The condition can be diagnosed with X-rays that will reveal whether there is loss of cartilage between the joints or bone spur formation.

Symptoms vary from patient to patient, but the most common symptom is pain, swelling, and stiffness in the affected joints. Some people have intermittent pain, and others very little, even when X-rays reveal a great deal of joint degeneration. Some of my patients tell me their pain is worse as the day wears on, which makes sense since they are using their joints more. Also, immobility can affect the pain; if you sit still for a long time, such as at a movie, when you move you might experience more stiffness and pain. A friend of mine is embarrassed to accept dinner invitations because she finds that she has to excuse herself to lie down flat on the floor after sitting at dinner for several hours.

> ### RHEUMATOID ARTHRITIS AND PREGNANCY
>
> Generally women with inflammatory or rheumatoid arthritis have a reduction in symptoms during pregnancy. There is some evidence that the DNA in the cells of the fetus get passed to the mother and helps reduce the symptoms of arthritis.[2] But a few months after delivery, the disease can flare up again.

Osteoarthritis of the knee, associated with obesity or repeated injuries, can lead to deformity, even to the extent that you limp. In some patients, medication does not relieve the pain and they require surgery, such as a knee replacement, in order to regain function. If you have osteoarthritis of the spine, your neck or low back can hurt. If spurs form along the spine, spinal nerves can be affected, which causes pain, numbness, and tingling. Osteoarthritis of the hand can lead to joints becoming enlarged and deformed and in the feet to the formation of bunions. Often women in the same family suffer from the same kinds of arthritis, especially of the fingers and toes, leading doctors to believe there is a genetic basis to the condition.

RHEUMATOID ARTHRITIS

Rheumatoid arthritis is an autoimmune disease that predominantly affects women. The immune system attacks the synovium, the inner membrane of tissue that lines the joint, which in turn causes the joint to be inflamed or destroyed. When that happens, the joint can become swollen, red, and tender. The most commonly affected joints are between the palm and the fingers, between the vertebrae, and in the hips, knees, and wrist. No one knows what causes rheumatoid arthritis.

TREATING ARTHRITIS

Most types of arthritis can't be cured, but the symptoms can be treated with medication such as ibuprofen (Advil, Motrin), which decreases inflammation. Sometimes steroids such as cortisone help, but there are side effects to taking steroids over the long term and it is most important to be supervised by a doctor. Physical therapy can help keep joints limber. For some people, splints may slow down the joint injury. In addition to splints, some patients use cotton gloves when they sleep to help with arthritis of the fingers by keeping them warm. Neck collars, a lumbar corset, and even a firm mattress can help to reduce symptoms as well. If these treatments are unsuccessful, surgery can be done to replace joints, fuse the joints, or take pressure off the nerves in the spine.

What can you do if you have arthritis?

- Physical exercise can reduce joint pain and stiffness.
- Lose weight—extra weight puts pressure on the joints.
- Try medication to reduce pain and inflammation.
- Heat therapy (warm baths, warm towels) increases blood flow and flexibility.

- Cold therapy numbs the nerves and relieves inflammation.

- Relaxation therapy helps to reduce muscle tension.

- Use splints, braces, and other physical devices to rest the joint and support weakened joints.

If you are overweight, try to lose the weight. Even losing a little bit of weight can help to decrease symptoms of osteoarthritis of the large joints, such as the knees and hips. Recently one of my patients told me that her knees were killing her. I told her that's what happens when you put twenty pounds of additional pressure on the joints. She was able to diet and lose the weight and now doesn't have to take the pain medication that she had been taking.

If you have arthritis, avoid activities that put too much stress on the joints, such as using a high elevation setting on the treadmill for your aerobic activity or too high a resistance on a stationary bicycle. Water exercise, swimming, and water aerobics put less stress on the joints. Usually the goal of treatment is to reduce the pain and inflammation. Because pain medications have side effects, especially on the stomach, take them only when you have pain. If medication does not help with the pain, talk to your doctor about a limited treatment of cortisone or surgery.

The NIH is studying the effectiveness of the supplements glucosamine and chondroitin (see page 300) for osteoarthritis, but the studies are not yet conclusive. Patients who are on blood thinners should be careful with chondroitin because it can cause bleeding.

TAKING CARE OF YOUR MUSCLES

BACK PAIN

I hardly know anyone over the age of forty who doesn't complain of back pain at some time or another. I get it too. Happily, most back pain lasts only a few days or a week.

There are many reasons for your back to hurt. As you age, you lose bone strength and muscle elasticity. Also, the discs in the spine begin to lose fluid and flexibility. Or you could have a muscle spasm, where the muscle cramps and locks up because of a simple sneeze or some awkward motion. If you do something that strains your back, such as lifting too

heavy a load in an awkward manner, a disc may rupture or bulge out-
ward, which compresses the nerves and causes pain. Back pain symptoms can be mild discomfort or shooting pains. Some of my friends can't
stand upright when their back pain flares up.

According to the NIH, back pain is the second most common neurological ailment in the United States, second only to headache. In addition to injuries to the back, pain can be caused by various conditions,
such as arthritis, osteoporosis, or viral infections. Certain lifestyle factors can contribute to back pain: being overweight, smoking, stress, lack
of exercise, poor posture, or poor sleeping position.

So since your back will likely hurt one of these days, you might as
well know what it is. The back is composed of bones, muscles, and other
tissue, going from the neck to the pelvis. At the center is the spinal column, which supports the weight of the upper body and protects the
nerves in the spinal cord. The spinal column is made up of a stack of
thirty bones, called vertebrae. There are discs between the vertebrae that
help keep the back flexible. Ligaments and tendons help to maintain the
vertebrae and attach muscles to the spinal column.

The vertebrae can be divided into four regions. Starting from the
top are the neck or cervical vertebrae, then the upper back or thoracic
vertebrae, the lower back or lumbar region, and finally the coccyx or
sacrum at the base of the spine. The lumbar region, or the lower back,
supports the bulk of the weight of the upper body.

TREATING BACK PAIN

Medications are used to treat both short-term and chronic back pain.
Over-the-counter pain relievers and anti-inflammatory medication, such
as aspirin and ibuprofen, help reduce the inflammation. Stronger prescription drugs that may incorporate opiates (such as codeine) may offer
more relief. Cold and hot compresses may relieve pain.

The National Institutes of Health recommends applying a cold compress, such as an ice pack, several times a day after an injury for up to
twenty minutes each time. After two to three days of cold treatment, you
should use heat (such as a heating pad) for brief periods, which will help
to relax the muscles and increase blood flow. Warm baths may also help
to relax the muscles. When I had my own back pain, which was related to

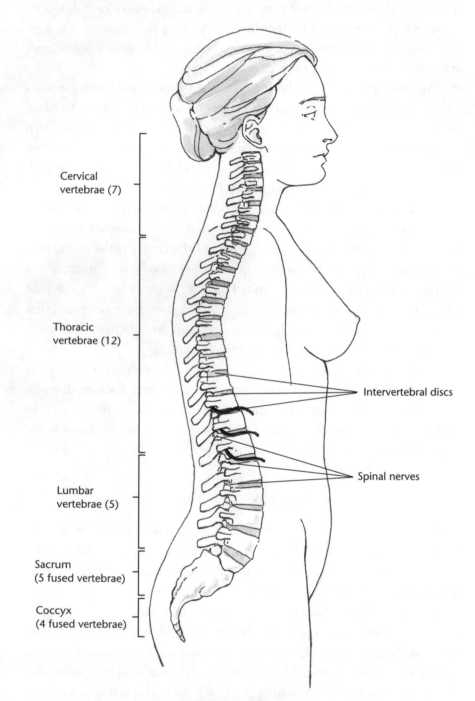

Cervical
vertebrae (7)

Thoracic
vertebrae (12)

Intervertebral discs

Spinal nerves

Lumbar
vertebrae (5)

Sacrum
(5 fused vertebrae)

Coccyx
(4 fused vertebrae)

THE SPINAL COLUMN

stress, I took warm baths and used a heating pad in addition to taking medication to relax the muscles.

Doctors used to recommend bed rest, but now it is thought that too much immobility can make the symptoms worse. Low-impact exercise such as walking and swimming can help strengthen the muscles and reduce low back pain. If all else fails, surgery can be done to correct skeletal injuries.

Strong back muscles actually reduce the incidence of vertebra fractures in postmenopausal women.[3] A routine of back-healthy exercises (see Chapter 18), and regular swimming, yoga, or walking exercise can improve coordination and help to ensure proper posture and muscle balance. I was thankful for my back-strengthening exercises after I slipped on a cobblestone street one rainy afternoon. Had I not been performing these exercises, my injury could have been a lot worse than the bruises I sustained.

Some people have recurrent back pain because they habitually are in positions that make their back vulnerable to injuries. This type of back pain can be prevented by doing muscle-strengthening exercises for the back and abdominal muscles, maintaining correct posture, and learning the proper way to lift and carry. Ergonomic furniture has been developed to protect the body from injury. I have a special chair and recommend that women who work at desk jobs request ergonomic chairs.

WHEN TO CALL THE DOCTOR

Even though back pain is so common and so many women simply live with it as normal, you should know that sometimes low back pain can signal a serious medical condition. If you have pain when coughing, tingling or weakness in the legs, or pain that is accompanied by loss of bowel or bladder control, it could be a symptom of compression of a nerve due to arthritis of the spine. If you have any of these symptoms, you should contact a doctor, who can take action to prevent permanent damage.

PREVENTING BACK PAIN

What's the best way to prevent back pain?

- Exercise regularly, two to three times a week, to strengthen and stretch the muscles. (See Chapter 18 for specific exercises.)
- Use good posture when sitting and standing.
- When you bend or lift, bend from the knees.

What About Muscle Loss?

If you are not physically active, after the age of thirty you begin to lose about 3 to 5 percent of muscle mass a decade, with a parallel loss of strength. Increasing age, being physically inactive, and having decreased hormone levels contribute to losing muscle mass and strength and can lead to a condition called sarcopenia, a Greek word meaning "poverty of the flesh." Women have a greater risk of developing sarcopenia than men because generally women have less muscle mass to start with and therefore muscle loss has a greater impact. It's one of the primary reasons that older women become frail and weak.

WHAT YOU CAN DO ABOUT MUSCLE LOSS

Getting tired of hearing that exercise is good medicine? It really is. An exercise program, especially one that involves resistance training, can help prevent and treat sarcopenia. When you do a high-intensity strength or resistance workout, such as lifting weights, the muscle tears microscopically; once torn, the muscle repairs itself by replenishing protein, which will make the muscle stronger. It's the same principle that so many people use to build themselves up. I am not recommending that you turn yourself into a bodybuilder, but resistance training exercise as you get older will help you maintain strength. Research done at Tufts University showed that when elderly, frail nursing home residents exercised by pushing weights with their legs, after only ten weeks their strength was increased by more than 100 percent.[4] Those are nice results. Strength training is good for you. Therefore, the sooner you start, the better. In addition to helping increase muscle mass and strength, the exercises can improve balance. Better balance means not falling and injuring yourself.

Proper nutrition, especially eating sufficient protein, is also important because it is necessary to take in enough calories and protein to feed your muscles.

Do Your Feet Hurt?

Shoes are responsible for most of the foot problems and deformities that doctors see in women.[5] As you get older, your feet get older too. That means that the padding on the bottom of your foot gets thinner and your arches flatten. When you wear high heels (and yes, I love them too), your foot slides forward, the toes cramp, your weight is redistributed, and your body is thrown out of whack. High heels have also been associated with osteoarthritis of the knee, low back pain, and ankle injuries. Wear sensible shoes as much as you can, and save those heels for special occasions. High heels are simply not good for your feet or the rest of you. If you love them and want to wear them, make sure not to wear them for hours and hours at a stretch; change into more comfortable and safer shoes often.

TAKE CARE OF YOUR TOES: PEDICURE SAFETY

You don't want to leave the salon with more than you came in with, such as an infection, a fungus, or worse! To be safe:

- Make sure your establishment has a state license on display.
- Make sure your pedicurist has her personal license on display.
- Check out the process used for disinfecting equipment. If someone resents the question, take your business elsewhere.
- Try to use a portable foot bath rather than a fixed one. Portables are easier to disinfect.
- Don't shave your legs before a pedicure. Research shows that doing so increases your risk of infection because small nicks can allow bacteria to enter the skin.
- Bring your own equipment.

Also, if you wear narrow shoes, your toes will suffer from being squeezed into the tips. Fashion can lead to corns and calluses, toenail problems, bunions, problems with your Achilles tendons, joint pain in your foot, and stress fractures, which are tiny cracks in a foot bone.

WHAT ABOUT YOUR KNEES?

Women athletes suffer from many more injuries than their male counterparts—depending on who's doing the reporting, between two and eight times more. There are many theories to explain this increased risk. The American College of Sports Medicine suggests that knee injuries may be more prevalent in women because women's knees have a smaller joint surface. Doctors at the American Academy of Orthopedic Surgeons found that women athletes move in a more upright position than men and that this could account for the greater damage done to women's knees. Other theories suggest that hip width may have something to do with greater knee damage, or that the way men train may strengthen their knees. Yet another avenue of research has suggested that estrogen, which helps the pelvic ligaments to loosen for childbirth, may have the effect of making the knee ligaments unstable as well and that women athletes frequently injure their knees during their ovulation.[6] Clearly there may be multiple reasons to explain the fact, but a fact it is: women are more vulnerable to knee injuries than men.[7] Therefore it is important to strengthen the muscles for protecting your knees.

OSTEOARTHRITIS OF THE KNEE

Many women, not necessarily athletes, suffer from knee pain, often due to osteoarthritis. Here's some good news: although being overweight increases the risk for knee osteoarthritis, weight loss reduces the risk. A decrease of about 5 pounds reduces the risk by over 50 percent.[8] In addition to weight loss, increasing bone density helps to reduce knee osteoarthritis as well. Not having enough vitamin D is also associated with an increased risk of knee osteoarthritis, as are hypertension, high cholesterol, and diabetes in women who were not overweight. Exercise is useful, as are pain medications.

TEN

You and Your Gut:
Understanding the Gastrointestinal Tract

CHERYL, AGE FORTY-TWO, CAME TO SEE ME AFTER SHE HAD BEEN to three other cardiologists. She was absolutely sure she had some kind of heart disease because she had been having chest pains for almost a year. They were scaring her and interfering with her life. Yet each of the cardiologists had done the same tests for heart function, and each had found that there was nothing wrong with her heart.

Nonetheless, Cheryl was sure that they were missing something and simply refusing to take her seriously. She continued to have chest pains and knew there had to be a reason for them. So she came to me—for a fourth opinion—because my practice focuses on women and she hoped I would take her more seriously. There was no need to repeat all the heart tests, which showed that her heart was normal. I told her that now that we had eliminated her heart as the cause for her symptoms, it was time to investigate the gastrointestinal or GI tract, because GI symptoms are often similar to heart problems. Both can produce chest pains.

When I made this suggestion, she rolled her eyes and was clearly annoyed. No doubt she thought of me as yet another cardiologist ignoring her symptoms and blowing her off with a casual diagnosis of heartburn. I assured her that I took her symptoms very seriously, and then took a careful history and physical, asking her a series of questions. Her answers reinforced my suspicion that she had gastroesophageal reflux disease (GERD), commonly known as acid reflux or heartburn.

Cheryl told me she often had an acid taste in her mouth, and her chest pain was worse when she was lying down. The symptoms never occurred while walking, however (heart symptoms do occur on exertion). The physical exam clinched the diagnosis: when I pushed down on her belly, the pain intensified, something typical of GERD. I recommended that she have an endoscopy, a procedure that would allow a direct look at the lining of the esophagus and confirm the diagnosis.

She was frightened of the procedure, which is actually not painful or difficult. I explained to her that if left uncontrolled, acid reflux could cause the lining of the esophagus to change and she could develop a condition called Barrett's esophagus, which would predispose her to esophageal cancer. I didn't want to scare her more than she already was, but I needed to convince her that ducking a diagnosis was really not in her best interests. Finally she agreed to have the endoscopy, which confirmed the diagnosis of GERD, and she began treatment.

Cheryl had been so convinced that she had heart disease that no other diagnosis felt responsible to her. Yet once she was correctly diagnosed and treated, her problems were solved and her chest pain stopped. The next time I saw her she was amazed at how good she felt. All her symptoms had disappeared and she felt just fine. I told her the most important question to ask a doctor the next time her tests are normal and she still doesn't feel well is "What else could it be?"

Cheryl's story is not unusual. Often when women come to see me with chest pain they are sure they are having a heart attack. Yet their heart tests come out negative. But they know there is something wrong because they don't feel well. One of the disadvantages of how specialized physicians have become is that patients are often sent away without an adequate explanation of their symptoms. Like Cheryl, the women feel that they are not taken seriously and end up going from doctor to doctor.

Many women live with a lot of pain unnecessarily because a doctor evaluates them with tunnel vision: for example, they are not asked whether their symptoms are provoked by certain types of stress or food or if they have the taste of acid in their mouth. The answers to these questions provide clues that their chest pain may not be heart-related. I know that symptoms are a sign of something, and once I know it's not the heart, I keep looking for causes. Often, I find that the GI tract is a likely suspect. Many gastrointestinal symptoms are easily treated with a combination of medications and lifestyle changes.

It's important that women have information regarding problems of the GI tract that can be useful in countering the barriers they often feel—shame, weakness—when they are in pain and being questioned by the doctor. I want to give you the inside track on the questions your doctor should ask. Knowledge really does give power.

GETTING TO KNOW YOUR GASTROINTESTINAL TRACT

The gastrointestinal tract refers to the approximately twenty-five-foot-long pathway that takes in nourishment and eliminates waste. It begins with the esophagus, the tube that helps to transport food from the mouth to the stomach, where acid breaks down the food; to the small intestine, where the food breakdown continues; and then to the large intestine (the colon) and rectum, which moves out the waste. The esophagus and stomach are considered to be the upper gastrointestinal tract, and the small intestine, large intestine, and rectum as the lower. Other organs are related to the functioning of the gastrointestinal tract, such as the liver, gallbladder, and pancreas, and are treated as part of the medical specialty called gastroenterology.

THE ESOPHAGUS

Let's start at the top, with the esophagus, the tube that connects the back of the throat to the stomach. The most common medical problem related to the esophagus is gastroesophageal reflux disease (GERD), otherwise known as acid reflux or heartburn.

If you have chest pain, go to your doctor. Your job is to describe what you are feeling, and the challenge for the doctor is to analyze those symptoms and make the correct diagnosis (heart, GI, other) in order to determine the appropriate treatment. After eliminating the heart as the cause

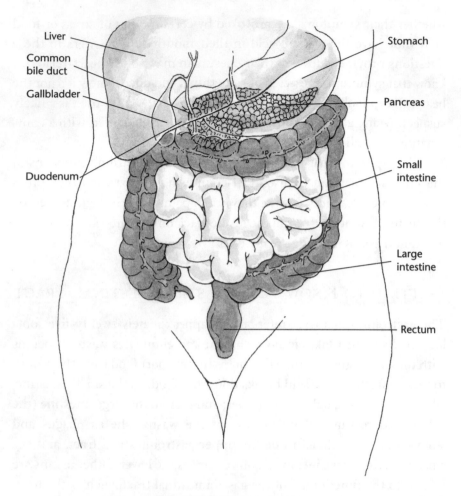

Liver
Common
bile duct
Gallbladder
Duodenum

Stomach
Pancreas
Small
intestine
Large
intestine
Rectum

THE GASTROINTESTINAL TRACT

of the chest pain, the doctor should ask you a series of questions based on the common symptoms for GERD.

- Do you have difficulty swallowing?
- Do you taste acid in your mouth?
- Are there foods that seem to make the symptoms worse?
- Are you on osteoporosis medication?
- Does pressing on your stomach make the pain worse?
- Are you nauseous?
- Have you recently lost weight?
- Do you have burning or pressure in the chest?

- Do you have regurgitation (liquid in the mouth) after eating?
- Do you have intermittent coughing?

GASTROESOPHAGEAL REFLUX DISEASE

Everyone experiences some acid reflux from time to time, and many people have occasional heartburn. The difference between what's normal and what's GERD is the persistence and intensity of the problem. GERD refers to a chronic condition where the liquid from the stomach, which contains acid, backs up into the esophagus and irritates and inflames its lining. Sometimes the liquid contains bile that has backed up from the duodenum (the beginning of the small intestine) into the stomach. Not only does the reflux occur more often than normal, but people with GERD have more acid in the refluxed liquid and it stays in the esophagus longer than normal, doing damage.

HEART ATTACK OR HEARTBURN?

One morning the phone rang. It was my sister Cindy calling to ask me a question about her friend Diane. Diane had had several days of chest discomfort that would come and go. The only thing that made it better was carbonated water. Although Cindy isn't a doctor, she has certainly been around me and others and has learned a few things. Especially since our father has heart disease, she knows that chest discomfort is not something that should be ignored. Before Cindy hung up, she said, "It's probably GI, right, because it got better with the carbonated water?" I said, "Maybe, but she still needs to be checked out. You never fool around with chest pain." She encouraged Diane to schedule an appointment with me.

You can't make a 100 percent certain diagnosis of the symptoms without a careful examination and some testing. With that said, here are some ways that I differentiate heart pain from esophageal pain.

WHAT RAISES THE RISK OF GERD IN WOMEN?

Hormones have an impact on women and GERD. Pregnancy makes a woman more susceptible to GERD because the higher hormone levels, especially when progesterone increases in the later months, may cause reflux. Also, the growing fetus can put pressure on the abdomen and stomach, which might make reflux worse. Premenopausal women are

HOW IS HEART PAIN DIFFERENT FROM ESOPHAGEAL PAIN?

Heart pain:

- Comes on with exertion
- Is relieved by rest
- May be associated with shortness of breath, light-headedness, or fainting
- Is usually not related to eating
- Pressing on the upper abdomen or lower chest doesn't increase symptoms

Esophageal pain:

- Not related to exertion
- Symptoms are worse when lying down
- Symptoms can be precipitated by pressing on the upper abdomen or lower chest
- Taste of acid in the mouth
- Sore throat or tongue
- Symptoms are worse after eating

If you have any of these symptoms, call your doctor and get checked out.

more at risk for GERD than postmenopausal ones, unless the latter group is taking HT, which puts them at risk also.

Weight affects GERD. Obese women are six times more likely to develop GERD than women of normal weight.[1] And not only being obese but simply gaining weight has been linked to increased risk. A recent study published in the *New England Journal of Medicine* found a relationship between weight gain and GERD in women.[2] The authors questioned women from the Nurses' Health Study about symptoms and concluded that even moderate weight gain and being somewhat overweight exacerbated the symptoms of reflux. The risk of having GERD was more than doubled among women whose weight increased by three points on the BMI scale (see page 346) over a fourteen-year period as compared with women whose weight remained constant. The study also found that women with frequent symptoms of GERD were more likely to take hormone therapy, medications for asthma or blood pressure, eat more than others, and be less active than women with fewer symptoms.

What Causes GERD?

People can get GERD for several reasons. There may be problems with:

- The lower esophageal sphincter
- Hiatal hernias
- Esophageal spasms
- Slow emptying of the stomach

The *lower esophageal sphincter,* a ring of muscle connecting the esophagus to the stomach, is designed to prevent reflux by contracting and closing the passage between the stomach and the esophagus. When food or saliva is swallowed, the sphincter relaxes for a few seconds and then closes. In patients with GERD, the sphincter contracts weakly or relaxes for an abnormally long time.

Hiatal hernias also can cause GERD. The hernia is a small tear that occurs in the diaphragm between the stomach and the esophagus. The tear allows a piece of the upper stomach to push through the diaphragm, letting stomach acid into the esophagus.

Esophageal spasms cause refluxed acid to remain in the esophagus rather than being pushed into the stomach.

Slow emptying of the stomach leads to problems as well. The stomach normally empties at a certain rate after a meal. Patients with GERD have slow-emptying stomachs, which increases the time that reflux can occur.

Diagnosing GERD

Generally the easy way to diagnose GERD is to take medication to reduce stomach acid and see if the patient has less heartburn. If the symptoms improve, you can usually assume that the diagnosis of GERD is accurate. The problem with this approach is that other conditions, such as ulcers, can also respond to medication, but really should be treated differently.

If medication is not effective, many doctors suggest a procedure called an upper gastrointestinal endoscopy, which allows the gastroenterologist to look directly into the esophagus and stomach through a tube. Many patients with GERD have a normal-looking esophagus, but sometimes inflammation, small lesions, or ulcers can be seen. During the endoscopy, biopsies or samples of the tissue in the esophagus are taken to see if there is damage from the acid and cultures can be taken to test for *Helicobacter pylori* (*H. pylori*), a bacterium that many people have but which under some circumstances damages the stomach and is associated with GERD and ulcers. An endoscopy is useful in diagnosing another complication of GERD, called Barrett's esophagus. Barrett's is a condition where the cells lining the esophagus change. Between 5 and 10 percent of people with Barrett's esophagus develop esophageal cancer.

UNDERSTANDING ENDOSCOPY

I always believe that if my patients understand what will happen to them in any procedure, they are less anxious and more comfortable. So let me tell you about having an endoscopy. The word *endoscopy* means "looking inside." It is a minimally invasive, usually outpatient medical procedure that is done in order to evaluate the condition of the lining of the esophagus (or other places). The doctor inserts a scope, a small flexible tube with a camera and an internal light, and looks at the lining for any abnormalities. If there are lesions, biopsies can be performed during the procedure. Usually patients are mildly sedated and the short procedure, which lasts about half an hour, is painless. Sometimes the back of the throat is sprayed with anesthetic to numb it and no sedation is used. You may be asked not to eat before the test. You may also be asked to discontinue blood thinners such as aspirin prior to the procedure, to avoid excess bleeding if biopsies are performed.

TREATING GERD

There are some lifestyle changes that you can make. For example, if the reflux is worse at night:

- Raise the head of the bed to keep the esophagus above the stomach.
- People who sleep on their left sides seem to do better than on their right.

If the reflux is worse right after meals:

- Eating smaller meals will decrease stomach bloating.
- Eating earlier in the evening will allow the stomach to empty before you lie down to sleep. Don't eat after 8:00 P.M.
- Sitting upright with good posture while eating may help symptoms as well.

Certain foods seem to be worse for patients with GERD and should be avoided. These are:

Chocolate

Peppermint

Alcohol

Caffeinated drinks

Citrus juices

Carbonated beverages

Tomato juice

Fatty foods

A number of years ago when I was starting my practice, working on a research project, and generally juggling several heavy balls simultaneously, I was drinking a great deal of coffee. One morning, after a cup of coffee, I felt a really sharp pain and started to feel sick as well. I was pretty sure it wasn't my heart, as I have none of the risk factors for heart disease. The pain was intermittent, but it was not going away. I went to my doctor, who diagnosed acid reflux and suggested appropriate medication. I got better, but having the pain of acid reflux made me more aware of how frightening such chest pain can be.

Let's say you have been diagnosed with acid reflux and have made serious lifestyle changes such as cutting out fatty meals and chocolate, decaffeinating yourself by phasing out tea, cola, and coffee but you still are not feeling better. Sometimes lifestyle changes are not enough. If you continue to have symptoms, you may require medication.

Here are two examples of how medication improved symptoms and quality of life.

My patient Margaret called my office and said she needed to come in because she was once again having chest pain. The last time I'd seen her was two years earlier, when she had a normal heart evaluation. I had recommended a consult with my colleague, a gastroenterologist, because I suspected her symptoms might be GERD, but she never made the appointment because she was too busy. Margaret tried lifestyle measures, but the symptoms never improved. Someone prescribed a medication, but she only took it for a week. When she came to see me and again had normal cardiac testing, I started her on a medication for acid reflux and said she had to take it for at least a month. Her symptoms improved, and I told her it was important to follow directions before deciding on her own that the medication was unsuccessful.

I had lunch with my friend Ginny, who was plagued with a dry cough and throat soreness and could no longer eat because she had so much pain. She could not, however, stop drinking coffee. She was a walking example of severe acid reflux. I sent her to a gastroenterologist because her symptoms were so severe. Luckily her stomach lining and esophagus did not look too inflamed, and she too is improving on medication.

Medications are prescribed to reduce the symptoms of acid reflux and the release of acid from the stomach. Antacids can give immediate relief of the symptoms, but they are short-acting and don't take care of the acid production. Also, they do not heal the inflammation of the stomach or esophagus caused by the acid. But for mild cases, antacids may be enough.

The most common medications, both prescription and over-the-counter (OTC), reduce the release of acid from the stomach. Generally the OTC medication is a lower dose than the prescribed medication. Whatever you do, it is important to work with your health care provider on any therapy that you are taking, particularly if your symptoms are not clearing up. Symptoms that don't tend to diminish with OTC remedies are coughing, hoarseness, difficulty swallowing, sore throat, and anemia. Prescription medications (see below) may help. If prescription medication doesn't work, an endoscopy should be performed to help determine the most effective treatment.

ANTACIDS

Antacids that can be purchased over the counter, such as Mylanta, Maalox, Tums, and Rolaids, are usually the first treatment that is recommended. They work by neutralizing stomach acid so that there is less acid in the reflux. The best way to take them is an hour after you eat a meal and then a second dose an hour later.

Antacids may cause constipation. Some antacids contain magnesium (read the package or ask the pharmacist) and should not be taken by patients with kidney failure because there is a risk of magnesium toxicity. Antacids with calcium carbonate contain 400 mg of calcium per dose so make sure you are not taking too much calcium (see page 197). Too much calcium is associated with an increased risk of kidney stones.

Many people don't realize that OTC products are actual medications, with side effects and interactions with other drugs. For instance, make sure to let your doctor know you have been taking antacids because they can inhibit the absorption of your other medications. Better yet, call her and discuss it with her before you take the antacids.

HISTAMINE-2 RECEPTOR BLOCKERS

Histamine-2 receptor blockers (H2 antagonists) such as cimetidine (Tagamet), ranitidine (Zantac), nizatidine (Axid), and famotidine (Pepcid), which are also available without prescription for lower doses and with a prescription for higher ones, work to relieve heartburn by blocking histamine, which reduces the acid. H2 antagonists are best taken a half hour before meals and at bedtime. Although H2 antagonists work effectively to relieve heartburn, they are not effective in healing inflammation.

Side effects can include headaches, dizziness, and constipation. These drugs can also inhibit the metabolism of other medications you might be taking, such as blood thinners or blood pressure medications.

Again, let me warn you to take these OTC remedies seriously and talk to your doctor if you need them. Also, make sure that if one doctor is prescribing medication for blood pressure and another for GERD, each knows about the other medications you are taking.

PROTON PUMP INHIBITORS

Proton pump inhibitors (PPIs), such as omeprazole (Prilosec), lansoprazole (Prevacid), rabeprazole (Aciphex), pantoprazole (Protonix), and esomeprazole (Nexium), are available by prescription. They reduce acid more effectively and more quickly than H2 antagonists by blocking the secretion of acid into the stomach for a longer period of time. They help relieve heartburn and also protect the esophagus from acid, which aids in healing inflammation. After eight weeks of therapy with these medications, there is an 83 percent improvement in acid reflux symptoms and a 78 percent healing rate of the erosion of the esophagus.

PPIs should be taken an hour before meals so that they function at peak levels after the meal. PPIs are used when there are complications of GERD, such as ulcers. A combination medication that includes the proton pump inhibitor, Prevacid, and antibiotics is prescribed for GERD caused by the *H. pylori* bacterium.

Side effects are similar to other medications for GERD: nausea, constipation, headaches, and dizziness. And they can interact with other medications, specifically antibiotics (ampicillin), iron, and digoxin. A recent study showed an important interaction for women taking PPIs: there was a 40 percent higher hip fracture rate in women who took PPIs for over a year. The fractures might have been related to decreased calcium absorption caused by the PPI.[3] PPIs are generally prescribed for four to eight weeks; it's important to take medication for a limited amount of time.

FOAM BARRIERS

Foam barriers, such as Gaviscon, are OTC tablets containing both an antacid and a foaming agent. The foam floats to the top of the stomach liquid, as the tablet dissolves, forming a physical barrier to the reflux. Simultaneously, the antacid works to neutralize the stomach acid. These tablets are most effective when taken right after meals and when lying down.

SURGERY

If lifestyle changes and medication do not reduce the symptoms of GERD, or if the medication needs to be taken in such massive doses that it seems unreasonable to maintain that regime for a lifetime, surgery may be an option. However, the recently revised guidelines for treating GERD point out that controversy exists about whether or not surgery is more effective than chronic medical therapy.[4]

The procedure is called reflux surgery (technically, fundoplication), and it can be performed laparoscopically (a procedure where a small incision is made in the abdomen and the doctor inserts a small tube with a camera to see what's going on). This procedure can be used to repair a hiatal hernia, or if the GERD is caused by a weak esophageal sphincter, the upper portion of the stomach can be wrapped around the esophagus, creating a kind of artificial esophageal sphincter so that the stomach acid is blocked from refluxing.

> **ENDOSCOPY WITH RADIOFREQUENCY ABLATION**
>
> New endoscopy techniques have been developed for treating GERD, but because they are so new, it is unclear how effective the treatment is for the long term. Three procedures have been developed: using radiofrequency waves to tighten the sphincter, decreasing reflux through endoscopic sewing, and injecting material into the wall around the sphincter.

Although usually very effective for relieving symptoms and treating the complications of GERD, especially for patients whose regurgitation is not controlled by drugs, half of the people who have the surgery have to continue taking medication. People under fifty years of age seem to have better surgical results than older people.

PROBLEMS WITH THE STOMACH AND INTESTINES

If you are experiencing stomach or upper abdominal pain, your doctor will probably ask you questions designed to locate the source of the problem.

- Does the pain get worse if you press on your stomach/abdomen?
- Are your stools black?
- Are your stools bloody?
- Do you smoke?
- How much coffee do you drink a day?
- Is the pain worse during the day or at night?
- Have you been vomiting?
- Do you feel better after you eat?
- Do you have relief from taking antacids?
- How much aspirin or other blood thinners do you take?
- Do you take arthritis medications?

PEPTIC ULCERS

If you have the following symptoms, you may have a peptic ulcer:

- Pain in the upper portion of the abdomen (between the breastbone and belly button)
- Pain that occurs after meals
- Nausea
- Pain that persists after taking acid reflux medication

WHAT IS A PEPTIC ULCER?

An ulcer is an open sore that develops in the lining of the stomach or duodenum (the beginning of the small intestine). These ulcers are called peptic because an enzyme produced by the stomach to help break down foods, pepsin, is present in both places. A peptic ulcer that occurs in the stomach is called a gastric ulcer; when it's in the duodenum, it's called a duodenal ulcer.

WOMEN AND PEPTIC ULCERS

Four percent of the women in the United States will develop a peptic ulcer at some time in their lives. Ulcers are more common in older women (over age sixty) than in younger ones. Years ago, men were thought to have twice the incidence of ulcers than women, but over the last decade research has shown that the incidence of ulcers in men and women is similar, with men developing more duodenal ulcers than women and women developing more stomach ulcers than men. This is yet another example of medical problems that have been underdiagnosed in women.

CAUSES OF ULCERS

It used to be thought that stress, spicy food, and alcohol caused ulcers to develop, and therefore doctors recommended treating ulcers with bed rest and bland diets. However, in 1982, it was discovered that a bacterium, *H. pylori*, caused an infection that weakened the lining of the stomach and small intestine and was the cause of 80 percent of peptic ulcers. Also long-term use of aspirin and other nonsteroidal anti-inflammatory drugs (Advil) can cause ulcers to develop. If you take these medications for arthritis, for example, ulcers can be prevented by prescribing H2 blockers.

If your doctor suspects your pain is from a peptic ulcer and doesn't test you for an *H. pylori* infection, ask why!

HISTORY OF *H. PYLORI*

Sometimes doctors have to go to unusual lengths to convince others about their ideas. Although several researchers had suggested the existence of a bacterium that caused gastric diseases, they were by and large ignored. In the early 1980s, this same bacterium was rediscovered by Drs. Robin Warren and Barry Marshall who were able to get specimens of the bacterium from the stomach and culture them. They were the first to suggest that stomach ulcers were not the result of spicy food or stress but caused by this bacterium.

However, the medical community was committed to the notion that no bacterium could live in the acid produced by the stomach and didn't believe them until Marshall drank a petri dish full of *H. pylori* bacteria, developed gastritis, and had the bacteria retrieved from his stomach. Happily, his problems were not long-lasting—Marshall and Warren also showed that antibiotics could effectively manage the bacteria. They were awarded the Nobel Prize for medicine in 2005 for their work on *H. pylori*.

DIAGNOSING ULCERS

It is important to identify the underlying cause of the ulcer in order to determine the most effective treatment. If the ulcer is caused by aspirin or ibuprofen, the treatment would be different from treating an infection caused by *H. pylori*.

Some diagnostic procedures used to diagnose an ulcer are:

- *Upper GI series,* an X-ray procedure where an ulcer of the esophagus, stomach, or duodenum is made visible by drinking barium (a hiatal hernia can also be diagnosed with this test)

- *Endoscopy,* a procedure in which the doctor uses a small camera to see the esophagus, stomach, and duodenum

- *Blood test* for the presence of the *H. pylori* bacterium

- *Breath test* for the *H. pylori* bacterium

TREATING ULCERS

The first goal of treatment is to relieve the painful symptoms. Then you want to heal the ulcer and prevent a recurrence. There can be serious complications from untreated ulcers, such as bleeding or perforation of the wall of the stomach or duodenum.

Treatments include:

- Discontinue the use of nonsteroidal anti-inflammatory drugs, if possible.

- Stop smoking.

- Use medications to reduce stomach acid.

- Take antibiotics for ulcers caused by *H. pylori* bacteria.

- Try laparoscopic surgery if all else fails.

GASTRITIS

Gastritis is a catch-all term for various conditions that inflame the lining of the stomach. The stomach can become inflamed by drinking alcohol, by taking aspirin or ibuprofen for prolonged periods, or as the result of an infection, such as that caused by *H. pylori*. Certain injuries or surgery, or conditions such as autoimmune disorders or chronic reflux, can result in gastritis as well.

Symptoms of gastritis include:

- Bloating

- Feeling full

- Belching

- Nausea

- Vomiting

- Vomiting blood

DIAGNOSING GASTRITIS

Your doctor may order the following:

- Endoscopy (to examine the stomach lining for abnormalities and to allow for biopsies for *H. pylori*)

- Blood tests (to check for anemia, which might be caused by stomach bleeding)

- Stool tests (to check for blood)

TREATMENT FOR GASTRITIS

Obviously the treatment should address the cause of the gastritis. If the lining of the stomach is inflamed due to excess acid, medication to reduce stomach acid is prescribed. Lifestyle changes, such as avoiding certain foods, drinks, and medicines, may also be recommended to reduce the stomach irritation. If the gastritis is caused by an infection such as by *H. pylori*, antibiotics would be prescribed.

GALLSTONES

If you have pain after eating, especially after eating foods high in fat, you might have gallstones, a disease of the gallbladder. The gallbladder is a small, pear-shaped organ located under the liver in the right upper section of your abdomen. It serves as a conduit for bile, which it stores from the liver where it is produced until it is needed for the digestion of food. Bile helps in the digestion of fats and oils and is composed of several chemicals, including cholesterol. Gallstones are caused by concentrations of cholesterol that form as the gallbladder absorbs water from the bile. You can't really prevent gallstones from forming by doing anything special or even by eating a low-fat diet, although that might help control symptoms.

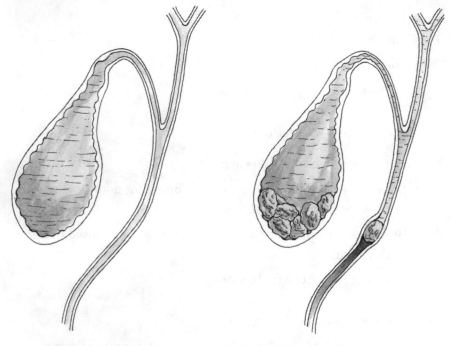

NORMAL GALLBLADDER   STONES IN GALLBLADDER AND STONE IN DUCT

The pain that people with gallstones experience, usually in the upper right side of the abdomen, is caused by gallstones getting stuck in the neck of the gallbladder or in the main bile duct to the intestine. Pain can be severe and last from minutes to hours or there can be no pain at all.

If a gallstone lodges in the main bile duct and blocks the flow of bile to the intestine, bile can back up into the liver or bloodstream and cause jaundice. If your skin turns yellowish, your urine very dark, and your stool very light, it is possible that you have jaundice. If you have any of these symptoms, talk to your doctor, who may ask the following questions:

- Do you have more pain after eating fatty foods?
- Are you overweight?

- Are you over forty?
- Where is the pain located?
- Are you on oral contraceptives or taking HT?
- Are you Native American?

DIAGNOSIS AND TREATMENT OF GALLSTONES

Gallstones cause upward of eight hundred thousand hospitalizations in the United States each year, with over half a million people a year undergoing surgery to remove them. The most reliable way to diagnose gallstones is with an ultrasound of the gallbladder. If the gallstones are not producing any adverse symptoms, many physicians decide on a "wait and see" course of action.

When treatment is called for, a common procedure is to remove the gallbladder with the gallstones laparoscopically through a small incision at the belly button. Some patients, especially those who are overweight, may require general surgery, which involves a hospital stay of several days and a three-to-six-inch incision in the abdomen (another reason not to be overweight). It turns out the body can function just fine without a gallbladder. There are also drugs that can be used to dissolve small stones, but this treatment can take up to a year. Most people opt for the surgery.

COMPLICATIONS OF GALLSTONES

Sometimes gallstones can obstruct the duct that leads from the gallbladder to the common bile duct, resulting in a sudden inflammation of the gallbladder, called acute cholecystitis. The symptoms of acute cholecystitis are severe abdominal pain and fever. It can be brought on by illness or alcohol abuse. In cases of acute cholecystitis, surgery to remove the gallbladder is recommended.

WOMEN AND GALLSTONES

There is a classic, if offensive, mnemonic about who develops gallstones: those who are fat, female, fertile, forty, and flatulent. Women develop gallstones two to three times more frequently than men in the same age groups. One explanation for this gender difference is that estrogen increases the amount of cholesterol excreted from the bile. Therefore, women who are pregnant, who take oral contraceptives, or who are on HT are at increased risk for gallstones.

Genetics can play a role too. In certain Native American tribes, especially the Pima, almost 100 percent of the middle-aged women have gallstones.

In addition to being female, research from the Nurses' Health Study that tracked women ages 39 to 50 revealed that being even slightly overweight can increase the risk of gallstones.[5] Obese women have seven times the risk of gallstones as women who are not overweight.[6] Even if you are not obese, if you have belly fat—the so-called spare tire around your middle—you have an increased risk for gallstones. Losing the extra weight has been shown to improve these risks. However, losing too much weight too rapidly (three pounds a week) can actually cause gallstones to form. And as with everything else, moderate exercise (a total of three hours a week) is good for you and decreases the risk of gallstones significantly. The typical gallstone sufferer may also suffer from flatulence because indigestion and colicky pain are symptoms.

IRRITABLE BOWEL SYNDROME

If you are suffering from diarrhea or constipation, abdominal pain, nausea, and bloating, you may have irritable bowel syndrome, or IBS. To diagnose this, your doctor may ask you:

- To describe the pain you experience. Is it crampy? Sharp? Intermittent?
- Do you feel bloated?
- Do you have alternating bouts of constipation and diarrhea?
- Are the symptoms worse after eating roughage, such as salads?

Irritable bowel syndrome, or IBS, is a gastrointestinal disorder where the nerves that control the muscles of the GI tract become overly active and sensitive. Typically symptoms are changes in bowel habits, diarrhea, constipation, nausea, gas, and bloating, and the condition is often associated with abdominal pain. IBS used to be called "spastic colon."

It's not known what causes IBS, and there is no cure, only manage-

OTHER REASONS FOR INTESTINAL PROBLEMS

It's important to remember that there are many reasons for intestinal problems, and they are not necessarily IBS. As always, common sense will tell you if you have a problem or not. If you are three days out of surgery, you may have unusual bowel movements. Some medications—codeine, for example—stop the bowels. I prescribed a medication for a patient I was treating for an irregular heartbeat. When I told her the medication may be constipating, she was delighted because her IBS symptom was diarrhea. Eating too much fiber can cause diarrhea in some people. You are the person who knows your body best. If after a few days, the symptoms remain, talk to your doctor. If you have diarrhea with fever, talk to your doctor.

ment of symptoms. Stress and anxiety are known to increase the incidence and severity of IBS attacks.[7] IBS is called a "functional disorder" because it is not associated with any disease of the colon and does no permanent harm to the intestines. For example, if you have IBS, you do not have a greater risk of intestinal bleeding or of intestinal or colon cancer. Symptoms vary in severity, from mildly annoying to disabling. Mild symptoms respond quickly and easily to over-the-counter medications for constipation, gas, or diarrhea, but people who experience more severe symptoms may find that they have to limit their lives; they can't travel long distances or go to certain social events because they always need to be near a toilet.

WOMEN AND IBS

Since IBS is related to stress, you won't be surprised to learn that women suffer from IBS three times more than men, and people of middle age, ages forty-five to sixty-four, have the highest incidence, according to a survey done by the Second National Health and Nutrition Examination Survey, 1976–1980. Data from the survey show that 3 percent of the population of the United States suffers from IBS.

HOW WE TREAT IBS

The best way to manage symptoms of IBS is through a combination of diet, medication, and stress management.

There have been several studies on Chinese herbal formulations and irritable bowel symptoms. The studies have been small and the results mixed. A 1998 study used capsules prepared by Chinese herbalists and found some symptomatic relief for IBS sufferers. Yet another study published in 2006 in the *American Journal of Gastroenterology* found no benefit for IBS symptoms.[8] The bottom line with Chinese herbs and IBS is that the treatment is not yet ready for prime time. More research needs to be done.

INFLAMMATORY BOWEL DISEASE

Ulcerative colitis and Crohn's disease are chronic inflammatory diseases of the intestines collectively called inflammatory bowel disease (IBD). Over a million people in the United States have IBD, with women and men being equally susceptible. Both colitis and Crohn's are different

---

FOODS TO AVOID IF YOU HAVE IBS

Certain substances can lead to cramps, diarrhea, flatulence, and abdominal bloating.

- *Dairy products.* If you have trouble digesting dairy products, it might be a sign of lactose intolerance, which means you have a deficiency of lactase, the protein necessary to digest lactose, the sugar found in dairy.

- *Beans.* For many people, beans are hard to digest and produce gas.

- *Sugar-free gums and candies.* Sorbitol, a sugar substitute, is incompletely absorbed in the intestine.

- *Onions.* Many people have trouble digesting onions.

- *Chewing gum, smoking, carbonated beverages.* Swallowing too much air results in intestinal gas.

- *Laxative abuse.* Too many laxatives result in diarrhea.

from IBS because IBS does not involve intestinal inflammation. Crohn's disease causes inflammation of the small and large intestine; colitis causes ulcers of the colon and rectum. Ulcerative colitis affects only the innermost lining of the colon, whereas Crohn's disease can affect the entire thickness of the bowel wall.

People with IBD have an abnormal response of the immune system. Instead of protecting the body from infection, if you have IBD the immune system reacts inappropriately, mistaking food, bacteria, and other materials in the intestine for foreign substances. To protect against these foreign substances, white blood cells rush to the lining of the intestines, where they produce chronic inflammation. Sometimes the white blood cells generate harmful products that can lead to ulcerations and bowel injury.

The causes of both Crohn's disease and colitis are not known, and they are easily confused because they have similar symptoms. Although there is no cure, medications are most often prescribed to control the symptoms of IBD.

Symptoms of IBD are:

- Abdominal pain

- Fever

- Rectal bleeding

- Diarrhea

- Poor appetite

- Weight loss

- Anemia

WOMEN AND IBD

IBD can cause irregular menstrual periods because inflammation can affect hormone production. Women with IBD may have decreased absorption of iron because of the inflammation. Generally, having IBD does not affect pregnancy, but medications for IBD may do so. Therefore, if you are pregnant and stop the medications, the symptoms will probably get worse.

WOMEN, IBD, AND OSTEOPOROSIS

IBD also affects osteoporosis (see Chapter 9). According to the Crohn's and Colitis Foundation of America, 30 to 60 percent of people with IBD have a significant risk for osteoporosis because the treatment used to reduce the inflammation of IBD involves steroids, which can have an impact on healthy bones, causing bone loss. Also, severe inflammation of the small bowel can result in difficulty absorbing calcium and vitamin D, which also has an impact on bone health. If you have IBD, it's a good idea to eat a diet rich in calcium and vitamin D and participate in an appropriate exercise program. Your doctor may prescribe calcium and vitamin D supplements. Not smoking and avoiding excessive use of alcohol are also important.

DIAGNOSIS AND TREATMENT OF IBD

IBD can be diagnosed via several types of tests:

- Blood tests (to check for anemia and a high white blood cell count)
- Stool sample (to reveal white blood cells, indicating inflammation, and blood)
- Colonoscopy (where a thin, lighted camera on a flexible tube is inserted through the rectum and into the colon to examine the lining of the entire colon) to confirm the diagnosis of ulcerative colitis and to rule out Crohn's disease

Various drugs are used to treat the inflammation, such as sulfasalazine (Azulfidine), antibiotics, and steroids. Patients who have severe ulcerative colitis may require surgery.

DIVERTICULITIS

Diverticulitis refers to an inflammation or infection of the diverticula, which are small sacs that form and protrude from the lining of the intestine, usually the lower part of the intestine, called the sigmoid colon. The presence of these sacs is called diverticulosis, and it is very common, especially in Western developed countries because, most doctors think, of the prevalence of eating a low-fiber diet. More than half the people in the United States over sixty have diverticulosis. There are generally no symptoms of this condition, and it is most often diagnosed when a doctor has ordered tests for an unrelated reason.

Having diverticulosis is not considered a medical problem. The problem comes when these sacs become infected, probably due to stool and bacteria in the sacs, and diverticulitis develops. About 20 percent of people with diverticulosis develop diverticulitis.

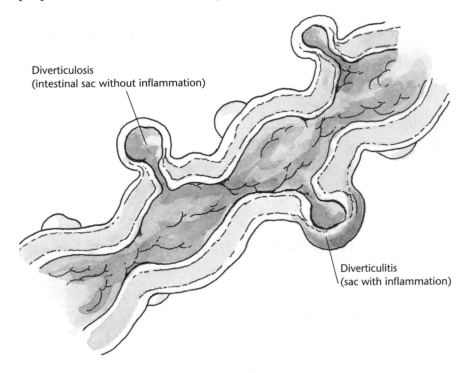

Diverticulosis
(intestinal sac without inflammation)

Diverticulitis
(sac with inflammation)

SECTION OF LARGE INTESTINE, SHOWING DIVERTICULOSIS AND DIVERTICULITIS

If you are having lower abdominal pain, it might be a sign of diverticulitis. Symptoms of diverticulitis can come on suddenly and be intense or mild. Typical symptoms are:

- Lower abdominal pain, especially on the left side
- Fever
- Chills
- Nausea
- Vomiting
- Diarrhea
- Constipation
- Cramping
- Rectal bleeding

Abdominal pain can be a symptom of a number of different illnesses and conditions, such as irritable bowel syndrome, ulcers, appendicitis, or gynecological problems, as well as diverticulitis. The questions the doctor will ask are designed to differentiate among them. (This is what doctors call making a differential diagnosis.) In addition to your symptoms, the doctor will ask about your bowel habits, your diet, and your medications.

WHAT CAUSES DIVERTICULITIS?

No one knows what causes diverticulosis to develop into diverticulitis, but some of the factors that are thought to increase your risk of having this condition are:

- Eating a low-fiber diet
- Having chronic constipation
- Being over age fifty
- Increasing pressure in the bowel from straining to pass a hard stool

DIVERTICULITIS AND WOMEN

Diverticulitis occurs with equal frequency in men and women. But in women the condition can easily be mistaken for gynecological disease, especially if the diverticulitis results in a pelvic mass.

One night my friend Anne Marie, a fifty-two-year-old stockbroker, called, obviously upset. For the past few weeks she had been having intermittent pelvic pain. She also had diarrhea and now was complaining of a low-grade fever. Her primary care physician sent her to the gynecologist, who did a sonogram and told her that everything was okay. But it wasn't okay. My friend didn't feel well. I suggested that she ask her primary care physician for a referral to a gastroenterologist because I suspected that her symptoms were those of diverticulitis, not a gynecological problem. She needed a CT scan to diagnose this properly.

She had the CT scan and was diagnosed with diverticulitis. Her symptoms improved with a course of antibiotics and a modified diet. I have so many opportunities to see how important it is to listen to a patient. In Anne Marie's case, listening would have brought about more efficient health care.

DIAGNOSING DIVERTICULITIS

If after taking a careful history and doing a physical exam, including a rectal exam, the doctor suspects that the cause of your abdominal pain is diverticulitis, she or he may order tests to confirm the diagnosis. Initial tests may include:

- Blood tests to reveal infection, inflammation, or bleeding
- Stool sample to examine for blood
- X-rays of the abdomen to look for a rupture
- CT scan to locate an inflamed area and pouch in the colon

Once the episode of inflammation is improved, the doctor may recommend other tests that would better reveal the condition of the colon. These include:

- Colonoscopy
- Barium enema, where dye is injected into the rectum and an X-ray shows the condition of the colon and any abnormal pouches
- Flexible sigmoidoscopy, where a thin, lighted camera is inserted into the rectum to examine the rectum and the lower colon

TREATING DIVERTICULITIS

A mild case of diverticulitis often resolves without medical treatment. But if not, the doctor will try to treat the condition in order to:

- Reduce the inflammation
- Cure the infection
- Allow the colon to rest
- Avoid complications

If the inflammation is mild, drinking clear liquids for the first two to three days of the attack will rest the colon.

If pain medication and a liquid diet do not relieve symptoms, antibiotics might be prescribed to eliminate the infection. Usually once the antibiotics start to work, the infection, and therefore the pain, will subside.

However, if the infection is so severe that outpatient antibiotics don't resolve the problem, it might be necessary to treat the infection with intravenous (IV) antibiotics, and if so, it is likely that you would be admitted to the hospital.

And if IV antibiotics don't work, it may be necessary to have surgery to remove the involved part of the colon.

COMPLICATIONS OF DIVERTICULITIS

Serious complications of diverticulitis require surgery. A tear or perforation of the intestinal wall can occur from a weakening of the colon due to diverticulitis and waste material can spill into the abdominal cavity. If this occurs, you can develop:

- Peritonitis (if a diverticulum breaks and the infection goes into the abdominal cavity)
- Abscesses (if the diverticula fill with pus)
- Fistula (an abnormal connection between two organs, such as bladder and colon, colon and vagina, or an organ and skin)
- Blockage of the bowel (caused by scar tissue)
- Rectal bleeding

WHAT CAN BE DONE TO PREVENT DIVERTICULITIS?

The best way to prevent diverticulitis is to maintain good health, which will contribute to good bowel health.

- Eat a diet high in fiber. That means eat whole grains, fruits, and vegetables (see Chapter 16). A high-fiber diet improves the movement of stool through the bowel and prevents constipation.
- Doctors often recommend that you avoid eating certain foods, such as nuts, corn, and seeds.
- Certain medications should be avoided: those that are constipating, and also laxatives and enemas, which could make the pain worse.
- Drink water every day.
- Exercise regularly.

COLORECTAL CANCER

Colon or rectal cancer, together called colorectal cancer, is the second leading cancer killer in the United States (lung cancer is the first). One out of twenty people will develop it in their lifetimes. In fact, the prevalence of colon cancer is so great that everyone over the age of fifty is considered at risk.

PREVENTING COLON CANCER

The good news is that colorectal cancer is preventable if you have colonoscopy screening to help identify polyps (noncancerous growths) on the lining of the colon before they become cancerous. You are at increased risk of developing colon cancer if you have a family history of polyps or colon cancer or a personal history of other cancers, such as breast, uterine or ovarian, or if you have IBD (ulcerative colitis or Crohn's disease).

WOMEN AND COLON CANCER

In the United States, colorectal cancer is the second most common cancer diagnosed in women of Hispanic, American Indian/Alaska Native, or Asian/Pacific Islander ancestry and the third most common cancer in white and African American women. Colorectal cancer is the third leading cause of cancer deaths in American women, after lung and breast cancer.

According to a 2003 study that followed seventy-five thousand women from the Nurses Health Study for twelve years, women who ate a typical Western diet of red meats, refined grains, sweets, and desserts were more likely to develop colon cancer than women who didn't.[9] Obesity and smoking have been linked to greater risks of developing this cancer too. There are some studies that suggest that estrogen HT may reduce the risk.

SYMPTOMS OF COLON CANCER

The colon is very long and depending on where the tumor is located in the bowel, symptoms vary. The right side of the colon (or right colon) is spacious, and if the tumor is located in that area, there may not be any symptoms until it is very large. Symptoms of right-sided colon cancers are anemia, fatigue, and shortness of breath.

Because the left side of the colon is smaller than the right, tumors that are located in this area are associated with blockage. Bowel obstruction can cause symptoms of constipation, narrowed or bloody stool, diarrhea, and abdominal pain.

TREATMENT FOR COLON CANCER

The most common treatment for colorectal cancer is surgery to remove the tumor and sometimes the adjacent lymph nodes. Then the healthy areas of the bowel are reconnected. If the cancer is in the rectum, the rectum is usually removed and an opening, called a colostomy, is created in the abdomen for the elimination of solid waste. Patients whose cancer has infiltrated the lining of the colon or where there is evidence that the cancer has spread (metastasized) may need chemotherapy.

THE COLON CHECKUP

Just as with mammography, checking your colon can catch some problems before they become big ones. It's not comfortable; most people don't like to take laxatives or enemas, or to have tubes inserted in their rectums. Nonetheless, do it! It could save your life.

Traditional colonoscopy. A colonoscopy is a diagnostic procedure that allows a doctor to examine the colon for various abnormalities and diseases, such as ulcers, bleeding, intestinal inflammation, colitis, diverticulitis, colon polyps, and cancer. Since most colon cancers develop from polyps, removing them while they are benign is recommended as normal preventive health care. Therefore, after age fifty, or earlier if there is a family history of colon cancer, it is in the best interest of your good health to have this procedure. If the first one is okay, it should be repeated in five years.

For a colonoscopy, the patient has to cleanse the entire bowel. This involves drinking a laxative liquid or taking laxative pills, using enemas, and fasting. For many people, the preparation is the worst part of the procedure. During the colonoscopy, which takes under an hour, you are generally mildly sedated.

An advantage to this procedure is that the doctor can view the entire length of the colon and if there is any abnormality, such as a polyp, the doctor can remove it and take tissue samples for analysis.

There is a small risk of perforation (tearing) of the colon wall or bleeding at the site of a polyp that was removed. These complications are generally rare and treated either with surgery (for a perforation) or antibiotics.

Virtual colonoscopy. Many people were enthusiastic about the development of the virtual colonoscopy procedure, because they believed that the new form of the procedure would eliminate much of the unpleasantness of the traditional colonoscopy. But as with most medical tests, there are always downsides as well as upsides. The advantage with the virtual colonoscopy is that it doesn't involve a colonoscope (the tube) and thus requires no sedation and there is no risk of perforation. Also, it takes less time than the traditional procedure.

But you have to prep the same way because the bowel has to be cleaned out. During the virtual colonoscopy, the doctor inserts a tube into the rectum and pumps in air so that the colon will be inflated. Then, for the CT scan, the table moves through the scanner and you are asked to hold your breath. The doctor views the picture of the colon on a video screen. If there are any abnormalities found, the doctor can't do anything about removing or analyzing them; you have to undergo the traditional procedure.

Because the unpleasant preparation is identical with both procedures, and because abnormalities can't be treated with the virtual colonoscopy procedure, and because insurance companies do not pay for virtual colonoscopies, many physicians recommend that their patients stick to the traditional version. Sometimes the virtual colonoscopy doesn't visualize the colon as well, which means that you will have to do the preparation all over again for the colonoscopy. Also remember that the virtual colonoscopy uses radiation to image the colon, while the traditional colonoscopy does not.

COMPARING METHODS OF COLON CHECKUPS		
Type of Test	**Upside**	**Downside**
Barium enema	No anesthesia	Drinking the cleansing fluid Radiation If there is an abnormality, need to have a traditional colonoscopy
Traditional colonoscopy	Can be done in a doctor's office or as an outpatient at the hospital Direct view of the colon Doctor can perform biopsies during the same procedure, so you don't have to come back and start the whole cleansing process over No radiation	Sedation—need to bring someone with you to drive you home Risk of tears in the colon May need to stop aspirin or blood thinners before the procedure
Virtual colonoscopy	Better pictures than the barium enema Does not require sedation Don't have to stop aspirin or blood thinners	Requires the same preparation as colonoscopy Radiation Any suspicious findings will need to be followed up with a traditional colonoscopy

Barium enema. A barium enema is a procedure used to examine the in-testinal lining for abnormalities, such as polyps, diverticulosis, or tu-mors, and is especially important for people for whom colonoscopy is not appropriate. In order to do a proper examination, the colon must be empty and your doctor will explain how to prepare for the test. Usually you take strong laxatives and use enemas as well as fast.

For the procedure, you are given an enema of barium fluid through a tube inserted into your rectum. A series of X-rays are taken, and then you are instructed to go to the restroom to pass the barium fluid out. After this, a second set of X-rays is taken after air inflates the intestines.

You can take care of your gut by eating a high-fiber diet, keeping your weight down, and drinking plenty of water. For additional diet tips, see Chapter 16. If you are a woman fifty and over, remember to schedule a colonoscopy and never ignore your symptoms.

ELEVEN

The Endocrine System and Your Health

D ID YOU EVER WONDER WHY YOU SWEAT? OR WHY YOUR HEART starts racing when you are scared or excited? Or why your periods are getting irregular? Or why you have less energy than you used to? Or why you have more or less interest in sex? The answer is hormones. Our hormones are highly sensitive to our environment and respond to our physical, emotional, and psychological condition. When it's hot, hormones make us sweat; when it's cold, they make us shiver. The adrenaline rush of the fight-or-flight response that kicks in when you are frightened or alarmed? Hormones again. Your heart starts racing because special hormones are released to help you cope with danger and stress.

Hormones are communicators. They are chemical messengers that are produced by the endocrine glands and carry information to the cells throughout the body. They are highly specialized communicators too, transferring information only to those cells (called target cells) that are designed to receive their message and to no other. The information transfer works on a kind of feedback mechanism. Think of how you heat your house. You set your thermostat to a desired setting, and when the house gets cold, the heat kicks on. When the temperature is reached, the heat shuts off. Same with hormones. When there is enough hormone to do the job, the feedback mechanism alerts the endocrine gland to stop producing the hormone, and when there is insufficient hormone, the feedback mechanism spurs the gland to kick in and start producing more. The seven endocrine glands—the pituitary, hypothalamus, thyroid, pancreas, parathyroid, adrenals, and ovaries (or testes)—are considered to be a system because they function in similar ways, producing hormones that control a great deal of the body's activities. When the system works, it's great. When something goes wrong, it makes a big difference in the way you feel.

WHAT CAN GO WRONG?

The word *hormone* comes from Greek and means "to set in motion" or "to urge on," and that is exactly what hormones do—get your body going. That is, when all systems are working properly. Since your homeostasis or physiological balance is regulated by the level of the different hormones in the body, endocrine-related problems can occur if there is:

- Overproduction of a hormone
- Underproduction of a hormone
- A problem with the target cell receptors

The good news is that most endocrine problems can be treated. But they have to be diagnosed first! Thanks to the miracles of modern pharmaceuticals, most hormones can be replaced synthetically if the body's production is inadequate, or blocked if there is an overproduction; there is also medication to make the cells more sensitive to the hormone. As always, the correct diagnosis is crucial to solving the problem.

THE PITUITARY GLAND

A cardiac patient of mine, Barbara, thirty-seven, came to see me because she had started fainting and was very worried. She knew she was overweight and had high blood pressure, and she also had started to get frequent headaches. She assumed that the stress in her high-powered life was causing her blood pressure to be out of control, which was in turn causing her to faint, and that she needed an adjustment to her medicine. She "knew" all this because she had researched her symptoms on the Internet.

Sometimes patients don't understand why doctors ask them to come into the office rather than communicate by phone or via e-mail. But doctors are trained to use visual clues to see what is going on. Just by looking at her, I could make an educated guess at her problem. Her skin had red streaks, called stria, that looked a bit like stretch marks. Also, she had a fatty lump on her upper back. These observations, together with her other symptoms and her apple shape (her weight was concentrated around her middle) made me pretty sure she was suffering from a pituitary problem.

To confirm my diagnosis, I ordered a CT scan of the pituitary. The scan revealed that Barbara had a benign pituitary tumor, which was interfering with the normal feedback mechanism and causing an overproduction of the hormone cortisol. She had surgery to remove the tumor, and her troublesome symptoms went away.

For anyone out there who still believes that size matters, consider the pituitary. This pea-sized gland, located at the base of the brain, makes a huge difference in how you feel and how your body functions. The pituitary is a kind of "command central," controlling several other endocrine glands (thyroid, adrenals, and reproductive glands). The pituitary itself is controlled by and attached to the hypothalamus, which is just above the brain stem.

The hypothalamus, located immediately above the pituitary, serves as a kind of translator, taking information from the brain and passing it along to the pituitary, which then either stimulates or suppresses its hormone secretions. Pituitary hormones affect metabolism, blood pressure, sexuality, reproduction, and balance of water in the body. This very important gland is affected by light and temperature as well as by feelings and emotions. It will hardly come as a surprise to most women that physical well-being is tied to how we live.

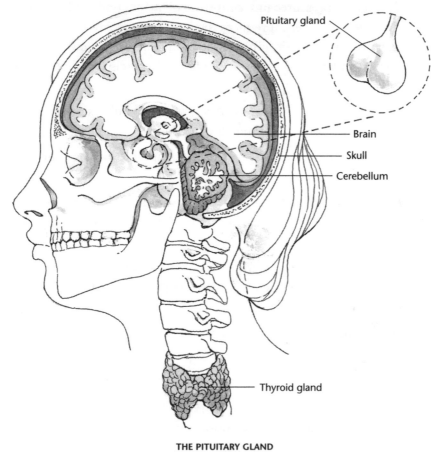

Pituitary gland

Brain

Skull

Cerebellum

Thyroid gland

THE PITUITARY GLAND

Pituitary Hormones

Pituitary hormones affect almost all of the body's physiological processes. You'll see, as you read through this list, how important this little gland is and how critical it is that its hormone production is normal.

The pituitary gland consists of three sections: the anterior, intermediate, and posterior lobes. Each of these sections produces specific hormones that regulate various aspects of the body.

The anterior or front lobe of the pituitary gland secretes six hormones:

- *Thyroid-stimulating hormone* (*TSH*), which stimulates the thyroid gland to regulate the body's metabolism. TSH also has an impact on energy, growth and development, and nervous system activity.

- *Adrenocorticotropic hormone* (*ACTH*), which stimulates the adrenal glands (situated just above the kidneys) to produce cortisol, a so-called stress hormone that is vital to survival. Cortisol helps maintain blood pressure and cardiovascular function and regulates blood glucose levels. It reduces the immune system's inflammatory response, balances the effects of insulin in breaking down sugar for energy, and regulates the metabolism of proteins, carbohydrates, and fats.

- *Follicle-stimulating hormone (FSH)*, which stimulates the ovaries to enable ovulation and promotes sperm production in the testes.

- *Luteinizing hormone (LH)*, which stimulates the ovaries to produce estrogen or the testes to produce sperm.

- *Prolactin*, which stimulates milk production after giving birth and affects sex hormone levels of the ovaries in women and the testes in men.

- *Growth hormone (GH)*, which stimulates growth in children and helps to maintain muscle mass and bone mass in adults, as well as fat distribution in the body.

The intermediate or middle lobe secretes:

- *Melanocyte-stimulating hormone*, which affects skin pigmentation.

The posterior or back lobe is responsible for:

- *Antidiuretic hormone (ADH)*, also called vasopressin, which regulates the rate of water absorption into the blood by the kidneys. ADH maintains water balance, particularly during times of dehydration, preventing urination and further water loss.

- *Oxytocin*, which helps the uterus contract during childbirth and stimulates milk production after birth. It also reduces stress.

WHAT CAN GO WRONG?

When the pituitary doesn't function properly, you don't get a pain in your pituitary. Rather, the malfunction is reflected in various other systems of the body. Because the pituitary is not easily accessible and can only be reached through surgery, pituitary problems are typically diagnosed by way of symptoms, physical examination, blood and urine tests, and MRI findings. If you have problems with your pituitary gland, you may want to see an endocrinologist, who is a specialist in hormone-related conditions.

PITUITARY TUMORS

Pituitary tumors or adenomas are common in adults. Although they are most often benign, they can interfere with normal hormone production. Often, people with pituitary tumors have headaches and eyesight trouble and take themselves to an ophthalmologist, who (if they are lucky and the doctor is well trained) will recognize the underlying problem. Another common symptom of a pituitary tumor is irregular periods, which are caused by excessive amounts of prolactin. Even small elevations of prolactin can cause women to stop having periods altogether and can result in a milky discharge from the breasts and reduced sex drive.

Pituitary tumors can be treated with medication, radiation, or surgery. Surgery is the best option for tumors that are large and compress the optic nerve (the nerve that connects the eye to the brain), or if the sinuses have become invaded, or tests reveal pituitary hormone deficiency. In addition to tumors, inflammation, infections, and injury can cause the pituitary to malfunction. With treatment, improvement is often immediate and dramatic. Therefore, if you have any of the symptoms related to the pituitary, don't hesitate to talk to your doctor and get treatment.

TOO MUCH OR TOO LITTLE ACTH

If you don't have enough ACTH, you can become tired, light-headed, and weak. It's easy to ignore or overlook these symptoms, but you should certainly have them checked out by a doctor. The ACTH deficiency can be treated with hydrocortisone, which is a synthetic version of the hormone cortisol.

On the other hand, you can have too much ACTH, which causes too much cortisol to be released into the body. This is the hormone that helps you respond to stress. Therefore, if you have too much cortisol, you are in a state of high stress (physically) all the time. There are times when you need extra cortisol: women in their last three months of pregnancy and highly trained athletes often have high levels of the hormone. But you can have cortisol levels that remain high for too long. People suffering from depression, alcoholism, malnutrition, and panic disorders have increased cortisol levels. Even lack of sleep can upset cortisol production and cause you to feel anxious and stressed. Too much cortisol is also associated with obesity and high blood pressure and can lead to insulin resistance (where you don't process insulin properly) and the risk of diabetes; it can also lead to Cushing's syndrome.

CUSHING'S SYNDROME

Too much cortisol can lead to Cushing's syndrome, a disorder that affects women five times more frequently than men. It is usually caused by a pituitary tumor. Sometimes called hypercortisolism (too much cortisol), Cushing's is characterized by increased weight gain, facial changes such as redness and roundness, mood swings, feeling tired and depressed, and increased body hair. Some women with Cushing's find that their periods become very irregular or stop altogether (amenorrhea), and therefore women with Cushing's may have trouble getting pregnant. Cushing's is also associated with high blood pressure and muscle weakness. Women with Cushing's syndrome can develop osteoporosis (see Chapter 9) because they have trouble maintaining normal amounts of estrogen, an essential ingredient for preserving bone mass.

Cushing's is diagnosed through blood and urine tests to check cortisol levels and MRI or CT scans to confirm the presence of a tumor. Surgery to remove the tumor is usually performed by a neurologist, who gets to the hard-to-reach pituitary gland through a nostril (called transphenoidal surgery). Because this is a delicate procedure and requires an experienced and highly trained surgeon, often women who are diagnosed with pituitary tumors are referred to hospitals that specialize in the surgery. Once the surgery is performed and the cortisol levels returned to normal, the symptoms go away.

DIABETES INSIPIDUS

Almost everyone has heard of diabetes, a chronic and common condition that affects the way your body processes sugars (see page 263). That form of diabetes is called diabetes mellitus. However, there is another condition, quite rare, that is unrelated to sugar diabetes, called diabetes insipidus (DI). It occurs when the hormone responsible for regulating the water in your body, called antidiuretic hormone or ADH, is low. When that happens, the kidneys don't process fluids normally. The condition is characterized by extreme thirst and frequent urination, sometimes to the point of bedwetting. Since thirst and urination are also symptoms of diabetes mellitus, a blood test is used to distinguish between the two.

If you have DI, you can suffer from dehydration, sunken eyes, unintentional weight loss, rapid heart rate, headaches, irritability, and fatigue. Treatment involves taking a medication called desmopressin, which mimics your own ADH and restores fluid balance.

> **GESTATIONAL DIABETES INSIPIDUS**
>
> There is a type of DI that occurs during pregnancy, in which the placenta affects the ADH of the mother. Treatment is the same, desmopressin.

DEFICIENCY OF LH AND FSH

In women, the gonadotrophins, LH and FSH, control ovulation, the menstrual cycle, and fertility. Therefore, having low levels of these gonadotrophins causes problems with the menstrual cycle, fertility, and sex drive. Other symptoms can be fatigue, decreased vaginal secretions, and osteoporosis due to low estrogen. The way that LH and FSH deficiency is treated is somewhat dependent on whether or not fertility is an issue. If it is not, then hormone replacement, such as for menopause, helps to restore estrogen, improving libido and avoiding bone loss. If you want to become pregnanct, then usually injections of LH and FHS are used.

DEFICIENCY OF GH

Growth hormone influences energy levels in adults and is also necessary to maintain normal muscle and bone mass. Therefore a deficiency in GH has an impact on energy levels and can lead to an increased risk of osteoporosis and heart disease.

Childhood GH deficiency, which can cause dwarfism, has been recognized since the 1960s, but adult GH deficiency was largely ignored until the early 1990s. GH deficiency in adults is usually the result of some type of damage to the pituitary gland, such as from a pituitary tumor or pituitary surgery. Adult GH deficiency is now a well-recognized clinical syndrome that includes symptoms of:

- Increased body fat
- Decreased muscle and bone mass with reduced strength and endurance
- Impaired psychological well-being
- Reduced vitality
- Poor quality of life

Treatment is with injections of synthetic growth hormone.

PROLACTIN

Prolactin levels normally vary throughout the day, but a pituitary tumor can cause these levels to be too high or too low. Prolactin is responsible for stimulating the breasts to make milk and affects ovulation. Low levels of prolactin may prevent women from successfully breast-feeding. A high level of prolactin has an impact on ovulation and menstruation and can result in infertility problems and a reduced sex drive. Regulating prolactin can be done fairly easily with medicines prescribed by a specialist.

THE THYROID GLAND

Recently, my friend Cathy, a forty-year-old nurse, called to tell me about what had been going on with her. For the past six months she had been gaining weight despite being on a careful diet and maintaining a vigorous exercise program. She had no energy at all, and she felt sleepy all the time. It was driving her crazy. She just didn't feel like herself. Also, uncharacteristically, she was sometimes so depressed that she had no interest in doing anything. When she went to her doctor, he told her that she should exercise more. Cathy felt that his response was a quick brush-off and that he wasn't taking her symptoms seriously. So, being the good nurse she is, she took her own advice and went for a second opinion.

The new doctor checked out her thyroid and found that it was underactive. After a few weeks on medication to replace her thyroid hormone, her doom and gloom turned into her usual high-energy state and she had started to drop her excess weight. Such a simple test to do, and so often overlooked.

The thyroid is a small, butterfly-shaped gland located in the front part of the throat at the base of the neck just over the trachea, or windpipe. It produces hormones (thyroxine, T4, and triiodothyronine, T3) that control your metabolic rate, that is, the rate cells burn food calories for energy. You know those people who seem to be able to eat huge amounts of whatever foods they want and never gain weight? They are not morally superior to the rest of us; it's just likely that they have a faster metabolic rate. My patients often ask me why the diet business hasn't found a pill to increase our metabolic rate so that we could all be lithe and lovely, but it turns out that it is dangerous to try to chemically manipulate metabolism.

Diane, forty-eight, came to see me because she had been having palpitations and sweating a great deal. She had also lost weight but had not made any changes in her diet. She had gone to a cardiologist with her concerns; he did an ECG and told her that her heart was just fine. But his response didn't do it for her. She felt vaguely dismissed and worse, as if she had been faking her symptoms. As her palpitations continued, she got more and more worried and decided she needed a second opinion. That's why she came to see me. She wanted to know, understandably, why suddenly her heart was acting up. She knew it wasn't normal, and she wanted to find out what was wrong.

When I examined her I found that her thyroid was enlarged and somewhat tender. I drew blood for testing and the results revealed an overactive thyroid. Diane was relieved when I told her that heart palpitations were a typical symptom of a thyroid disorder. I referred her to an endocrinologist who prescribed medication, and she recovered from her symptoms completely.

Like so many women, Diane thought she might have brought this condition on herself, and she blamed herself for feeling sick. She thought that maybe she had done something, or hadn't done something, and her illness was her fault. Of course not! There is nothing anyone can do or not do to regulate thyroid function. All anyone can do is exactly what Diane did: notice when something is wrong and find out what it is. Get it checked out. Find a doctor who wants to get to the bottom of the symptoms, and don't settle for anything less.

In my cardiology practice, I see a great deal of thyroid disease because so often it can be associated with heart symptoms, such as palpitations.

When my patients complain of feeling tired, or just generally not feeling well, I am quick to check their heart, blood pressure, and thyroid function. If the problem is thyroid, appropriate medication helps quickly. It is very important for patients to tell the doctor their symptoms, even if their description doesn't sound scientific or, as many patients say, important. It is! You shouldn't feel that you need to study before you go to the doctor.

WOMEN AND THYROID DISEASE

- Thyroid disease is five times more prevalent in women than in men.
- One out of five women will get thyroid disease in their lifetime.
- Most thyroid disease remains undiagnosed.
- Postmenopausal women who are prescribed thyroid replacement therapy may require higher doses if they are also on hormone therapy.
- Thyroid cancer is three times more common in women than in men.
- Female hormones (estrogen) and diet may influence the development of thyroid cancer.

WHAT CAN GO WRONG?

The first step in diagnosing a thyroid problem (or any medical problem, for that matter) is to go to a doctor, who will take a careful history and physical. The doctor examines the thyroid by feeling (palpating) the gland in the neck in order to see whether it is enlarged and whether it is smooth or bumpy. If it's enlarged, the doctor may order a sonogram to get a better look and to assess for thyroid cancer.

Usually, thyroid function is reflected by blood levels of thyroid-stimulating hormone (TSH) (see page 249). When the thyroid is underactive, called hypothyroidism, TSH levels will be high; when the thyroid is overactive, called hyperthyroidism, TSH levels will be low. If the TSH is abnormal, your doctor will order additional blood tests.

Two common thyroid disorders, Hashimoto's and Graves' diseases, can be diagnosed through blood tests for thyroid antibody as well. Some people develop an enlarged thyroid or a growth or nodule on the thyroid, called a goiter, and their physician may recommend a scan, sonogram, or biopsy to rule out cancer.

Because the endocrine system is a set of interrelated rather than isolated systems, sometimes thyroid disease is related to other glands. For example, thyroid disorders can be caused by a malfunction of the adrenal glands (also known as "adrenal fatigue"), which can produce too much cortisol and impair thyroid function.

HYPOTHYROIDISM

The majority of women who suffer from thyroid disease have an underactive thyroid. Hypothyroidism may be more common in women than in men because hormonal imbalances can act as a trigger. Stress, perimenopause, menopause, and pregnancy, all associated with hormonal changes, are also associated with hypothyroidism. Women with hypothyroidism who are pregnant or who are on estrogen therapy may require more thyroid medication than women who are not. Regardless of the underlying cause, an underactive thyroid can make you feel as if you are walking knee-deep in molasses. Unfortunately symptoms of hypothyroidism may be easily dismissed as typical of middle age.

Symptoms of hypothyroidism:

- Fatigue
- Forgetfulness
- Dry skin
- Reduced libido
- Weight gain
- Depression
- High cholesterol
- Brittle nails
- Constipation
- Muscle aches
- Heart failure (weakened heart muscle)
- Slow heartbeat
- Edema (swelling)
- Heavy menstrual periods

The disease can also cause irregular ovulation; therefore women who are untreated may have trouble conceiving and have a higher-than-normal rate of miscarriage and premature delivery.

As noted, hypothyroidism can also cause depression. A study conducted at the University of North Carolina found that women who had a slightly decreased thyroid level suffered depression at a rate that was almost three times as great as among those with normal thyroid function.[1] Unfortunately patients who are treated for depression often do not get their thyroid tested as a first line of defense.

FOR PREGNANT WOMEN

Levothyroxine, sold under the brand names Synthroid and Levoxyl, is the preferred thyroid replacement medication for pregnant women.

A common form of hypothyroidism is Hashimoto's disease, named for the Japanese physician who first recognized it in 1912. Hashimoto's disease can occur at any age but is most common in middle-aged women, especially in those women with a family history of thyroid disease. You can also develop thyroid problems if you have trouble metabolizing glucose (sugars) or are insulin resistant (a condition where the body does not respond to insulin properly). Insulin resistance can be related to poor nutrition. Therefore it's a good idea for women who have been diagnosed with an underactive thyroid to be evaluated for insulin resistance as well.

Causes of an underactive thyroid gland include:

- Autoimmune disease
- Thyroid surgery
- Treatment with radioactive iodine for an overactive thyroid gland
- Iodine deficiency
- Treatment with iodine-containing contrast
- Medications (such as amiodarone, lithium, interferon)

An underactive thyroid is usually treated with thyroid hormone replacement to restore normal concentrations of thyroid hormone to your body. The medication provides relief for the symptoms of hypothyroidism, such as weight gain, fatigue, and hair loss. But it's critical to accurately determine the correct medication and dosage. If you get too much thyroid hormone, it increases your risk of bone loss, osteoporosis, and cardiac arrhythmia; if you take too little, it can lead to mild high blood pressure and elevated cholesterol levels. Your doctor should measure the blood level TSH (thyroid-stimulating hormone) every six weeks until normal thyroid function is detected. If the TSH is too high, you will need more thyroid replacement; if the TSH is too low, you will need less thyroid hormone.

Dietary fiber supplements, iron supplements, and antacids may decrease the absorption of thyroid medication, resulting in low levels of the thyroid hormone. Levels may be lower if you are taking phenytoin (Dilantin), a medication that prevents seizures. Make sure the doctor who prescribes your thyroid medication is aware of what else you are taking.

SUBCLINICAL HYPOTHYROIDISM

When the thyroid gland is not producing sufficient thyroid hormone, the pituitary starts sending out more TSH to try to stimulate hormone delivery. Subclinical hypothyroidism is diagnosed when the TSH is either mildly elevated or high normal. Five percent of the adult population has mild thyroid failure, or subclinical hypothyroidism. It is more common in women, particularly those over sixty-five. There are several studies that show that women with this condition benefit from thyroid hormone replacement. Also, women who have this condition are at a higher risk for heart disease.[2] If you are among the group of women at higher risk, then you and your doctor can take steps to ensure better heart health, such as a healthy diet, cholesterol monitoring, and an exercise program.

Recently a patient came to me complaining of feeling tired, and said that she was having trouble losing weight, although she was dieting, and her hair seemed to be falling out more than usual. She had gone to several doctors who had told her to go on a diet and to hit the gym. I checked her labs and her TSH was in the high normal range. Because of her symptoms I put her on thyroid hormone replacement, and her fatigue and hair loss have improved. This is yet another example of how important it is to listen to the patient and interpret the labs in the context of the patient's symptoms.

HYPERTHYROIDISM

Hyperthyroidism occurs when there is overactivity of the thyroid gland. More thyroid hormone is produced than the body needs and the over-production can cause Graves' disease, named for the nineteenth-century Irish physician who was among the first to describe it. A simple blood test of thyroid hormone is usually the best way to diagnose it.

Among the typical symptoms of hyperthyroidism are weight loss and rapid heartbeat, trouble sleeping, and irritability. Hyperthyroidism can also result in eye problems—redness, irritation, dryness, or swelling. Some patients get increased pressure on the optic nerve, which can cause eyes that bulge from their sockets. "It's like having size-ten eyes in size-seven sockets," says Nancy Patterson, executive director of the U.S. National Graves' Disease Foundation.

Graves' can be caused by many factors, including infection, certain medications (such as amiodarone for heart arrhythmias), and heredity. Also, there is some evidence that emotional stress might contribute to developing the disease and that postpartum women are particularly susceptible to it. It can be treated with medication or in some cases surgery. The condition is more common in young and middle-aged women than in men.

Because there are several options for treating thyroid disease, you and your doctor need to discuss the advantages and disadvantages of each and decide which option is best for you. Each type of therapy has its own pluses and minuses and the decision is based on the needs of the individual patient.

Once the underlying cause of an overactive thyroid is determined, you can treat it. For example, if the overactive thyroid gland is caused by inflammation, then nonsteroidal anti-inflammatory medication, such as ibuprofen, can be used. In some cases the inflammation requires treatment with steroids. Medication can be used to stop the excess production of the thyroid, but the medication needs to be carefully monitored because there is a risk of having a low white blood cell count, inflammation of the liver, and fever. Therefore, if antithyroid medication is prescribed, blood tests for liver function and white blood cell count need to be monitored regularly. You also treat the symptoms. So if one of my patients has a rapid heart rate, I might prescribe beta-blockers (see page 190) until the thyroid problem is cleared up.

POTENTIAL
MEDICATION INTERACTIONS

Medications for hyperthyroidism can interact with ACE inhibitors, angiotensin receptor blockers, and potassium-sparing diuretics. There is a risk of an elevated potassium level when these drugs are used with potassium iodide. Blood levels of potassium should be carefully monitored.

The supplements kava and black cohosh should be avoided when taking antithyroid drugs because they increase the risk of liver function abnormalities.

More frequent monitoring through blood tests for patients taking Coumadin may be required because antithyroid medication interferes with the blood-thinning effects of warfarin (Coumadin; see page 184). This is done by blood testing. Medication side effects can be minimized by following blood tests for liver function, blood count, and blood thinning.

If you are taking medications such as Coumadin, digoxin, or beta-blockers, dose adjustments may be required.

Still another alternative is to have surgery to remove the thyroid, followed by thyroid hormone replacement. Surgery is performed for those individuals who are unresponsive to medication. Also, sometimes radioactive iodine is used to inhibit overproduction of the thyroid hormone, especially in older patients or those who have had previous surgery.

GOITER

Because the body requires a certain level of thyroid hormone, when it isn't produced, the pituitary will make additional thyroid-stimulating hormone in an attempt to lure the thyroid into producing more hormone. High levels of TSH can cause the thyroid gland to become enlarged and form a goiter. A goiter is usually a benign enlargement of the thyroid gland.

Being female, being over forty, having an inadequate amount of iodine in your diet, or a family history of goiter increases the risk of developing one. Four times as many women as men have goiters. In the

United States, where we have adequate iodine consumption from food, goiters are usually caused from a disruption of normal thyroid hormone production. A goiter can grow very slowly and over many years. It can press on the larynx or esophagus, and patients with goiters often complain of cough, hoarseness, or nighttime choking episodes. Over time, hypothyroidism may develop because the normal thyroid tissue is destroyed. Occasionally, a goiter may begin making thyroid hormone on its own, causing hyperthyroidism.

If your doctor feels that your thyroid is enlarged, he or she might recommend a sonogram, a radiological test that shows soft tissue rather than bone and does not use radiation. If the results reveal a goiter, it is possible that your doctor may want to do a simple office biopsy to rule out cancer. Once confirmed as benign, you can leave a goiter untreated unless it gets so large that it begins to affect your breathing, compresses the nerves of the voice box, or just looks too ugly. If the goiter becomes so large that it needs to be removed, surgery is normally indicated. The operation is generally safe, but there is a risk of injuring the parathyroid glands (four tiny glands adjacent to the thyroid) or vocal cords.

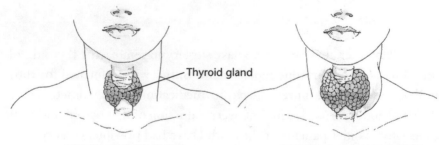

NORMAL THYROID GLAND   **THYROID GLAND WITH GOITER**

THE PANCREAS

The pancreas is a small elongated organ in the abdomen, located behind the stomach, which produces enzymes that break down food and hormones that help metabolize carbohydrates. The hormone-secreting cells of the pancreas produce insulin, and are located in the islets of Langerhans, named after the German pathologist who discovered them. Insulin enables the cells of the body to use glucose, which is necessary for them to function properly.

The pancreas regulates how much insulin goes into the blood in accordance with the body's needs and the amount of nutrients that the body has received from food. If the amount of insulin is not enough to process the glucose, the cells can starve, even if the glucose in the blood is high. In order to get an alternate source of energy, the body breaks down fats, which can lead to harmful by-products, called ketones.

Maintaining appropriate insulin levels is a full-time job for the body. Constant regulation and subtle calibrations are required. If there are problems with the level of insulin, it can wreak havoc on our health. In particular, if the pancreas malfunctions, the result can be diabetes.

DIABETES

People with diabetes have problems converting sugars (glucose) from food into energy. You are diagnosed with diabetes if your blood glucose levels are above normal when tested after a six-hour fast. Recently the defining level for diabetes has been lowered from a blood glucose level of 126 to 100 mg/dl because people are showing complications and symptoms of diabetes even at that lowered level.

TYPE 1 DIABETES

Type 1 diabetes is most commonly diagnosed in people under twenty years old, which is why it used to be called juvenile diabetes. Today, however, we realize that people at any age can develop type 1 diabetes. People who have type 1 diabetes cannot produce any insulin because the cells that produce insulin have been damaged or destroyed. No one really knows why the cells become damaged, but doctors believe that there may be some heredity involved, that is, there may be a genetic predisposition to getting it, and that viruses might be responsible. Because the body cannot function without insulin, people who have type 1 diabetes must take insulin in order to control their blood sugars.

Symptoms that signal type 1 diabetes can occur quite suddenly and can be quite severe. Ask your doctor to do a glucose tolerance test if you experience:

- Increased thirst
- Unexplained weight loss

- Frequent urination
- Fatigue
- Vision problems

Because of the necessity of taking insulin medication, people with type 1 diabetes may be particularly susceptible to hypoglycemia, which means low blood sugar, and which can occur when the sugar levels fall (usually below 70). If you use too much insulin, or exercise too much or don't eat enough food, you can get hypoglycemia, which is why I recommend a snack before exercise for my diabetic patients. Symptoms of hypoglycemia are headache, sweating, nervousness, and weakness; doctors usually recommend eating something with sugar until the symptoms subside.

TYPE 2 DIABETES

People with type 2 diabetes do produce insulin, but either they do not make sufficient insulin or their bodies are not able to use the insulin they do make to convert glucose to energy. Without adequate utilization of insulin, the amount of glucose in the blood increases while the cells are starved of energy. Although the underlying cause is unknown, there are certain risk factors that may predispose people to type 2 diabetes. These include having a family member with diabetes, being overweight, being over forty, or having had gestational diabetes during pregnancy.

Type 2 diabetes used to be termed adult-onset diabetes, and this is the most common form of diabetes in this country, affecting almost eighteen million people. But due to the epidemic of obesity in children in this country and their poor nutrition, type 2 diabetes is on the increase in younger people.

It is important to diagnose and treat type 2 diabetes because having high blood glucose levels can damage nerves and blood vessels, leading to complications such as:

- Heart disease
- Stroke
- Blindness
- Kidney disease

- Nerve problems

- Gum infections

Symptoms of type 2 diabetes are similar to those of type 1, but sometimes they occur very gradually and sometimes there may be no symptoms at all. In addition to the symptoms listed for type 1 above, symptoms of type 2 diabetes may include:

- Weight fluctuation

- Slow healing of sores or cuts

- Numbness or tingling of the hands and feet

- Increased thirst

- Increased hunger

- Fatigue

- Increased urination, especially at night

- Blurred vision

The sooner you are diagnosed and regulate your blood sugar, the less damage there will be to your body. If you have any of these symptoms, ask your doctor to do a blood test.

How Do You Know If You Have Diabetes?

The only way to be certain about diabetes is to be tested. The most common test is a blood test taken after a six-to-eight-hour fast, called a fasting plasma glucose test (FPG). The American Diabetes Association recommends that a fasting blood sugar be done in healthy men and women every three years, starting at the age of forty-five. A normal glucose level is less than 100 mg/dl.

If there is a mild elevation or if you are considered at risk for diabetes, an oral glucose tolerance test (OGTT) is performed. This test measures how well your body metabolizes glucose and is done over a two-to-five-hour period after you ingest a special glucose-containing drink in a laboratory or your doctor's office. This test is useful in distinguishing diabetic patients from prediabetic patients.

A blood test I find very useful in my practice is one that tests hemoglobin A1C, which reveals the effectiveness of diabetes treatment. A recent study has shown that this test may also be effective in screening for

COMMON ORAL MEDICATIONS FOR TYPE 2 DIABETES

Class	Brand	Generic	Frequency	Side Effects	Potential Interactions
Sulfonylureas	Glucotrol, DiaBeta, Amaryl	Glipizide, glyburide, glimepiride	1–2 times per day 30 minutes before meals Take with full glass of water	Weight gain, low blood sugar, low sodium, gastrointestinal upset	Alcohol; diuretics; beta-blockers; flaxseed
Meglitinides	Starlix, Prandin	Nateglinide, repaglinide	3 times per day 15–30 minutes before meals	Low blood sugar, liver test abnormality, headache, diarrhea	Alcohol, gemfibrozil, insulin
Biguanides	Glucophage	Metformin	1–3 times per day with meals	Abdominal discomfort, anorexia, metallic taste	Cimetidine; must hold before IV contrast for radiology procedures
Glitazones (these drugs should be avoided in people with heart disease)	Actos, Avandia	Pioglitazone, rosiglitazone	Once daily	Weight gain; liver abnormality, fluid retention	Moderate to severe heart failure; decreases effectiveness of oral contraceptives
Alpha glycosidase inhibitors	Precose, Glyset	Acarbose, miglitol	1–3 times a day, taken with first bite of the meal and a full glass of water	Bloating; flatulence; diarrhea; constipation; jaundice	

patients who have a greater than normal risk of developing diabetes.[3] Patients who have an elevated hemoglobin A1c test should have more rigorous monitoring of their glucose levels, especially if they are overweight.

It is also important to have your cholesterol and thyroid function tested if you are being evaluated for diabetes because diabetes can affect both.

Generally type 2 diabetes is treated with lifestyle changes and medications. In addition to diet and exercise, if you are diagnosed with type 2 diabetes, most likely you will be treated with oral medications to control your glucose levels; some people with type 2 diabetes take more than one medication. Insulin may be prescribed for some people who don't respond to other medications, and it is the drug of choice during pregnancy. The objective is to treat the glucose so that levels stay around 100 mg/dl and the three-month hemoglobin A1c test is less than 6 percent.

If the dose of diabetes medications is too high, then the side effects are the same as that of low blood sugar (fatigue, dizziness, rapid heart rate); if the dose is too low, symptoms are the same as high blood sugar (thirst, frequent urination). The side effects of low blood sugar are more common if you are elderly, have kidney or liver disease, or skip meals.

Pam, a fifty-year-old woman, came in because she was feeling constantly tired. She had heard that fatigue could be a symptom of heart disease and thought she should be checked over. In taking her history, I saw that she was overweight, with weight concentrated around the middle. This put me on alert. I asked her if she was urinating a lot. She said she couldn't stop; she also said she was very thirsty. Frequent urination and thirst are common symptoms of diabetes. Also she said she craved sweets, another typical symptom. When I took her blood pressure, it was mildly elevated.

Since I suspected that her symptoms were related to diabetes, and since diabetes affects so many other body systems, I ordered various blood tests, including hemoglobin A1c; an electrocardiogram; and a urinalysis. These tests confirmed that she had diabetes. Her glucose level was high at 140, her "good" cholesterol was low, her "bad" cholesterol was high, and her triglycerides were high. The hemoglobin A1c, which shows the concentration of sugars in the blood for the past three-month period, was elevated.

There is no cure for diabetes. It requires control for a lifetime. And this does not mean simply controlling the glucose levels in the blood. Because diabetics are at increased risk for heart disease and other complications, the entire body has to be carefully monitored. Pam was already showing signs of high cholesterol, high triglycerides, and high blood pressure—not good.

I started her on oral medication for diabetes. As her blood sugar becomes reduced, her triglyceride levels should go down as well. I also needed to control her high blood pressure, so I prescribed medication for that. I wanted to see her blood pressure at 120/80. Pam also had to begin cholesterol-reducing medication, and I put her on statins, a class of drugs that are effective in reducing cholesterol (see page 185). Diabetics should have even lower cholesterol levels than those recommended for the general population because complications of vascular diseases are so common. I wanted to see her LDL at less than 100.

> If you are diagnosed with diabetes, you need to:
> - Control glucose levels through careful diet and medication
> - Lose weight
> - Exercise regularly
> - Reduce cholesterol and triglyceride levels
> - Get regular checkups from an ophthalmologist
> - Get regular foot care from a podiatrist

But medication, even a lot of medication, is only the beginning of treating diabetes. I recommended that she go to an ophthalmologist because diabetes can affect the blood vessels in the eyes. I also recommended that she establish a relationship with a podiatrist because diabetics can develop neuropathy, which is a loss of sensation in their nerve endings. Therefore, foot injuries can occur and remain unnoticed and untreated. For the same reasons, I told her to be very careful if she wanted to get pedicures; she had to be sure that all the instruments were sterile. I see a number of infections every year due to lack of sterility of pedicure equipment.

Since the best thing for managing diabetes is reducing excess weight, eating a special diet low in carbohydrates and sugars, and getting regular exercise, I had to evaluate her ability to do vigorous exercise. I gave her a stress test to assess her heart function under exercise stress, and the results were normal. Exercise is most important for diabetics because it improves insulin sensitivity and therefore sugars get metabolized more efficiently. Exercise also lowers blood pressure. Remember that the body is an interconnected system and improving one part can lead to improvement in others.

Pam, like many of my patients, reacted strongly to learning that she had a disease that could make a tremendous impact on her health. Who wants to hear that she would have to make some dramatic lifestyle changes if she wanted to control the progress of the disease? Although she was understandably upset to receive this diagnosis, there is good news here too. One of the cruelest aspects of having a disease is how powerless a patient can feel. However, with diabetes, the patient can actually take an active role in her care, controlling and even improving the situation by making changes in diet and exercise patterns. Of course the patient has to take her medication; that goes without saying. But in many cases, losing weight, exercising, and a careful diet can lead to requiring less medication and improved health all around.

Pam was the one in her household who was primarily responsible for food shopping and preparing the family meals. As I followed her over a period of months, I learned something about her family. She confided to me that her husband had very little interest in her diabetic diet and wanted what he had always had for dinner—lots of pasta, starches, and fats. He also liked desserts, and Pam was finding it difficult to stick to her low-sugar, low-carbohydrate diet in the face of daily temptation, not to mention the lack of support from her husband. She was, in fact, close to despair that she would ever be able to control her diet the way she wanted to, and knew she should, in order to stay healthy.

It was not until her husband was diagnosed with diabetes himself that the eating habits in the family began to change. He was scared, and he wanted to take better care of himself. His commitment to his own well-being helped her to control her eating too. There is a lesson in here somewhere: it's hard to take good care of yourself without the support of family members. I wish I had the cure for that condition!

WOMEN AND DIABETES

According to the American Diabetes Association, more than nine million women over the age of twenty in the United States have diabetes, and one-third of these women do not know they have it. Not knowing and not being treated can cause serious harm to your body. Obviously the sooner you are diagnosed and treated, the safer you are. The prevalence of diabetes in African American, Hispanic/Latina, American Indian, and Asian/Pacific Islander women is two to four times higher than among white women. African American women have the highest death rates associated with diabetes compared to any other group.

Women who have diabetes and who have had a heart attack have double the risk of having another heart attack compared to men with the same medical history. Women with diabetes develop cardiac failure four times more often than women who don't have diabetes. Postmenopausal women with diabetes are at a higher risk for falling and for hip fractures than nondiabetic postmenopausal women. And women with diabetes have more urinary tract infections (UTIs) than women without diabetes. Women over sixty-five with diabetes have a lower level of cognitive function than women in the same age group. The list goes on: depression is twice as common among women with diabetes as in the general population.[4]

GESTATIONAL DIABETES

Some women develop gestational diabetes during the late stages of pregnancy. Usually sugar levels return to normal after the birth of the baby, but having gestational diabetes puts you in a higher risk category for developing type 2 diabetes later in life. In fact 50 percent higher than women without gestational diabetes. Gestational diabetes can affect as many as 4 percent of pregnant women. The causes are unknown, but it seems to be related to placental hormones blocking the mother's ability to properly use insulin.

PRE-DIABETES

If your blood glucose is higher than normal but lower than the diabetes definition, you have what is called pre-diabetes, which means that you are at risk for getting type 2 diabetes. If you are pre-diabetic, it is important to have your blood glucose checked annually. The good news is that with modest weight loss and moderate physical activity, you can delay or even prevent the onset of type 2 diabetes.

A major federal study followed 3,234 people who were at high risk for diabetes because they were overweight and had pre-diabetes. Results showed that eating a healthy diet and getting regular exercise that led to a 5 to 7 percent weight loss could delay and possibly prevent type 2 diabetes. People who modified their lifestyle by exercising or walking thirty minutes daily and lowered their consumption of fat and calories reduced their risk of getting type 2 diabetes by 58 percent. For people over sixty, the risk was reduced by 71 percent.

METABOLIC SYNDROME

Metabolic syndrome is a cluster of risk factors that indicate that you may be at increased risk for type 2 diabetes, stroke, and heart disease (see Chapter 8). More than fifty million Americans are estimated to have the syndrome. Research indicates that women who have premature coronary artery disease had more than twice the prevalence of metabolic syndrome than men and had significantly more components of the metabolic syndrome than men.[5] The metabolic syndrome includes hypertension, diabetes, and central obesity. Women with polycystic ovary syndrome frequently have metabolic syndrome and are at increased risk for heart disease.[6]

The American Heart Association and the National Heart, Lung, and Blood Institute recommend that metabolic syndrome be identified as the presence of three or more of the following symptoms:

- Blood pressure higher than 130/85

- Low HDL (good) and high LDL (bad) cholesterol

- Glucose level greater than 100

- Triglycerides greater than 150

- Waist size 35 inches or greater for women, 40 inches for men

Being physically inactive, getting older, having hormonal imbalances, and having a genetic predisposition to diabetes are also associated with the metabolic syndrome. As with diabetes, the first line of defense against this syndrome is to lose weight, increase the amount of exercise you do, and reduce the fats and carbs in your diet.

How to Manage Diabetes

Diabetes cannot be cured; it can only be treated and controlled. Taking good care of yourself can help you avoid getting diabetes or reduce its severity if you have it. I can't say it enough: maintain a healthy weight,

WHAT TO DO TO TAKE CARE OF YOURSELF IF YOU HAVE DIABETES

- Have your physician monitor your blood sugar several times a year.

- Have your cholesterol, triglyceride levels, and kidney function evaluated at least yearly. If you are on cholesterol medication, your physician may want these tests done more frequently.

- Visit your ophthalmologist (preferably one that specializes in diabetic retinopathy) at least once a year, more frequently if signs of diabetic retinopathy develop.

- Have a thorough dental cleaning and examination every six months. Inform your dentist and hygienist that you have diabetes.

- Monitor your feet every day for early signs of injury or infection. Make sure your health care provider inspects your feet at each visit. Ask for a referral to a podiatrist. Avoid potentially unsterile pedicures.

- Stay up to date with all of your vaccinations (including pneumococcal), and get a flu shot every year in the fall.

exercise as part of a daily routine, moderate your intake of sweets and starches, don't smoke, and take any medicine that's been prescribed. You might be surprised how many people are not careful about medication, dosage, timing, and so on. It makes a difference.

Parathyroid

Many times when friends call and ask me questions they really are asking if they are being nutty or hypochondriacal or if there is something to worry about. I always tell my friends, and my patients, that they know their body best, and to trust their instincts. Usually if something seems wrong, it probably is.

Sandra, a friend, called me one evening, clearly scared. She told me her fingers were in spasm and that these spasms had happened a few times. What could cause this? Was something seriously wrong?

I told her that it would be a good idea to call her doctor, explain about the hand spasms, and ask for a consultation. She could expect the doctor to examine her and do some lab tests. I said that the doctor would probably do tests for calcium levels. I didn't want to scare her with unnecessary information, but I wanted to make certain that she could facilitate her own care. High calcium levels sometimes manifest as hand spasms. Sometimes knowing what to look for and ordering the correct test is the hardest part of the diagnosis.

If the calcium levels were indeed high, as I suspected, it would be a symptom of some underlying issue. It could be a tumor on the parathyroid, a sign of kidney disease, or aluminum toxicity (dialysis patients are at risk for this). It could be simply an overuse of calcium supplements.

I also knew that she had had a recent bout with kidney stones, a condition related to high calcium. Also, she was usually cranky, which is another symptom—often ignored—of high calcium levels. I remember reading in some book that the symptoms of high calcium were summed up as "bones, stones, groans, and psychic moans." I reminded her to tell her doctor about the kidney stones and the moods.

I told her to encourage the doctor to test for parathyroid hormone, which no doubt the doctor would have ordered, but just in case. She said jokingly she didn't even know she had a parathyroid (we have four), never mind that it made a hormone.

I suspected that the doctor would also order a sonogram of her neck to look at the parathyroid and see whether it was enlarged.

Good thing she called and saw her doctor. The doctor did find that her calcium levels were high due to an enlarged parathyroid. The cure would be surgery and then taking hormone replacement medication. She would be fine. The spasms would stop. Her mood would improve. She would feel like herself again.

WHAT IS THE PARATHYROID?

The parathyroid consists of four pea-sized glands in the neck, located behind the thyroid. Other than name and location, and the fact that they are both part of the endocrine system, the parathyroid is unrelated to the thyroid.

The parathyroid glands control the calcium level in our blood by releasing parathyroid hormone (PTH) to maintain optimal amounts of calcium through a continuous feedback system. If the calcium levels are not within a very small range, the glands secrete more or less PTH. A steady calcium level is critical for proper brain function. If the calcium in the blood is low, PTH calls on the bones to release the calcium stored there, increases our intestinal absorption of calcium or reduces the amount of calcium excreted from our kidneys. If the level is high, the parathyroid releases less hormone, or none at all, which then allows the blood calcium level to decrease.

Although most women are familiar with the role of calcium in maintaining bone health, that really is secondary to the major function of calcium regulation. Calcium maintains the electrical energy in the nerves and provides the muscles with energy.

WOMEN, BONES, AND PARATHYROID

Having excess parathyroid hormone, being middle-aged, and having low estrogen can cause osteoporosis, and currently more than twenty million women suffer from osteoporosis (see page 199). Postmenopausal women with parathyroid disease will generally develop osteoporosis more quickly than their peers, up to two to five times faster.

Calcium is the mineral responsible for making bones strong. If the osteoporosis is caused by a problem with the parathyroid gland, which is releasing too much PTH and leaching calcium from the bones, surgery to remove the gland will reverse the problem and bone density can increase.

WHAT CAN GO WRONG?

Calcium levels affect the nerves and how they communicate information to each other. If there is too much calcium in the blood, called hyperparathyroidism, the symptoms—depression, tiredness, irritability—are easily misdiagnosed or ignored. Hyperparathyroidism is generally caused by a benign tumor on one of the parathyroid glands.

If your parathyroid is underactive and does not produce enough

PTH, calcium levels can be low. Low calcium can alter your electrolyte balance, affecting levels of sodium, potassium, and magnesium in your body. Having low levels of calcium can also affect heart rhythms. Since calcium levels also have an impact on our muscles, when levels are off, people can feel weak and have joint problems or muscle spasms.

Diagnosis and Treatment of Parathyroid Problems

The best way to diagnose a parathyroid disorder is to have a blood test to determine calcium levels and parathyroid hormone levels. Normal calcium levels are considered to be between 8.5 and 10.5 (measured in miligrams per deciliter mg/dl). Most parathyroid problems are easily resolved with surgery to remove the gland that is not doing its job properly. If surgery is indicated, you take PTH replacement so that the levels are normal.

Adrenal Glands

The adrenal glands are two small, orange-colored, triangular glands located near the top of both kidneys. The word *adrenal* means "near the kidney." Each adrenal gland consists of two parts: the adrenal cortex, which is the outer region, and the adrenal medulla, which is the inner region. The two parts of the adrenal glands have separate functions. The adrenal cortex secretes hormones (corticosteroids, aldosterone, and androgen hormones) that affect the body's metabolism, blood chemistry, and certain body characteristics. The adrenal medulla helps us cope with stress, both physical and emotional. Two hormones are secreted: epinephrine (also called adrenaline) and norepinephrine (also called noradrenaline), which are responsible for the fight-or-flight response people have when frightened.

Adrenal Glands and Women

Since the primary task of the adrenal glands is stress management, when adrenaline and other hormones are released your heart rate increases, your digestion slows down, and your senses are sharpened. This emergency response to stress takes priority over other metabolic functions, but it is not meant to last for long periods of time.

ADRENAL HORMONES	
Hormone	**Function**
Hydrocortisone or cortisol	Helps the body use fats, proteins, and carbohydrates effectively Aids in digestion
Corticosterone	Suppresses inflammatory reactions Affects the immune system
Aldosterone	Controls sodium levels secreted into the urine Maintains blood volume and blood pressure
Epinephrine (adrenaline)	Increases heart rate Facilitates blood flow to the muscles and brain (fight-or-flight response)
Norepinephrine (noradrenaline)	Increases blood pressure by constricting the blood vessels

Most of us live with a great deal of stress in our lives. With increased emotional or physical stress, the adrenal glands stay on red alert, which can result in adrenal fatigue. When cortisol remains at a high level, it is not good for the body, affecting muscle, bones, normal cell regeneration, digestion, and metabolic and mental functioning. It interferes with other endocrine functions and can cause your immune system to weaken. Poor adrenal function can cause fatigue, depression, hormone imbalance, skin problems, high blood pressure, weight gain, and other symptoms.

What Can Go Wrong?

As with other hormones, problems occur if there is too much or too little hormone. If the adrenal glands don't produce enough hormones, that is, are underactive, you can develop Addison's disease, with symptoms of low blood sugar and a weakened immune system. Overactive adrenal glands can cause Cushing's syndrome (see page 252). Cushing's syndrome is the result of the excessive production of corticosteroids by the adrenal glands, which are stimulated by the pituitary gland. Other causes include benign or cancerous tumors on the adrenal glands. If there is an overproduction of the androgen hormones (such as testosterone), women can have increased male characteristics, including hairiness and a deeper voice.

Because corticosteroids help the body respond to stress, elevated levels of these hormones are often found in pregnant women, athletes, and people suffering from depression, alcoholism, malnutrition, and panic disorders. An overproduction of the hormone aldosterone can lead to high blood pressure and to those symptoms associated with low levels of potassium (weakness, muscle aches, spasms, and sometimes paralysis).

ADDISON'S DISEASE

Addison's disease occurs when an underactive adrenal gland produces inadequate amounts of corticosteroid hormones, called adrenocortical failure. The cause of Addison's is not always known, but in some instances drugs, such as prednisone, which is a corticosteroid treatment, or infection can have an impact on the adrenal glands.

Symptoms of Addison's disease are:

- Darkening of the skin, especially on pressure points (elbows) and scars
- Lack of appetite
- Muscle aches
- Dizziness
- Low blood sugar
- Low blood pressure
- Kidney failure and shock, especially during times of stress

Addison's is diagnosed by blood tests to determine levels of corticosteroid hormones and kidney function tests.

Treatment usually involves medication to replace the hormone. A study reported in the *Journal of Clinical Endocrinology and Metabolism* suggests that in addition to improving physical symptoms, there is also a significant psychological impact to maintaining appropriate hormone levels.[7] Study participants reported that self-esteem was enhanced, and they had a sense of overall well-being; mood improved and fatigue was reduced as well.

CONN'S SYNDROME

If your adrenal glands are producing too much of the hormone aldosterone, you can develop Conn's syndrome. Conn's is associated with high blood pressure. Investigations have shown that 15 percent of patients with hypertension may have this condition. Among the causes of Conn's are benign tumors (adenomas) of the adrenal cortex. These tumors are five times more common in women than men. Conn's is difficult to diagnose, but a careful evaluation by an endocrinologist can usually confirm the diagnosis. Treatment, either medication or surgery, is usually effective in curing this condition.

The complex endocrine system affects every part of our body. As I have said repeatedly in this section, if you don't feel right, if something feels like it has changed, talk to your doctor. Medications are available for most endocrine problems. There is no reason to be uncomfortable or to suffer unnecessarily. Get checked out.

TWELVE

The Mind-Body Connection

Y OU'RE NOT REALLY CRAZY! STRESS, ANXIETY, DEPRESSION, AND moodiness can take a terrible toll on the body as well as on the mind. And you know when you are upset, just as you know when you are sick. All you need to do is look at Edvard Munch's painting *The Scream* to imagine what a woman might look like at the end of her rope. I've been there, you've been there, and now I want to help you understand it and contain it.

For a long time, doctors ignored stress, thinking that emotions, and especially women's emotions (women were thought of as the "hysterical" sex), were medically benign and something that existed apart from the physical self in some limbo. But this separation of mind and body turns out to be medically incorrect. Unfortunately many of my colleagues still ignore the mind-body connection, although the impact of emotions on health and disease has been well established.

Complaints of fatigue, shortness of breath, or upper chest discomfort can be signs of problems that are all too often ignored or written off as something that will go away with a vacation. But if not treated, stress, depression, and anxiety can have a negative impact on your quality of life and on your health. Being overworked, stressed, anxious, exhausted, and depressed can lead to self-soothing techniques that are really not good for your body, such as overeating and drinking, sitting in front of the TV, not exercising, smoking, and generally not taking care of yourself. Stress, depression, and anxiety often surface together and are interrelated; physical symptoms of these states are often similar.

STRESS

My practice is in New York City, and I know that many people think New Yorkers are pushy, angry, and rude. And on the surface, Candace seemed like a typical stereotyped New Yorker, arrogant and thinking she was entitled. Fran, my office manager, told me that when Candace first called for an appointment she made all kinds of demands: if she came in and someone was put in ahead of her, she would leave; she insisted that she be the first patient of the day, that the appointment be scheduled for 8:15, and that she could only come in on a Wednesday. She also told Fran that, if necessary, another patient should be canceled so that her demands could be accommodated. Fran, who is the most level-headed person I know, wanted to send her to another doctor instantly. But instead of turning her away, I got on the phone myself and offered her a choice from the available appointments. Finally she chose one.

Candace came in on a Thursday morning at 8:30. As she sat in my office, I noted that she was leaning rigidly forward and that she appeared anxious and spoke quickly. She told me that she had a racing heartbeat, had gained thirty pounds over the past year, and had started to smoke again after having quit for more than five years. In response to my questions, she said that her mother had recently died of a heart attack, and her company was having financial problems and she was worried about losing her job. Candace was an only child and had few friends. She told me she hated doctors, but the palpitations really worried her, and that's why she had scheduled the appointment.

After examining her, I determined that her weight, smoking, and borderline high blood pressure were more of a problem than her palpitations. Her anger and stress were taking over her body, resulting in overeating, weight gain, and high blood pressure. I encouraged her to join the 92nd Street Y's Women's Heart Plus program, which holds a group exercise class targeted for heart disease prevention.

I developed this class several years ago with my friend and colleague Mirabai Holland, the director of fitness and wellness at the Y. We had recently completed a research study that showed that women who exercised in a group had lower anxiety, less anger, and a better quality of life than women who exercised alone on exercise machines. There is something about being part of a community rather than working on your own that helps to reduce a woman's stress. Since Candace lacked supportive family and friends, this would be of extra benefit to her.

Candace also joined Weight Watchers and has again quit smoking with the help of nicotine patches (see page 43). I remarked at one of her follow-up visits that she seemed more relaxed sitting in the chair and was even scheduling afternoon appointments! It was no surprise to me that her palpitations had stopped and her blood pressure was normal. Stress can have a terrible impact on the body.

SHORT-TERM STRESS

Stress refers to the body's response to stressors. During stress, adrenaline is released to prepare us physiologically to handle what lies ahead. This fight-or-flight response, which helps us confront danger, involves physical changes, such as quicker heart rate, elevated blood pressure, and dilated pupils. Stress can be good and adaptive, such as when you see a bear while hiking and you need all your energy to make a quick getaway. In other situations, "good" stressors provoke physical changes that help us respond appropriately to the environment. For example, good stress can help athletes who are competing in an event to perform optimally, or help a public speaker keep up energy to hold the audience's attention. I can feel a fluttering in my chest right before I give a big speech and I know my body is readying me to handle my nervousness. Good stress can even stimulate the way we think, helping students to do well on a test, scientists to work, or artists to accomplish their creative goals. But—and this is most important—after the "red alert" passes, the body should return to normal.

CHRONIC STRESS

Many of us live with chronic or long-term stress, however, and this can take a terrible toll on body and mind. Chronic stress, with the body constantly aroused and ready to confront danger, is very wearing and damaging to your health. Taking care of a parent with Alzheimer's, living in poverty, coping with a miserable marriage, or feeling trapped in a despised job can lead to physical and psychological symptoms. Chronic unrelieved stress—distress—can lead to depression, anxiety, IBS, high blood pressure, overeating, alcohol or drug abuse, social isolation, even suicide.

Some of us type A personalities also live with a kind of self-inflicted stress. We feel pressured, always rushing, always needing to be early, always trying to do too much. This can cause symptoms associated with acute stress: headaches, high blood pressure, stomach and bowel problems, even heart disease.

Both short-term and chronic stress can cause:

- Arthritis flare-ups
- Asthma problems
- Constipation
- Diabetes
- Diarrhea
- Headaches
- High blood pressure
- Irritable bowel syndrome
- Irritability
- Low libido
- Lower immunity
- Skin problems, such as hives
- Stomach cramps

SYMPTOMS OF STRESS

Many people don't realize that some of the things we do unthinkingly, such as grinding our teeth or chewing our fingernails, or physical feelings that we take for granted and live with, such as neck pain or chronic indigestion, can be symptoms of stress. The first step toward helping yourself feel better is to recognize some of these common signs and symptoms of stress. After that, you can take some steps to relieve it.

IF YOU HAVE. . . .	YOU MAY FEEL. . . .
Frequent headaches	Anxious, lonely, forgetful
Teeth grinding	Frustrated, angry, unable to concentrate
Fatigue	Nervous, unproductive
Insomnia	Sad or depressed, guilty
Backaches	Worried, confused
Stomach problems	Tense, lethargic
Frequent colds	Mood swings
Neck pain	Bored, discouraged
Shoulder pains	Crying spells

WOMEN AND STRESS

Some researchers believe that women handle stress differently than men. When confronted with stress, women have the instinct to protect their children and loved ones and to reach out for social support. This "tend and befriend" response to stress is a unique characteristic of women.

There may be a physiological reason for these responses. Women's bodies make a chemical called oxytocin, the chemical released during childbirth and found in breast-feeding mothers at higher levels than non-breast-feeding mothers. Oxytocin is thought to have a calming effect during periods of stress. A 2005 study showed that when women had warm contact from their partners, such as hugs, they produced higher levels of oxytocin compared to men.[1] Estrogen also boosts the effects of oxytocin. Men, on the other hand, have been found to have high levels of testosterone during stress, which blocks the calming effects of oxytocin and can cause hostility, withdrawal, and anger.

Researchers from Arizona State University have studied the way different personality traits interact with stress and women's health.[2] They concluded that women who were not assertive and who were unable to express their feelings when confronted with stressful situations reported more and stronger negative physical symptoms than women who were able to express their feelings. Anger, and especially holding in your anger, is not good for your heart health, and in fact predicts heart disease in postmenopausal women.[3,4] Since so many of us live with stress, and since so many of us have been trained from childhood to be polite, to be seen and not heard, not to make a scene, and so on, as adults we are vulnerable to health problems. Forget all those lessons! As Madonna says, express yourself, don't repress yourself.

MARITAL DISTRESS IS NOT GOOD FOR YOU

Too much stress over too long a period of time is called "distress." Most women will not be surprised to learn that having problems in a relationship or in a marriage is not good for you. It seems that relational stress is worse for your health than work stress (which we all know can get pretty bad). Research has shown that women who live with marital distress over time have elevated blood pressure when they are home but not when they are at work, even if the work they do is highly stressful.[5] Women who have had heart disease have an almost threefold increase in risk of recurrence if they live with marital stress.[6]

STRESS AND SICKNESS

The pioneering work being done by Dr. Esther Sternberg, director of the Integrative Neural Immune Program at the National Institutes of Mental Health, over the past decade has led to an increased understanding of the association between the brain and the body's immune system. When you get sick, such as when you have an infection, your immune system is designed to rush to the rescue by fighting off the invader to your normal good health. When cells from the immune system do their normal work, they coordinate their activities by signaling the brain that the body needs to fight some disease or other problem—and to stop fighting (that is, suppress the immune system) when the danger is past.

If you are chronically stressed, stress hormones flood the body, and these hormones affect the immune system, "telling" them to relax and stop fighting. Therefore when you are stressed, your immune system is less able to respond normally to fight off infection or disease, and you are easy prey for sickness.

The interrelationships among physical symptoms, hormones, and psychological issues are numerous, yet poorly understood. For example, more than 50 percent of people who have Cushing's syndrome (see page 252), a disease of the adrenal system that is associated with the release of cortisol, have depression and anxiety. Chronic stress, anxiety, or panic attacks can have a direct impact on breathing, and in asthma patients this can bring on an attack. The higher cortisol levels associated with stress can lead to the buildup of fat around the middle, resulting in the apple-shaped body type most at risk for heart disease and type 2 diabetes. Stress can affect your ovaries, causing menstrual irregularities and ovarian failure, with resulting lower levels of estrogen. This increases the risk for premenopausal women to develop atherosclerosis.

STRESS AND YOUR HEART

If you have unregulated and constant stress, the excessive amounts of adrenaline that are produced can cause palpitations and increase blood pressure. Stress can have a terrific impact on the heart as well. For example, there is "broken heart syndrome," related to the death of a loved one, which can actually mimic the symptoms of a heart attack. Shock can stun your heart, and it's not until weeks after the event when the heart function returns to normal that it becomes clear that the problem was stress (see page 280).

TAKE CONTROL

Empirical studies show that having some sense of control over your life is essential for good health. Stress related to being without control can increase blood pressure and cause elevated cholesterol levels, which can lead to an increased risk of heart disease. Interestingly even if you have high-stress work, having a sense of control makes a difference. Women who work in jobs with little control, such as in clerical positions, are at higher risk for heart attack, whereas women who work in managerial positions have no increased risk. Women who work in high-stress jobs who have low levels of support from co-workers have a higher risk of hypertension than those who have support.

MANAGING STRESS

For most of us, stress is simply part of life and we can't easily change who we are or how we live. The best way to manage stress is to recognize the triggers that you react to and then to put some interventions in place to manage your stress. Exercise is an excellent destresser. Try to eat well and get enough sleep. Many of my patients enjoy yoga, meditation, crafts, and gardening. Whatever works for you is what you should do. Find some fun in your life. Laugh, watch silly movies, do whatever tickles you. Studies have shown that laughter is very good medicine for many ailments, including stress.

FIVE STEPS TO MANAGING YOUR STRESS

1. Try to get some control over some of the pieces of a stressful situation.
2. Talk to someone you trust—a friend, counselor, or loved one.
3. Find a way to relax—meditate.
4. Get enough sleep. No one does well on empty!
5. Increase your physical activity. Exercise reduces stress hormones.

COPING STYLES

Some people are able to handle more stress than others and to handle the stress they have better than others. I also think that stress is different for different people. For example, I freak out at the thought of driving. Some people become anxious very easily; others are able to go with the flow. Often we are not even aware of what our coping style is. When I ask my patients how they emotionally handle difficult situations, they invariably say "Just fine." Yet my observations and their test results suggest stress and anxiety. I don't think they are lying, only trying really hard to cope—or, even worse, are used to the high level of stress in their lives, which they think is normal. They remain calm and cool on the surface, but inwardly they are in a state of acute stress.

I had a patient I was seeing as part of my research on cardiac rehabilitation who didn't come in for her one-year checkup. I didn't know why

at the time, but later I found out that she had gone into a de
sion after losing several friends in the World Trade Cente
2001. When she finally did come to see me, she was almost ı
able because she had gained so much weight. Her stress, depression, and
anxiety had resulted in chronic overeating. For a woman with heart disease, being overweight is especially not a good thing. After we talked and
she realized what she was doing to her health, she agreed to make some
lifestyle changes and started cognitive behavioral therapy. Information,
for both the doctor and the patient, can make a huge difference in being
healthy.

DEPRESSION

Here are some depressing facts about depression:

- Depression is the fourth most disabling illness in the world, ac-
  cording to the World Health Organization.
- Depression is twice as common in women as in men.
- Depression in women is misdiagnosed approximately 30–50 per-
  cent of the time.
- Women of color are at greater risk for depression than white
  women.
- Immigrant women have a higher risk of depression.
- Asian American women over the age of sixty-five have the highest
  female suicide rate among all ethnic and racial groups.
- The prevalence of major depressive disorder in women is about 21
  percent as compared to about 13 percent in men.
- About seven million women in the United States are clinically depressed; depression occurs most frequently between the ages of
  twenty-five and forty-four.

Clinical depression—a serious illness, and distinct from feelings of
sadness—is currently the leading cause of disability in the United
States, and the World Health Organization expects it to be the second
leading cause of disability in the world, second only to heart disease, by
the year 2020.

There are many theories about why depression should affect so many more women than men. Most likely there are social and biological factors that predispose women to depression, such as hormone fluctuations, a disadvantage in social status, and the greater rate of violence and abuse that women suffer.

THE IMPACT OF DEPRESSION ON HEALTH

Depression can make blood more likely to clot, which can cause heart attacks and stroke. Patients who are depressed are less likely to take their medication properly or to follow a healthful diet or to stop smoking, all of which can have an impact on heart disease. Women who are depressed and have heart disease or have suffered a heart attack need to treat the depression just as they would any other complicating factor. Yet very few doctors even assess for depression, never mind offer treatment.[7]

Stress and depression can trigger a heart attack, and depression and anxiety are associated with poor outcomes following a heart attack. Some people think that often women wait longer than men to seek medical help when having a heart attack, and this delay may account for their poorer outcomes. The antidepressants sertraline (Zoloft) and citalopram (Celexa) can be used to treat depression following a heart attack.

DEPRESSION AND PREGNANCY

Low birth weight associated with preterm delivery can cause a host of problems for the infant, and there is evidence that depression in the mother can lead to preterm delivery. Depressed women and women who seem to have a pessimistic disposition (the glass is always half empty) have babies who weigh significantly less than babies born to women who are positive and optimistic. Low birth weight can also be caused by having a great deal of stress during the pregnancy.[8] As if that isn't bad enough, pregnant women who are depressed and anxious have an increased risk of preeclampsia (see page 60), a serious condition that can affect the mother's and the baby's health.[9] Of course, it's possible that women who are not depressed take better care of themselves—by exercising, for example—which may lower the risk of preterm delivery.[10] Getting regular exercise really does make a huge difference in your health.

POSTPARTUM DEPRESSION

The "baby blues" is a very common experience for new mothers. More than 70 percent of women experience this feeling within three or four days of delivery. They find themselves crying for no reason, or worrying and anxious; as my friend Linda and others say, they just don't feel like themselves.

However, the baby blues are different from postpartum depression, which is thought to affect one in ten women and can begin anytime within a year of delivery. Women who experience postpartum depression are often sad or depressed, have very little energy to do ordinary tasks, may have sleep and eating difficulties, and feel that their lives, and even themselves, are worthless. They have mood swings and are irritable and sometimes take little interest in their babies.

No one is really sure what causes postpartum depression, but most people believe that the dramatic hormone fluctuations that occur during pregnancy and after delivery can affect the chemistry of the brain. Social and psychological factors may also contribute. Many new mothers are isolated, sleep-deprived, overwhelmed with new responsibilities, and generally stressed. Postpartum depression should be treated by a doctor, like any other serious medical problem. Most women recover with medication, therapy or counseling, or a combination of both.

SOCIAL SUPPORT AND DEPRESSION

It is important for everyone, but especially for women who are at risk of depression, to develop and maintain close and nourishing relationships. Women who have emotionally supportive social relationships are at substantially less risk of major depression than men, which is especially important when you consider that depression due to social isolation has been associated with higher death rates in women.[11] Social support acts as a buffer against depression. In fact, not only do women who don't have strong social support and live with a great deal of stress have a greater risk of becoming depressed, but their depression is more severe. Of course, you can't put an ad in the newspaper for a best friend, but you can join an exercise group or get involved in a cause that you admire and meet like-minded people. If you sit alone watching TV, it's hard to maintain friendships and relationships. It's good for your health to get out.

ANXIETY

There is a difference between normal fears and an anxiety disorder. Anxiety disorders are very common and can affect anyone. Here are some facts:

- General anxiety disorders afflict approximately forty million people in the United States.

- Women are twice as likely to be afflicted with anxiety as men.

- Panic disorders, which often have symptoms similar to having a heart attack, affect about six million people.

- Women are twice as likely to be afflicted with panic disorders as men.

- Panic disorders often are associated with depression.

If you feel the following symptoms, it may be a sign of an anxiety disorder:

- Unrealistic worry

- Fear that has no apparent reason

- Constantly checking actions for safety (unplugged appliances)

- Nightmares

- Uncontrollable, obsessive thoughts

- Gastrointestinal problems

Anxiety can take many forms: panic attacks, phobias, obsessive behavior, post-traumatic stress disorder, and other kinds of problems, even eating disorders. People who have panic attacks, which are defined as uncontrollable terror, have heart palpitations, dizziness, sweating, shaking, and shortness of breath. There is also a condition called generalized anxiety disorder, which is anxiety that is long-lasting (at least six months) with excessive worry that manifests in physical or behavioral symptoms. Physical symptoms can include fatigue, headaches, muscle aches, difficulty swallowing, sweating, hot flashes, and irritability. A phobia—an excessive fear of some situation, object, or activity, including social phobia and agoraphobia (fear of leaving home)—can cause women to lead limited and restricted lives.

Anxiety is related to fear or panic, and people who have generalized anxiety fear situations that most people would find unthreatening. Of course there are normal feelings of apprehension, such as when you're waiting for the results of a biopsy, but anxiety disorders are responses to situations that are not normally anxiety-producing. A panic attack caused by high anxiety is a terrible thing, mimicking many of the symptoms of a heart attack. Anxiety can cause palpitations, high blood pressure, sleeplessness, stomach cramps, and GERD; worsen irritable bowel syndrome; and cause hyperventilation that can lead to dizziness and fainting.

How to Treat Anxiety

First of all, anxiety must be properly diagnosed, which it often isn't, since the physical symptoms that are associated with anxiety can look like other conditions. Also, patients don't come in saying "I have anxiety"; they say "I have palpitations" or "I have an upset stomach," as they should. It's the patient's job to describe symptoms and the doctor's job to make a diagnosis. If your doctor cannot find a physical cause that explains your symptoms, anxiety or depression could be a possible source and should not be overlooked.

Anxiety is nothing to be ashamed of, yet so many women are reluctant to share these feelings with their doctors. Telling your doctor is the first important step in taking care of this serious condition.

POST-TRAUMATIC STRESS DISORDER (PTSD)

Research sponsored by the National Institute of Mental Health found that women have twice the risk of developing PTSD after a traumatic event than men. Reactions to traumas such as rape, violence, war, sexual abuse, natural disasters, or serious accidents can include nightmares, terror, depression, anger, irritability, and being easily startled or distracted. Women with PTSD are more likely to have higher rates of medical and psychiatric problems than men.

Once anxiety has been correctly diagnosed, cognitive-behavioral therapies have been successful in reducing and controlling anxiety disorders. Medications such as SSRIs (selective serotonin reuptake inhibitors) alter chemicals in the brain; other antidepressant medications help to relieve symptoms. Medication is especially effective when coupled with cognitive-behavioral therapy. There is no reason to be needlessly suffering because of lack of treatment. It's available.

Medications commonly used for anxiety and panic attacks may be the same as those prescribed for depression, such as the antidepressants paroxetine (Paxil) and escitalopram (Lexapro). However, you need to be carefully monitored because they can cause side effects, such as weight gain and raised blood pressure. The benefit of using SSRIs such as Zoloft, fluoxetine (Prozac), or Celexa to treat depression is that they can be used safely in the elderly and in patients with heart disease. However, SSRIs have side effects, such as irritability, decreased libido, difficulty sleeping, weight gain, and increased blood pressure. If you start on a low dose and gradually increase the dosage, side effects can be minimized. These medications take a few weeks to work, and your doctor may be able to prescribe a second medication that works quickly to relieve anxiety until the SSRI level is therapeutic.

> You should talk to your doctor if you:
> - Start doing poorly at work or at school
> - Feel overly anxious
> - Begin using alcohol or drugs to feel better
> - Feel overwhelmed by the ordinary chores of daily life
> - Have fears that are interfering with your life
> - Become overly preoccupied with food
> - Hate the way you look
> - Can't sleep
> - Don't feel well physically
> - Don't feel that life is worth living
> - Begin to hurt yourself (for example, cutting) or have other self-destructive behaviors
> - Feel withdrawn or disconnected from everyone

Stress, anxiety, and depression pose serious health problems and shouldn't be ignored or thought of as a normal part of life. Talk to your doctor. Exercise, eat well. Take medication if necessary. Don't accept feeling bad as okay. It isn't.

THIRTEEN

Complementary and Alternative Medicine

COMPLEMENTARY AND ALTERNATIVE MEDICINE (CAM) REFERS TO several different kinds of practices and products that are not considered—at this time—to be part of conventional medicine. The reason I stress "at this time" is because at one time many of the practices we are entirely comfortable with today as being "scientific" began as something "alternative." For example, the importance of exercise for good health was mocked as quackery years ago, as was acknowledging the effects of depression, stress, and anxiety on physiology, but now both are entirely part of mainstream medicine. Digitalis and penicillin, once eyed with suspicion, have been completely adopted into conventional health care practices. Once thought to be alternative and out there, these practices and substances are now completely traditional and uncontroversial.

Some definitions may be useful. When used in conjunction with traditional medical practice, CAM is considered "complementary." When used alone, without traditional medicine, it is labeled "alternative."

The National Center for Complementary and Alternative Medicine (NCCAM) of the National Institutes of Health defines "integrative medicine" as a combination of conventional medical practices and those CAM therapies that have been proven safe and effective. CAM techniques and products are constantly changing.

WHO USES CAM?

Surveys show that about 62 percent of adults in the United States have used at least one form of alternative medicine within the previous year. Generally white women with high socioeconomic status use CAM more than other groups of both women and men. More people make use of CAM for chronic conditions, such as HIV or inflammatory bowel disease, than for episodes of acute sickness. Often people try CAM when traditional medicine has failed them.

HOW SAFE IS CAM?

The answer to this critical question is that it's hard to know. There are very few clinical trials, and even fewer rigorous ones, about the safety and

---

CAM CATEGORIES

The National Center for Complementary and Alternative Medicine has classified CAM practices into five categories:

- Alternative medical systems, such as Chinese and Ayurvedic medicine and homeopathy

- Mind-body interventions, such as biofeedback, hypnosis, meditation, and prayer

- Biologic-based therapies, including herbal medicine, dietary supplements, and aromatherapy

- Manipulative and body-based methods, such as chiropractic, massage, acupuncture, and acupressure

- Energy therapy, such as therapeutic touch and Reiki

efficacy of CAM. In dietary supplements, the most popular CAM therapy, there is no standardization; therefore it is difficult to evaluate and compare the components of supplements. Recently, I gave a talk on heart health and a woman asked me why doctors didn't recommend turmeric instead of aspirin. I said I didn't know of any studies that showed that turmeric was either safe at high doses or effective at preventing heart attacks, nor were there studies about what dosage might prove to have either risks or benefits. Be very careful of swallowing (literally) what the press touts as magic cures. Look to see whether there is scientific evidence behind the claims.

DIETARY SUPPLEMENTS

The term "dietary supplement" can cover a great deal of ground. They are defined as vitamins, minerals, herbs, or other botanicals that are intended to supplement (that is, add to) a normal diet. They come in various forms, such as pills, liquids, and powders, and can be sold in department stores, food stores, via TV or the Internet, or through magazine ads.

There are so many supplements on the market that the FDA has serious trouble regulating their safe use; for the FDA, safety is based on food safety rather than pharmaceutical standards. Supplements have become a billion-dollar business, and representatives lobby doctors and health care organizations and inundate the public with advertisements in order to sell their product, using the same techniques as the pharmaceutical companies. Remember ephedra, an herb that for years women used to lose weight? People had to die before the FDA decided to ban its use. Recently claims are being made that bitter orange extract is an alternative to ephedra for weight loss. However, studies show that this extract can cause high blood pressure and lead to heart attacks.[1] Furthermore, there is no evidence that it helps with weight loss. Yet people can't buy it fast enough.

On the other hand, lack of standardization can work to make doctors and the public wary of what might in fact be a useful product. For example, one of the difficulties in evaluating whether the plant echinacea is really effective in treating upper respiratory tract infections, as many people believe, is that there is so much variation in products available for sale that it is hard to conclude anything definitive. What exactly are you evaluating? It's hard to know because you don't know what part of the plant was used, how concentrated it is, what methods were used to extract the product from the plant, how the product was manufactured, or what else has been added to the product. Without standardization, all these factors vary.

Not only is there very little research on these products, probably because there is no financial advantage to anyone to do this research, but the research that is being conducted is often flawed, and therefore the results are suspect. As supplements are increasingly being studied, it is important to keep up to date with the most recent information. Just as with new medication, I generally wait for time to pass and evidence to amass. Ignorance is often bliss, because when studied, much of what initially is thought to be helpful and valuable turns out not to be.

ALWAYS TELL YOUR DOCTOR WHAT YOU ARE TAKING

Often patients don't even think of the vitamins they take as worthy of mentioning when their doctor asks them about medication. But in many cases there can be negative effects from mixing traditional medication with certain vitamins. For example, one of my patients was taking vitamin E to keep her skin looking young. She was also a heart patient and was taking a blood thinner. When she went for an angiogram, she had a serious bleeding episode because the combination of the prescribed blood thinner and the vitamin E caused her to bleed more than if she used the prescribed blood thinner alone.

Patients are not the only ones who forget the importance of remembering what to say. Many doctors never ask about vitamins, herbal supplements, or other forms of CAM; they just don't think of it. Nonetheless, it is most important that they know. For example, some supplements (such as taking over 10,000 IU of vitamin A) could damage a fetus or a nursing baby. If you don't tell your doctor what you are taking, even if it is only a multivitamin or a calcium tablet, she or he won't have the information needed to treat you properly and effectively.

Remember that supplements are chemicals that you are putting in your body. When my patients tell me they are only taking what's "natural," I remind them that arsenic is natural too, but we don't want to be eating it. Natural does not mean safe.

People take supplements for many reasons: because they think they will be healthier if they do; they feel that their regular diet is not adequate and want to ensure that they have more nutrients; or because their use feels somewhat traditional: take a pill and feel better. There are specific reasons people take supplements as well, such as to improve memory, to sleep better, to have more energy, to bolster the immune system. Ironically, a 1999 study reported in *Public Health and Nutrition* concluded that the people who take supplements are those people who are committed to a healthier lifestyle and are aware of their nutritional requirements. In other words, it is exactly the people who don't need supplements who take them![2]

> ## NATURAL DOES NOT MEAN SAFE
>
> Many poisonous mushrooms are natural and can kill you. Hemlock is natural but deadly. Maggots occur naturally and are gross, but they can help you heal from a wound (they help to reduce infection by feeding off dead tissue); nonetheless, you wouldn't want to eat them. You get the idea.

OF SPECIAL INTEREST TO WOMEN

Women are eager to find natural ways to cope with menopausal symptoms, especially now that HT is no longer readily prescribed for the long haul, and many have tried using herbal supplements to manage the symptoms. *Black cohosh* is a plant that has been used for ages by Native Americans to treat various problems, including symptoms associated with menopause. Some women swear that black cohosh helps to reduce their hot flashes, but I speak to many women who say they tried it and it didn't help. According to the NIH, studies about the effectiveness of black cohosh on menopausal symptoms show conflicting results, mainly because of poor study design and differences in the amounts of black cohosh being studied. A 2006 study reported in the *Annals of Internal Medicine* found that black cohosh, used by itself or as part of a multibotanical regimen, had no more effect in reducing menopausal symptoms than a placebo.[3]

Red clover has not been proven to have any impact on menopausal symptoms.

Folic acid is good for women who want to become or are pregnant. It prevents certain birth defects such as neural tube defects.

Ginger may be useful for reducing nausea and vomiting, although again there are no definitive studies that prove its value. But pregnant women in particular may want to use ginger because they are reluctant to take medication if they don't have to. Ginger tea or grating ginger into food seems harmless, but remember, there are no studies that prove it.

Think you have a handle on *soy*? There is so much contradictory information out there it's hard to know what to think. I am a scientist, and I want evidence that something works. So let me tell you about the research on soy. Soybeans, which contain isoflavones, have been used to reduce menopausal symptoms. There is research that does not support this claim and suggests that any benefit is a placebo effect.[4] Yet, other research shows that daily soy protein has helped to reduce hot flashes.[5] A 2002 study reports that although studies are inconclusive, soy may have a modest effect on reducing hot flashes but that isoflavone supplements are not as effective as soy foods.[6] Bottom line: we don't yet know about soy for menopause (although we do know that it has health benefits for blood pressure and cholesterol).

St. John's wort can compromise the effectiveness of oral contraceptives and blood thinners. Tell your doctor if you are taking it so she can adjust the dosages of your medications.

SUPPLEMENTS AND HEART HEALTH

The chemical *coenzyme Q_{10}* (CoQ_{10}) is found naturally in the body and is important for the proper functioning of cells. Levels of CoQ_{10} have been found to be lower in people with chronic diseases, such as heart disease, cancer, and diabetes. This fact makes some people infer that having more CoQ_{10} in your body would be good for you. If you take supplements of $CoQ_{10,}$ you will increase the levels of the chemical in your body, but there is no evidence that this is good for your health. Its use is controversial at best. For example, although there is no proof that it can prevent a heart attack, it might protect the heart in patients undergoing certain forms of chemotherapy. There is some evidence that this supplement may reduce the risk of muscle aches from taking statin medication, and I sometimes recommend it for this purpose. But more research needs to be done before we really understand any health benefits.

Folic acid supplementation is no longer recommended to prevent heart disease.

Although it used to be thought that *vitamin B₆* helped to prevent heart disease, a large study reported in 2006 has now disproved this claim.[7] The study showed that even though B vitamin supplements such as B₆, B₁₂, and folic acid reduced homocysteine levels (a protein associated with higher heart disease risk), heart disease risk was not lowered in women.[8]

Garlic is supposed to be good for heart health, but again, it has not been proven, and there are risks associated, such as gastrointestinal problems. Garlic supplements have not been studied for the prevention of disease. However, there is some evidence that people who eat half a clove per day have lower cholesterol than those who do not.[9]

Ginkgo can cause palpitations and should be avoided if you have heart problems.

A patient came to me not long ago after she heard me give a talk on women's health because she liked the idea of a woman doctor who focused on women's health. She had elevated cholesterol levels but no family history of heart disease, and her internist suggested that she increase her cholesterol medication. She asked me for advice, particularly because her husband—not a doctor—had told her to take *resveratrol,* an antioxidant found naturally in red grapes and blueberries, rather than increase her medication. I told her that although resveratrol helps with blood vessel flexibility it would not help lower her cholesterol and that there was no research to support that claim. I suggested she simply eat red grapes, and gave her a prescription for cholesterol medicine.

Vitamin C does not reduce death due to heart disease, nor does it reduce the risk of stroke. The role of vitamin C in reducing cholesterol has not been studied.

Vitamin E does not reduce the risk of death from heart disease, nor does it reduce stroke or cholesterol.[10] There is inconsistent research about the effect of vitamin E on Alzheimer's disease.

SUPPLEMENTS AND CANCER

Research suggests that *multivitamins* may reduce the risk for colon cancer, but the finding may be related to one or more of the components of the multivitamin, especially folic acid. Without studying it, no one knows which component it is.[11]

An antioxidant is a nutrient that prevents oxidation, which causes cell damage. *Vitamins A, C,* and *E* and *beta-carotene* are antioxidants, as is the mineral *selenium.* Most doctors believe that antioxidants are good for you. But it is most important to talk to your doctor about dosage. Something that's good in smaller doses is not always a good thing in larger doses. There is no recommendation that you should take these vitamin supplements. According to the Agency for Healthcare Research and Quality, which studied clinical trials involving *vitamins C* and *E* and *CoQ10,* there is no evidence that these supplements help in preventing or treating cancer.

OTHER SUPPLEMENT FACTS

Preliminary studies show that *CoQ10* may help slow down some of the symptoms of early-stage Parkinson's disease.

According to a 2005 study published in the *New England Journal of Medicine, echinacea* had no significant effect on either the intensity of the symptoms or the duration of the common cold. However, it may be that the dosage studied (900 mg daily) was too low. A December 2006 study reported in the *Journal of Clinical Pharmacy and Therapeutics* found that *echinacea* increased intestinal bacteria, diarrhea, and inflammatory bowel disease and was associated with an increased risk of colon cancer.

There is controversy about whether or not *glucosamine* and *chondroitin* help with symptoms of arthritis. There is some evidence that the combination may help relieve symptoms of mild knee pain.[12]

Studies have shown that *melatonin* is not effective for treating sleep disorders.

Genistein, an isoflavone in soy supplements, improved bone density in osteopenic post-menopausal women.

St. John's wort was not found to be any more effective for treating depression than a placebo, and is dangerous if you are pregnant.

Supplement	Conditions It Is Commonly Used to Treat	Cautions and Side Effects
Aloe vera	Diabetes	Doesn't lower blood sugar (although it is not bad if you want to use it to moisturize your skin)
Ascorbic acid (vitamin C)	Upper respiratory infections Urinary tract infections	Has no impact on infections once you acquire them
Black cohosh	Menopausal symptoms	No evidence that it is effective
Coenzyme Q_{10}	Heart failure	Doesn't prevent heart attack or heart failure, although it may relieve the muscle aches associated with statin medication
Comfrey	Gastrointestinal problems	Can cause liver damage
Cranberry	Urinary tract infections	There is no evidence of effectiveness; don't let these remain untreated
Echinacea	Upper respiratory infections	Gastrointestinal problems
Evening primrose	Menopausal symptoms	No evidence of effectiveness

Supplement	Conditions It Is Commonly Used to Treat	Cautions and Side Effects
Garlic	Cholesterol, hypertension	Doesn't lower cholesterol; doesn't work for hypertension and has the same side effects as statins
Ginkgo biloba	Dementia, tinnitus	Can cause palpitations
Kava	Anxiety	Can cause liver damage
Licorice root	Fatigue	Can raise blood pressure
Melatonin	Insomnia	No evidence of effectiveness
Red clover	Menopausal symptoms	No evidence of effectiveness
Soy	Menopausal symptoms	No evidence of effectiveness
St. John's wort	Anxiety, depression	Interferes with other medications; should not be taken if pregnant; compromises effectiveness of oral contraceptives
Valerian	Insomnia	No evidence of effectiveness
Zinc	Upper respiratory infections	No evidence of effectiveness

Valerian has not been proven effective in treating sleep disorders.

Vitamin C has not been proven to prevent colds, as many people believe.

Zinc can slow the progression of macular degeneration, an age-related eye disease.

SUPPLEMENTS ARE OFTEN NOT EFFECTIVE

There are several problems with using supplements, even when they are not directly harmful. In addition to the lack of clinical information and the potential risks involved, my real issue is that sometimes patients use herbal supplements to treat themselves. If so, then they may not be getting the appropriate and more clinically proven treatment. If you have any medical condition, it should be diagnosed by a health care professional and options for treatment discussed. Especially if there is no scientific evidence that supplements are effective, make sure you don't leave yourself without treatment.

ACUPUNCTURE

According to the NCCAM, acupuncture is one of the most common and oldest medical procedures used in the world. It originated in China more than two thousand years ago, but it took a *New York Times* reporter to introduce it to the United States. In 1971, James Reston, while traveling in China, needed surgery and wrote about how his pain after surgery was alleviated through the use of needles. Since then acupuncture has become popular in the United States. In 1997, the NIH reported that it was offered by thousands of practitioners for relief of pain and various other ailments. It is estimated that 8.2 million people in the United States have had acupuncture.

HOW DOES ACUPUNCTURE WORK?

The fundamental concepts of traditional Chinese medicine, which include acupuncture, are quite different from Western medicine. The basis of acupuncture is that balanced energy, *qi* or *chi*, is responsible for well-being. Illness results when the *qi* becomes unbalanced. It is believed that the *qi* travels through the body in certain pathways and that there are points on the body where this energy is accessible. The goal of acupuncture is to restore balance. This is accomplished through inserting needles into the points and redirecting the energy balance. Once in balance, the body will heal.

Today, many health professionals who practice acupuncture are not committed to the *qi* principles. Western practitioners are more comfortable with the notion that the acupuncture points match nerve junctions and other anatomical features. They understand referred pain, such as when a nerve in your neck has an impact on your arm.

What Is Acupuncture Used For?

Western medicine is not quick to embrace other kinds of practice, but there is so much evidence that acupuncture can be effective in certain circumstances that an independent panel of experts recommended it to the NIH.

In 1997, the panel issued a statement that acknowledged medical conditions that can be helped by acupuncture. These include:

- Addiction
- Adult postoperative nausea
- Asthma
- Carpal tunnel syndrome
- Fibromyalgia
- Headache
- Low back pain
- Menstrual cramps
- Myofascial pain
- Nausea and vomiting caused by chemotherapy
- Osteoarthritis
- Postoperative dental pain
- Stroke rehabilitation
- Tennis elbow

ACUPUNCTURE AND WOMEN

While I must stress that many studies may be inaccurate and inconclusive, there are various areas where acupuncture is known to be effective. In addition to those areas listed opposite, acupuncture has been shown to be useful in:

- Reducing morning sickness in pregnant women[13]
- Preventing recurring UTIs in women[14]
- Reducing low back pain in pregnancy[15]
- Reducing pain during labor[16]
- Reducing the intensity and number of hot flashes[17]

ACUPUNCTURE SAFETY TIPS

You need to make sure you go to a reputable, qualified, experienced practitioner. You need to make sure that the needles are disposable and taken from a sealed package. The FDA requires that acupuncture needles be labeled for single use. The sites that the needles go into should be cleansed with a disinfectant. You should feel no pain when the needles are inserted.

HYPNOSIS

Hypnosis involves an altered, relaxed state of consciousness that can be used to help people control bad habits, such as smoking or overeating, and to learn to reduce pain and stress. When you are hypnotized, a trained hypnotist (hypnotherapist) makes suggestions, often using mental imagery, to help you change certain behaviors or to teach you to alter physical sensations. For example, if you are suffering from migraine headaches, you might be trained to visualize the blood vessels in the brain opening from a constricted position, allowing the blood to flow more freely and thereby relieving the pain. Most people are capable of being hypnotized, but you have to be willing to trust the hypnotist enough to relax. You can also learn techniques of self-hypnosis.

Hypnotism has been used successfully to reduce pain, to help people who want to stop smoking, to learn relaxation techniques, to help reduce stress and anxiety, and to overcome phobias. Hypnosis and self-hypnosis have been used to reduce labor pain and pain from dental surgery. Patients who suffer from IBS have been helped with hypnosis; they find that their symptoms of pain and bloating are improved.

BIOFEEDBACK

Like hypnosis, biofeedback is a mind-body intervention that is a relatively recent CAM therapy, beginning only in the 1960s. The process of biofeedback involves learning to use your mind to control your bodily functions, such as heart rate, breathing, blood pressure, skin temperature, and muscle tension. By learning how to monitor these physiological functions, you can learn to have some control over them. By controlling them, you can learn how to reduce stress and relax. As with all CAM interventions, a biofeedback practitioner should be certified.

You learn to know your body's responses to stress and relaxation through a device that monitors electrical signals from the muscles and then translates those signals into beeps or other sounds or lights. By learning to recognize increasing tension, for example, you can learn to relax the muscles. When relaxed, you can hold pleasant images in your mind and reduce pain. Generally, once you learn the technique, the mechanical device is unnecessary, although small home machines have been introduced for use.

Biofeedback has been shown to be effective in treating:

- Anxiety
- Attention deficit hyperactivity disorder (ADHD)
- Binge eating
- Constipation
- Fecal incontinence
- Fibromyalgia (chronic pain)
- Improving circulation (especially useful for diabetics)
- Ringing in the ears (tinnitus)
- Stroke rehabilitation
- Tension and migraine headaches
- Urinary incontinence

CHIROPRACTIC

The word *chiropractic* comes from the Greek and means "done by hand." Chiropractic therapy is based on the idea that the structure of the body, especially the spine, affects the body's health. By manipulating the body, the relationship between structure and health can be restored and the body can heal itself. Chiropractors have specialized training and have to be licensed and certified by the state after passing examinations. Some chiropractors have done specialized residencies in sports injuries, neurology, orthopedics, pediatrics, nutrition, internal disorders, or diagnostic imaging.

Just as with any responsible health care practitioner, a chiropractor should ask a lot of questions, take a medical history, and do a physical examination and may order X-rays or other diagnostic images in order to diagnose a problem for correction. However, unlike medical doctors, they cannot prescribe drugs or perform surgery.

How Do Chiropractors Differ from Osteopaths?

Osteopaths also believe in the interrelationship of skeleton structure and health and also use manipulation, but they make greater use of arms and legs to align the body. Osteopaths are trained differently than chiropractors, although both disciplines believe in the power of the body to heal itself if impediments are removed. They are trained in both manipulation and in traditional medicine and can prescribe medicine and perform surgery. Called doctors of osteopathy (DOs), they are trained with a more holistic approach to health and disease than traditional medical training. Osteopaths are integrated into traditional Western medicine more than chiropractors, to which the medical establishment is quite hostile.

Chiropractic and Traditional Medicine

Historically the Western medical establishment rejected chiropractic as "quackery." In 1963, the American Medical Association (AMA) tried to eliminate chiropractors as "unethical," and in the 1970s the Joint Commission on Accreditation of Healthcare Organizations refused to accredit hospitals that had chiropractors on staff. Chiropractors brought a lawsuit against the AMA and won. Since 1974, Medicare has paid for chiropractic therapy.

Although doctors don't seem to like chiropractors, consumers of their services do. About 10 percent of the U.S. population goes to chiropractors annually, most commonly for back pain. Research is mixed about whether chiropractic is any better then traditional medicine at treating back pain. The *New England Journal of Medicine* reported that patients "had only marginally better outcomes" when treated with chiropractic or with an educational booklet.[18] However, in 1994 the Agency for Healthcare Policy and Research endorsed chiropractic for treating acute back pain. There is also some evidence that shows that patients have been injured when treated for neck pain.[19]

MASSAGE THERAPY

Many people believe that massages help relieve stress and anxiety. People also go to massage therapists for muscle aches and pains. There are many different kinds of massages: Swedish massage involves stroking and kneading, shiatsu massage focuses on manipulation of certain pressure points, Rolfing on deep tissue manipulation. There is also total body massage and neuromuscular massage. Often the therapist makes use of a combination of these massage techniques and may also use aromatic oils (aromatherapy) to enhance relaxation.

As with other forms of CAM, research about the effectiveness of massage is scant and inconclusive. There are several small studies that suggest that massage can help relieve body aches and headaches and help with anxiety. There is evidence that massage can help with chronic back pain. If a massage is properly done by a trained massage therapist, there should be no problems.

THERAPEUTIC TOUCH

Therapeutic touch is a technique for healing that uses the hands to influence, balance, and distribute energy throughout the body, but without actually touching the body. The technique was developed by a nurse, and many nurses make use of the technique for hospital patients, especially those suffering from arthritis, headache, and anxiety. There is very little evidence about whether or not therapeutic touch works, but it can't really hurt.

TRANSCENDENTAL MEDITATION

As I keep saying, stress is very bad for your health. We all live with a great deal of stress. Transcendental meditation (TM) is a relaxation technique used to reduce stress and induce calm. It has been proven to lower blood pressure that is moderately elevated and may have other health benefits as well. Generally, you get trained in TM, either through a course or with a professional instructor, and once the technique is learned, you can practice it by yourself.

YOGA

Yoga is another practice that many people use for relaxation, to reduce anxiety and promote a feeling of well-being. I recommend it to my patients as a means of relaxation leading to stress reduction. It is an ancient Indian practice that involves special postures and exercises combined with meditation to develop a positive relationship between mind and body. The very limited data regarding yoga and health suggests that it may help with carpal tunnel syndrome and symptoms (not causes) of asthma. It can help your posture and teach you breathing techniques for relaxation. I always tell my patients who practice yoga in local fitness centers that they should use their own mats to prevent fungal infection.

FOURTEEN

Plastic Surgery

EVERYONE WANTS TO LOOK GOOD. IN THE UNITED STATES TODAY, that usually means looking younger and being slimmer. Increasingly people are turning to plastic surgeons for cosmetic surgery or for procedures that are designed to improve their appearance and increase their self-esteem. The word *plastic* comes from Greek and means "to reshape"; it has nothing to do with the modern synthetic material.

Although plastic surgery has been performed since ancient times, it is becoming more and more popular as modern surgical techniques have made these procedures readily available. In 2005 more than ten million people had cosmetic surgery, a figure up 38 percent from 2000, with liposuction, nose reshaping, and breast augmentation among the top procedures. Millions of people have had nonsurgical cosmetic procedures as well, such as Botox treatments, chemical peels, and microdermabrasion. That's a lot of people electing to have treatment.

Physicians make the distinction between plastic surgery performed for cosmetic reasons—to improve appearance—and surgery performed because it is medically indicated. When surgery is done because of disease, birth defects, trauma such as burns, or other medically necessary reasons, it is called reconstructive surgery. Usually insurance companies will pay for reconstructive surgery but not for cosmetic. However, different companies may have different definitions of what is or isn't reconstructive; it pays to check in advance of the procedure.

If you're considering plastic surgery:

- Learn as much as you can about the specific procedure you are considering.

- Use a surgeon who is board-certified by the American Board of Plastic Surgery. Certification ensures that the surgeon has been trained in plastic surgery and has passed appropriate exams.

- Be sure that you tell your surgeon about all medications and drugs you are taking. Women who are taking oral contraceptives or hormone therapy should be sure to tell the doctor.

- Make sure that the surgeon takes a complete medical history. Sometimes for elective surgery patients don't realize how important it is to give complete and comprehensive medical information. For example, if you or your family has a history of blood clots, that information is critical for your surgeon, since there is a risk of blood clots with surgery. If you are subject to cold sores, you need to inform your doctor.

> ### SHOULD YOU HAVE PLASTIC SURGERY?
>
> It's good to have options and as long as we make informed choices and have reasonable expectations about what plastic surgery can accomplish, I am in favor of it. But not everyone is a good candidate for plastic surgery for physical, emotional, or psychological reasons. Changing the way you look has an impact on how you feel about yourself. In order to be properly evaluated it is important that you be honest with your surgeon about your hopes and expectations.

- Check out the facility where the procedure is to take place and be sure it conforms to safety standards. Especially if you are undergoing anesthesia, make sure that the facility is accredited by a recognized organization, such as the American Association for

Accreditation of Ambulatory Surgery Facilities or the Joint Commission for Accreditation of Healthcare Organizations, and that it is licensed in the state where the facility is located.

- Find out about expected complications.
- Learn about the recovery process.

COSMETIC PROCEDURES

There are many different cosmetic procedures for the face and for the body.

BOTOX

Botox is the brand name of a toxin that in large doses causes botulism. Injecting small amounts into the muscles causes paralysis of the muscles, which then causes frown lines and deep wrinkles to disappear. It is most often used to smooth out forehead wrinkles or wrinkles between the eyebrows. The effects of Botox last about six months. Side effects include bruising and headaches. Occasionally patients get droopy eyelids. It is important not to rub the area that was treated for twelve hours so that the Botox doesn't affect any other area.

Women who are pregnant or breast-feeding should not have Botox treatments. Also, if you have any history of neurological problems, you may not be a good candidate.

PLASTIC SURGERY ON THE BREAST

Many women are dissatisfied with their breasts, just as they are with their noses or their thighs, and many women seek surgery to change their appearance.

BREAST REDUCTION

Advertising to the contrary, many large-breasted women are not happy with the consequences of their big breasts. They experience back, neck, and shoulder pain, find that there are physical activities that they can't do comfortably, such as jogging, and have trouble finding clothes that fit well. For these women, breast reduction surgery provides help. According to the American Society of Plastic Surgeons, about 105,000 breast reduction surgeries are performed each year.

If you are considering plastic surgery to reduce your breast size, your surgeon will discuss with you how much breast tissue will be removed. You should also discuss the positioning of the nipple. If the breast is very large and sags, the surgeon may have to reposition the nipple and areola (the colored area around the nipple).

All surgery is serious and should not be undertaken lightly. You will have an anesthetic, and there will be scars from the incision that need to heal. After the surgery you may have drainage tubes under your arms. You may need pain medication and antibiotics so that you don't get an infection. You may be recovering for several weeks and unable to work.

> **IF YOU WANT TO BREAST-FEED**
>
> If you plan to have children, you should be aware that breast reduction surgery may decrease your ability to breast-feed.

On the positive side, you will be more comfortable, especially in your back, neck, and shoulders. Your bra straps won't dig tunnels into your shoulders. You will be able to exercise and do physical activities that might have been limited before the surgery. You may like the way you look much better. Most women who decide to have the surgery express satisfaction that they did it.

BREAST AUGMENTATION

According to the American Society of Plastic Surgeons, breast augmentation has become the second most commonly performed cosmetic surgical procedure after liposuction. More than 291,000 breast enlargement procedures were performed in 2005. Women have this surgery because they want to change the appearance of their breasts or as reconstruction following breast surgery.

Breast size is increased by surgically inserting an implant. Before 1992, there was a choice of implants, either silicone gel or saline (salt water). After 1992 the FDA restricted the use of silicone gel because women began complaining of serious side effects. For many years, they

BREAST IMPLANTS AND MAMMOGRAPHY

Breast implants can interfere with the effectiveness of mammography screening for breast cancer. If you are at high risk for developing breast cancer, probably breast implants are not a good idea. If you have implants, you should always alert your doctor as well as the technician doing the mammogram.

There are several reasons that implants can make the mammogram unreliable. Sometimes scarring or calcium deposits can mimic the way a tumor looks on a mammogram. Also, during a mammogram the breast needs to be compressed. If the compression is too severe, the implant can rupture; if the compression is too lax, the mammogram won't be effective.

were available only to women who needed reconstruction after having a mastectomy or women who had breast deformities. But in 2006, the FDA reapproved the use of silicone implants for cosmetic reasons. Although there was some media attention given to silicone implants leading to autoimmune disease, there is no evidence that this is true. Also, implants do not cause cancer.

There are risks to augmentation. Implants can leak or rupture. They can cause infection and pain. There may be a loss of feeling in the nipple or breast. Implants can interfere with breast-feeding. Mammograms may be unreliable. Scar tissue can form around the implant, which can cause hardening of the breast tissue. Sometimes the pain is severe from this hardening, and surgery is necessary to replace the implant. Breast implants can also get in the way of getting a good ultrasound of the heart.

CHEMICAL PEELS

Chemical peels improve the appearance of the skin of the face, reducing wrinkles, discolorations, and acne scars. A chemical is applied to the skin that causes the topmost layers to peel off, akin to what happens if you get a bad sunburn. The new skin is usually smoother, but it is also more sensitive to the sun; be careful to use sunscreen. Complications can include swelling, scarring, and blisters. Women who are taking oral contraceptives can develop brown discolored spots on the face. If you are subject to cold sores (herpes), chemical peels may increase their appearance. Tell your doctor if you get cold sores.

Collagen Treatments

Collagen treatments use fat (either from a cow or from you) or synthetic fillers to plump up facial wrinkles. As we age, skin loses elasticity and lines appear. Collagen injections are supposed to replenish the skin's lost collagen and give you a younger-looking face. Risks from collagen injections are allergic reactions, such as hives or a rash, and swelling. Collagen treatment has not been proven safe for pregnant women; if you are pregnant, discuss this with your doctor.

Dermabrasion

Dermabrasion uses a wheel or rough brush to remove the upper layers of skin. As with a chemical peel, the new skin has a smoother appearance, and the appearance of scars and heavy wrinkles is improved. Again, sunscreen should be used to protect the new skin. Complications include infection, scarring, and discoloration of the skin.

Eyelid Surgery

Eyelid surgery lifts droopy eyelids and removes excess fat "bags" from underneath the eyes. If the droop is interfering with normal vision, sometimes insurance covers the procedure to correct the problem. Complications from this procedure are rare but can include infection, dry eyes, blurry vision, and discoloration of the skin of the eyelids.

Face-Lifts

As we age, the skin sags and loosens, especially around the jowls, neck, and eyes. Face-lifts tighten these signs of age. But they don't last forever, usually about five to ten years. Risks include bruising, infection, numbness of the face and scarring. We have all seen bad face-lifts, where it looks as if a woman is wearing a plastic mask; the good ones are less noticeable. Get a very good recommendation before you have this procedure done.

LIP AUGMENTATION

Lip augmentation plumps up the lips, making them larger, by injecting fat or collagen. These substances get absorbed by the body over time, and so eventually the procedure has to be repeated. Sometimes synthetic material such as Gore-Tex or implants are used. Complications can include allergic reactions, nerve damage, or scarring. If you have a lot of swelling or develop a fever, you need to get medical attention right away.

LIPOSUCTION

Liposuction is the removal of fat, done with a kind of vacuum device, usually for the abdomen, buttocks, hips, thighs, neck, and upper arms. This procedure works best on women who are in good health and who are slightly above average weight. If you have lots of cellulite, liposuction can make it appear worse. Older women, who have skin that is not as elastic as it was, may not reap the advantages of the procedure. Some risks from the procedure are baggy skin, fluid retention, infection, and pain.

RHINOPLASTY

Rhinoplasty—what used to be called a "nose job"—reshapes the nose. If breathing problems are resolved by the procedure, it may be covered by insurance. The procedure is usually done from inside the nose. Some risks include nosebleeds, a weakened sense of smell, and trouble breathing. I confess that although I thought I had done my homework properly, I had a botched nose job and suffer from chronic sinus infections. After two procedures I still can't breathe out of the left side of my nose. When I went to an ENT (ear, nose, throat) specialist to evaluate my problem, he was critical of my decision to have the surgery in the first place. He said, "Can you believe you actually paid for someone to do this to you?" In fact, what I had was a complication of the surgery, and his job was to tell me how to correct the breathing problem, not to mock my original decision. Needless to say, I found a different doctor. Remember, if you are considering rhinoplasty, not only should your nose look good, it should also work well.

TUMMY TUCK

A tummy tuck, or abdominoplasty, removes excess fat and skin from the abdomen. Many women who have tummy tucks have had multiple pregnancies and hope to tighten their loose muscles and flabby skin. Others want this procedure because they may have lost a great deal of weight and feel that they have excess skin. It is not a good idea to have a tummy tuck if you plan to become pregnant because pregnancy will stretch the muscles that the tummy tuck tightens. The downside of a tummy tuck is that you can have noticeable scars. After the surgery, you may have pain for several months, numbness, and fatigue.

FIFTEEN

Taking Care of Your Skin

THE SKIN IS AN ORGAN THAT IS DESIGNED TO PROTECT THE INSIDE of your body by providing a barrier against germs and other irritants, keeping them on the outside of your body. In addition to keeping the inside in and the outside out, skin helps to regulate body temperature and has nerves that help us feel what's around us. An average-size adult has about twenty square feet of skin.

There are three layers of skin: epidermis, dermis, and subcutaneous fat. Each layer helps to protect the body in specific ways. The epidermis replenishes cells, making new ones every 28 days as the old cells get sloughed off. Also, the epidermis contains melanin, which gives skin its color (the more melanin, the darker the skin) and helps to protect the body from some of the sun's ultraviolet (UV) rays. The dermis contains sweat glands, nerve endings, blood vessels, hair follicles, collagen, and elastin; the last two give skin its flexibility and provide hydration. The subcutaneous (which means under the skin) fat layer helps maintain a constant temperature and provides protection against bumps and other injuries.

Just as with the other organs, skin health is dependent on lifestyle factors such as sun damage, genes, and hormones, especially estrogen. Because our skin is (literally) out there, many of us don't remember that it requires protection, just as our liver or lungs do. We hardly notice our skin unless we see something unusual, such as a mole, a bruise, a sunburn, a pimple, or a wrinkle.

For doctors, however, the skin is an important window on the rest of the body. Just as a skin rash alerted our mothers to the fact we were having chicken pox as children, rashes, black-and-blue marks, red streaks, or skin tone and color can provide clues for your doctor that you might be suffering from an autoimmune disorder, bleeding problem, dehydration, liver problem, or infection. Every physical examination, regardless of the doctor's specialty, should involve an examination of the skin.

Some skin problems are often pooh-poohed, even by doctors, as vanity, but in most cases they shouldn't be, certainly not without some investigation. I had a typical and unpleasant experience that brought this home to me. At the age of thirty, after I came back from a trip to the Caribbean, I saw a big reddish brown spot on my forehead. I couldn't understand what it was. I always use sunscreen, so I didn't think it was a burn. I went to see a dermatologist at the hospital where I was training, who told me that the brown spot was most likely sun damage. He suggested that I use sunscreen. What about the red rash? I asked. He said it was only cosmetic, and if it really bothered me, I should wear more makeup and cover it with bangs.

I wasn't happy with this advice, which was clearly unhelpful and also insulting. I was a doctor, I knew about sunscreen, and his response made me feel as if he thought I was not only vain but foolish. If I, a professional colleague, got treated that way, other women must experience this kind of treatment very often. Somewhat embarrassed, I talked to a friend and colleague about my brown rashy blotch, and he told me about a dermatologist at New York University who was actively doing research in hyperpigmentation, or brown spots, on the skin. He sent me for allergy testing and concluded that I was allergic to the sunscreen I was using. The brown spot was due to sun damage, and he prescribed a lightening cream that faded the discoloration. Of course, I now use a different sunscreen and always wear a hat. And I wear my hair with bangs because I like them.

Our skin changes throughout our life cycle, and we are concerned with different skin issues at different times of life. Most teenagers worry about acne; adults worry about the risk of skin cancer as well as the more benign wrinkles and jowls.

THE SUN AND SKIN

One of the major culprits of skin damage is the sun. Exposure to the sun speeds up the aging process of the skin, causing the early onset of wrinkles that are coarser than the ones you expect from the normal aging process. The sun also damages the collagen of the skin, so you have less elasticity and moisture. The sun is responsible for worsening the uneven pigmentation and brown spots that are associated with age. Most important, too much sun increases your risk for getting skin cancer.

SUN PROTECTION

There are two types of damaging sunlight: UVB rays and UVA rays. UVB causes sunburns, and UVA, which goes deeper into the skin, causes wrinkling and other skin damage and also increases the risk of cancer from UVB rays. You need to protect yourself from both kinds of rays.

But remember that sunscreen is only one of multiple ways you should protect yourself. Not long ago, I was at home putting on my

THE SUN IS NOT ALL BAD

Not all sunlight is bad for the skin. In fact, a little sunlight is necessary to allow our bodies to manufacture vitamin D, which is an important component of calcium metabolism and necessary for good health.
You need at least twenty minutes a day of sunlight to make sufficient vitamin D. In fact, if you don't get enough sunlight, you should take vitamin D supplements (see Chapter 9).

Some people suffer from seasonal affective disorder, a form of depression that is associated with low sun exposure in wintertime. If you have this, you need twenty minutes of sun a day, but choose the less intense hours of the day.

makeup, listening to a news report on the radio. The announcer said that rates of skin cancer had gone up even though people were using sunscreen. The implication was that sunscreen didn't prevent cancer. All I could think of was what a bad message that was and that people were going to go out into the sun thinking that it didn't matter whether or not they wore sunscreen. What the announcer didn't mention was the study's conclusion that the skin cancer rate had increased because people who did use sunscreen thought they were protected and stayed out longer in the sun. That's not about sunscreen use; it's about poor sun habits. Also, some of the participants in the study were not using enough sunscreen or weren't using sunscreens with UVA protection.

SUNSCREENS

There are two types of sunscreens: ones that contain chemicals to filter out UVB and UVA rays, and ones that use a physical barrier, such as zinc oxide and titanium dioxide, to form a thick visible layer on the skin and reflect light off the skin. There are a few sunscreens that combine both types. The physical sunscreens are not absorbed by the skin, but sit on the skin's surface—think lifeguard at the beach with a white nose. Today the physical sunblocks are produced in microfine particles so you don't have the heavy white buildup on the nose, making them less likely to cause acne. Physical sunblocks protect against both UVA and UVB rays.

You have to read sunscreen labels the way you read food labels (and many of the words on the labels are just as difficult to pronounce). When you read the front of the bottle, look for the SPF (sun protection factor) number. This is the number that measures how quickly your skin burns. You need at least an SPF of 15,which allows you to stay in the sun fifteen times longer than it would normally take you to burn. If you have a great deal of sun exposure, get one with a higher number; however, sunscreens with an SPF greater than 30 are no more effective than those with an SPF of 30. The SPF number applies only to protection against UVB rays.

Different chemical ingredients are combined in sunscreens in order to provide the broadest possible protection. PABA derivatives, octyl methoxycinnamate, and cinoxate help to filter UVB rays. For protection

Sunscreens that contain UVB filters should contain one or more of the following ingredients:

Octocrylene

Octyl salicylate

Homosalate

Octyl methoxycinnamate

Butyl methoxydibenzoylmethane

Cinoxate

Ethylhexyl-*p*-methoxycinnamate

Sunscreens that block UVA should contain:

Avobenzone (Parsol 1789)

Mexoryl SX (This is available in the United States in a product called Anthelios SX made by L'Oréal. It includes avobenzone and octocrylene, so it also protects against UVB rays. Mexoryl SX is considered to be the best UVA blocker.

Sunscreens that combine UVB and UVA filters contain:

Oxybenzone benzophenone-3

Avobenzone (Parsol 1789) and oxybenzone (available as Helioplex, patented by Neutrogena)

Physical sunscreens that block UVA and UVB rays contain either:

Titanium dioxide

Zinc oxide

against longer-wavelength UVA rays, sunscreens include benzophenones; for broader-range protection, they include avobenzone (Parsol 1789), ecamsule (Mexoryl), titanium dioxide, or zinc oxide.

Regardless of what it says on the package, most sunscreen is useless after two hours and should be reapplied. Try to put on sunscreen a half hour before you are exposed.

How to Protect Yourself from the Sun

Some people make the mistake of thinking that using sunscreen is enough to protect their skin from sun damage. You should try to do everything you can to minimize sun exposure. This means that in addition to sunscreen, wear appropriate clothing and a hat.

- Use sunscreen with UVB and UVA protection. Make sure to apply it liberally, and reapply after being in the water, sweating, or toweling off. Don't forget to cover the places you can't see, such as behind your ears and the back of your legs. Also, wear lip balm with SPF protection.

- Wear a hat with a wide brim.

- Wear sunglasses. Sun damage to the eyes increases the risk for cataracts.

- Avoid the strongest rays. If possible, stay out of the sun between 10:00 A.M. and 4:00 P.M., when the sun's rays are strongest.

- Cover up with protective clothing. Loosely fitting, tightly woven fabrics are most protective against sun damage to the skin. Hold your clothes up to the light and see how much comes through; choose the ones where minimal light is coming through. When I am snorkeling, I wear a surfing shirt; sometimes I wear it to swim as a bathing suit top. Sun-protective clothing with an ultraviolet protection factor (UPF) of 50 is even better than sunscreen, but this clothing is expensive.

> ### HOW TO PICK YOUR SPF
>
> 1. If you burn easily, never tan, or have red hair, blue eyes, and freckles, you need to wear SPF 15 routinely and increase the SPF to 25–30 when doing outdoor activities.[1]
>
> 2. If you burn easily and tan a little, use SPF 15 for routine activities and SPF 25–30 for outdoor activities.
>
> 3. If you burn minimally and tan easily, use SPF 6–8 for routine daywear and SPF 15 for outdoor activities.
>
> 4. If you are Middle Eastern or African American, use SPF 6–8 for routine daywear and SPF 15 for outdoor activity.

- Use self-tanning moisturizers rather than tanning parlors, which expose you to UV rays. Self-tanners do not give sun protection, so you still need to wear sunscreen even if you look tan.

SKIN CANCER

Ultraviolet rays from the sun are considered to be an environmental risk factor in the development of skin cancer. There are three basic types of skin cancer: basal cell, squamous cell, and melanoma.

Basal cell is the most common type and usually does not spread to other parts of your body. This accounts for 75 percent of skin cancers.

Squamous cell cancer is more serious and can spread through the lymph nodes to other parts of your body. Actinic keratosis is considered a precancerous condition and is caused by sun damage. Approximately 10 percent of actinic keratosis develops into squamous cell cancer. Both basal cell and squamous cell cancers have excellent cure rates when caught early.

Melanoma, the most serious form of skin cancer, usually develops within a mole; the risk is increased with sun exposure, but this cancer can occur in areas not exposed to the sun.

Chronic sun exposure is the most important cause of squamous cell skin cancer. Painful sunburns have been associated with basal cell carcinoma and malignant melanoma. Clearly it is important to protect yourself from the sun.

WHEN TO CALL A DOCTOR

One day a patient, Natalie, came in for a consultation about her high blood pressure. When I put my stethoscope on her back to listen to her lungs, I noticed a very dark mole with an irregular shape. I asked her if she knew about it and if a dermatologist had evaluated it. She said that another doctor had mentioned it to her, but she hadn't had time yet to see a dermatologist. Then she also told me that she had noticed blood on the back of her shirt a week ago. I didn't wait for her to call a dermatologist; I called one for her, and I was happy I did, because she was diagnosed with an early melanoma.

Call a dermatologist if:

- Moles change shape, become thicker, change color, or bleed
- Skin changes in color or thickness
- Sores don't heal
- Moles or spots become painful
- Moles or spots begin itching

If you have a lot of freckles and moles, it's a good idea to see your dermatologist yearly or even more frequently, the way you go to the gynecologist. Dermatologists should photograph your skin in order to track any changes to the moles and freckles. In certain cases computerized imaging, called MoleMax, is used to follow suspicious freckles or moles.

If You Have a Suspicious Spot

If the dermatologist suspects skin cancer, you will probably have a biopsy to see if it is cancer and if so, what type. Usually the biopsy can be performed in the doctor's office with just a topical anesthetic. The tissue sample is sent to a laboratory for analysis.

If you have skin cancer, the treatment is determined by the type of cells and size of the affected area. If the tissue sample shows precancerous cells, topical mediation can be used. Usually if there is cancer, the area of the skin is removed. Another way to treat cancer, especially basal cell, is to cauterize (burn) it or freeze the cells with liquid nitrogen. Squamous cell cancer responds to radiation therapy.

Normal Skin Aging

Even if you haven't had a great deal of sun damage to your skin from years of sunbathing or outdoor activity without sun protection, your skin will still change. This is normal. As you get older, you are likely to begin to see fine wrinkles. Your skin will feel drier; you may begin to see brown spots and other places of irregular pigmentation. As your skin becomes thinner, you may see the superficial blood vessels that lie just under the surface of the skin.

Also, as we age, the skin becomes more fragile and more susceptible to trauma. We bruise more easily. And if you are on blood-thinning medication, as many women are, you may see black-and-blue marks erupt easily. Sometimes my patients call me thinking they have blood clots because they see marks that they don't understand, but these marks are typically bruises from trauma to the small blood vessels under the skin, and not a serious problem.

As elasticity decreases, from reduced elastin, the protection that it provides also decreases, so if you brush up against a piece of furniture, you can break a blood vessel and get a bruise. Further, since sensitivity of the skin also decreases with age, you may not even notice the pain sensation of having injured yourself. Along these same lines, we don't heal as easily from wounds as we used to. Therefore recovery after surgery takes longer.

Smoking, which damages the body in all kinds of ways, also damages the skin. The more you smoke, the worse your skin will look. Smoking decreases the blood supply to the skin, increasing the appearance of superficial blood vessels. Also, smoking accelerates the development of fine lines around the lips, another sign of aging. There is some evidence that women who take HT have greater protection against skin aging than those who don't—unless they smoke.[2] If you smoke, you have three times the number of moderate to severe wrinkles compared to women who don't smoke, hormone therapy or not.

DEALING WITH WRINKLES

Believe it or not, men and women have the same wrinkling rate at any age. Maybe women talk about it more, or men don't mind it as much. But most of the women I know are not happy to see their faces aging. Wrinkles happen because as we get older our skin's fat layer thins out and the elasticity of our skin decreases. Frown lines between eyebrows and crows' feet appear because of chronic muscle contractions. That's why your mother told you to stop squinting. Gravity pushes down the facial skin and results in jowls and droopy eyelids. Sun exposure makes the situation worse, and smoking, air pollution, and rapid weight loss also contribute to this process.

If you don't feel ready for wrinkles, there are ways to treat them. The huge cosmetics industry spends zillions trying to help women camouflage aging skin and wrinkles. One of the most popular products is Retin-A, a prescription medication used for fine and coarse wrinkles, pigmented spots, and rough skin surfaces. It can be applied to face, legs, and body. For a couple of days after you first apply it, the skin surface can become red or rosy, and you can have itching and burning. If these symptoms are severe, you can treat them with a steroid cream. It takes two to six months of use to show improvement. Low-dose Retin-A may be less effective, but you will have less irritation. If you use this product, you need to wear sunscreen because it makes your skin more sensitive to the sun. Don't use Retin-A if you are pregnant because there is a risk of birth defects.

Many skin care products that are available over the counter contain retinol, which is a natural form of vitamin A. It claims to provide some of the skin benefits of Retin-A without the irritation. These products are not regulated by the FDA, so there is no standardization.

Wrinkle creams camouflage wrinkles temporarily by hydrating the skin. Under-eye creams reduce the appearance of wrinkles by constricting blood vessels under the skin and leaving a thin film on top of the skin. Yellow correcting creams reduce the appearance of dark circles under the eyes. It's better to use a light foundation rather than a heavy one if you have wrinkles; if you use a lot of makeup, it just makes the wrinkles more noticeable. Facial powder reflects light and makes wrinkles appear less prominent.

TOPICAL SKIN PRODUCTS WITH ANTIOXIDANTS

Many products claim to reduce the appearance of wrinkles and help heal sun damage to the skin. There are very few scientific studies to support these claims, but using them probably can't hurt. These products contain:

- Vitamin E
- Green and black tea extracts
- Coenzyme Q_{10}
- Vitamin C (there is some evidence that products with vitamin C reduce the appearance of wrinkles but may increase the potential for sun damage to the skin)

ALPHA HYDROXY PREPARATIONS

Alpha hydroxy acids (AHAs) remove dead skin cells and may boost the production of collagen and elastin. Over-the-counter products that contain AHAs have a concentration of between 2 and 10 percent. Stronger concentrations require a doctor's prescription and usually contain 12 percent AHAs.

Light chemical peels using AHAs, also called glycolic peels, are usually performed in the doctor's office. Even though many women buy these products on the Internet, if you are interested I would recommend that you see a dermatologist because there is a potential for skin irritation, infection, and sores. Chemical peels remove the top layer of the skin and promote new skin growth, reducing wrinkles, skin discoloration, and skin blemishes. Depending on the concentration (another reason to do this in the dermatologist's office, so you are sure of what you are getting), the skin will redden or scab. It usually heals in a week. Skin will be highly sun-sensitive, so don't get this done before a trip to the beach and wear sunscreen when you go out.

DERMABRASION

Dermabrasion is used to remove more of the top layers of skin, improving the appearance of deep wrinkles and deep skin scars secondary to acne. There are two types. Standard dermabrasion uses rotating brushes to remove surface skin. Since the deep skin layers are exposed, there is oozing, and a temporary scab forms. Microdermabrasion uses tiny crystals to polish the skin and a vacuum to remove them. This type of dermabrasion is more common and can be done over a lunch hour. The skin becomes slightly red. Most people spread out five or six procedures at two-week intervals.

LASER THERAPY

Another option for wrinkle removal is laser therapy, which uses a high-energy beam of light to remove the top layer of skin. This procedure should be done by specially trained dermatologists and plastic surgeons. Again, because the new skin is highly vulnerable to sun damage, make sure you wear sunscreen for months after the procedure. Many women use laser therapy to remove the appearance of wrinkles around the mouth and eyes. Newer lasers are used for dark circles under the eyes.

ADULT ACNE

Acne occurs when the oil-producing glands of the skin become clogged, promoting the growth of bacteria. The body responds by trying to kill off the bacteria with inflammatory substances that also produce swelling and redness, along with whiteheads, blackheads, and pustules. Acne triggers are stress, health conditions associated with increased testosterone such as polycystic ovary syndrome, and hormonal fluctuations. Although routine hormone testing for acne is not necessary, if the acne is associated with irregular menstrual periods, infertility, and increased hair growth or hair loss, I recommend hormone testing because in this situation the acne may be a sign of an underlying hormone problem.

Acne is not a problem reserved for teenagers alone. Many women develop adult acne. I did. As a teenager I was lucky and rarely had pimples. Yet when I was thirty-five, I developed acne—big painful red pimples. I tried to use heavy makeup for a cover-up and bought various over-the-counter acne medications, but nothing helped. When I was prescribed Retin-A by a physician, I was surprised to learn that it wasn't covered by my insurance plan because in my age group it was used for wrinkles, not acne. I told the pharmacist to look at my face; I had serious acne and very few wrinkles. I got the prescription covered, but I turned out to be allergic to it.

> **DO CERTAIN FOODS CAUSE ACNE?**
>
> Growing up, my friends used to say that eating a lot of chocolate or fried foods made their acne worse. Although my acne got better when I cut back on caffeine, there is no research that has shown a link between specific foods and acne. However, if you think a food is precipitating your acne, stop eating it and see if the situation improves.

Then I went to a dermatologist who prescribed the antibiotic minocycline. However, I guess he looked only at my skin, not at my size, because he gave me too large a dose. I didn't realize that initially, but after taking the medication, I felt light-headed and asked a nurse to take my blood pressure. She was shocked when my blood pressure was very low: 70/50. She got me a chair and gave me some water. I stopped the medication. Finally I went to my current dermatologist, who talked to me and told me to decaffeinate myself, that changing my coffee habit might help. At that time I was drinking a lot of diet cola and coffee. When I told my husband of this recommendation, he said he couldn't imagine what I would be like unplugged. Because my acne was so bad and I had been through a variety of therapies already, the doctor also advised me to use Cetaphil, a mild facial cleanser, on my skin, and she scheduled a follow-up for glycolic acid peels. I had several treatments, and they improved my acne. I guess the moral of this story is that you shouldn't give up. If one treatment doesn't work, there may be another that will.

There are some things you can do if you find yourself in the midst of an acne flare-up as an adult.

- Listen to what your mother told you as a child: don't squeeze your pimples. If you do, you just worsen the inflammation and spread the infection. She was also right when she told you to stop touching your face and to pull your hair back off your face. Having less oil on the face helps.

- Use a mild soap such as Cetaphil or Dove to clean your face.

- In addition to Retin-A and retinol, there are other medications that help stop inflammation and infection. Benzoyl peroxide kills bacteria and is found in over-the-counter acne medications. Antibiotics such as clindamycin and erythromycin are prescribed to treat the infection.

- If the acne is not responsive to topical medications, sometimes oral antibiotics are prescribed. The most effective are doxycycline and minocycline. The downside of the antibiotics is that the bacteria causing the acne may become resistant with repeated use. These antibiotics also cause sensitivity to the sun, so use sunscreen.

- Accutane (isotretinoin) is an oral medication used for severe and resistant acne. You must be on birth control to use this medication because it is associated with severe birth defects if you take it during pregnancy. Remember, you are considered to be of childbearing potential unless you have had a total hysterectomy (see page 79) or are one year past menopause (see Chapter 5). The medication can also cause depression and mood changes.

- If the acne is caused by hormonal imbalance, another option is oral contraceptives. Spironolactone, a medication that blocks testosterone production, can improve acne related to hormone imbalance. (This medication is also a diuretic used to treat heart failure.)

- Chemical peels have not yet been shown by research studies to be successful for the treatment of acne, but it worked for me. However, they are not covered by insurance, as antibiotics usually are.

- Many people believe that herbal remedies are successful in treating acne. But only one, tea tree oil, has been studied. Although the research found that it was successful for acne, it took longer to work than the other topical medications.

ACNE ROSACEA

A fifty-year-old friend of mine told me she was most upset when she started to see redness and acne-like bumps on her nose and forehead. Also, she was alarmed that she could see blood vessels right under the skin. She had no idea what had happened to her. She didn't think it was acne, and imagined that it was something weird, like she had walked into poison ivy or been bitten by an exotic spider. But no. This common condition is called acne rosacea and occurs in fair-skinned women between the ages of thirty and fifty.

The causes of rosacea are unknown, but stress, anxiety, or strong emotions (fear, embarrassment) can bring it on. If you have rosacea, don't use over-the-counter acne medication, as it can make the condition worse by irritating the skin. See your doctor. Treatment is oral antibiotics, such as tetracycline, and antibiotic creams. Sometimes cortisone (steroid) creams are also used. For very severe cases Accutane might be prescribed. The condition gets worse if you rub your face or get too much sun.

HAIR LOSS

Another friend called to tell me that she had been losing clumps of her hair for the past month. She said she was afraid to comb her hair. We all shed some hair as our hair follicles go through the different stages of the hair growth cycle, but her hair was falling out at an unnatural rate. Typically women's hair gets thin around the front, crown, or sides, but she said her hair loss was certainly not normal.

She had been to see two dermatologists; one thought it was a symptom of menopause, and the other suspected it might be related to stress. One doctor gave her a prescription for spironolactone, a medication that decreases testosterone production and can be used to treat hair loss. She was also given a prescription for Rogaine, a medication that is used to treat hair loss in both men and women.

I was a little concerned because I knew she was taking a blood pressure medication that could increase her potassium. If she was going to be taking spironolactone, which is a diuretic that increases potassium, her potassium levels had to be watched carefully. I assumed the doctor who prescribed it was following up, and I was absolutely shocked to learn that he had not even asked about her other medications and so wasn't even aware that she was on blood pressure medication.

Not asking about her medications was definitely not good medical care. Hair loss can be a side effect of several medications: beta-blockers, certain antidepressants, cholesterol medications, or ACE inhibitors (see page 189). Chemotherapy can also result in hair loss. Birth control pills and too much vitamin A can cause hair loss as well.

I asked her if either of the doctors had done any blood work. After medications, there are other reasons for hair loss that can be determined through blood tests—for example, an overactive thyroid or increased testosterone levels. Hormonal changes associated with menopause and pregnancy can also have an impact on hair. I would have tested her blood for lupus and diabetes, conditions that may cause hair loss.

Other possible causes of hair loss include stress, either emotional or physical. Some people experience hair loss after surgery; one of my patients started to lose her hair after her heart attack, but happily the excessive shedding stopped several weeks later, after she got back to her life.

I asked her if she changed her diet, because low-protein diets can cause hair loss.

Some women lose their hair due to their hairdos. If you wear tight rollers or cornrows, the traction on the hair causes hair loss. Hair chemicals or hot oil treatments may cause hair to fall out. Burns to the scalp from hot combs and hair dryers can also make a difference.

There is another form of hair loss, called alopecia areata, where the hair falls out from a particular location, usually a small area of the scalp, for unknown reasons. Usually it grows back again.

Another cause could be infection, especially fungal infections of the scalp. I asked if either of the doctors had taken a culture to test her scalp for infection, and she said no. It really was terrible that my friend had been given medications for hair loss without any investigation as to the underlying cause. This is certainly not what they taught us in medical school.

I told her to come to my office the next morning, and I did blood tests. I changed her blood pressure and cholesterol medications to see if the hair loss would improve. All of her lab work came back normal. Her hair loss improved after she changed medications.

HAIR DYES

Does hair dye cause cancer? People ask me this question all the time. About 33 percent of women and 10 percent of men worldwide use hair dyes. From time to time there are reports in the news that link hair dyes to certain forms of cancer. In 2005, researchers analyzed seventy-nine studies done over a twenty-year period that evaluated a potential link between cancer and the use of hair dye. The analysis revealed that there was no increase in breast or bladder cancer but there was a slight increase in blood cancers. The bottom line is that there is not a strong link between hair dyes and cancer.[3] Allergic reactions are more common than cancers.

Many women are also suspicious of using hair dyes when they are pregnant, although there are no studies that link hair dye and birth defects.

GOOD NAIL HEALTH

Our finger- and toenails are part of our bodies and require good health habits, just as other parts do. It's easy to overlook our nails, especially if they are covered with nail polish. But without polish, you can see changes in color to the nail that might indicate an infection. You should also examine your nails and the surrounding skin for allergy, trauma, and signs of disease.

There can be several reasons for nail color changes. For example, certain medications can affect nail color. Blood thinners can cause hemorrhaging under the nails. Chemotherapy makes nails more fragile and can increase pigmentation.

In addition to using nail polish, we further weaken our nails by exposing them to detergents and other harsh chemicals. Getting a manicure sets us up for infections. Cutting and buffing the cuticle can destroy a natural barrier and leave us vulnerable to bacterial, viral, and fungal infections. Acrylic nails with their associated chemicals are a source of bacterial infections; nail polish remover can dry our nails, making them more brittle, and can also cause allergic reactions. B vitamins may help to protect us against brittle nails.

Signs of nail infection include:

- Pain and swelling of the finger

- Pus released from the side of the fingernail

- Thickening and yellowing of the nail

Treatment of the infection is based on the type of infection. Bacterial infections are treated with antibiotics; fungal infections are treated with either topical or oral medications. The oral medications may be given for several weeks or months. You can also prevent infections by bringing your own instruments for your manicures and pedicures.

PART III

The Three Keys
to Four-Star Health

SIXTEEN

The Woman's Healthy-Eating Plan

EVERYONE HAS HEARD A ZILLION TIMES THAT IT IS IMPORTANT TO eat a balanced diet, but what exactly does that mean? It means eating from different food groups—carbohydrates (breads, grains, cereal), fruits and vegetables, proteins (meat, fish, eggs), dairy, fats and sugars—and making intelligent choices about what you eat and how much to eat from each food group. You have heard that certain foods are better for you than others, that, for example, whole grains have more nutritional value than processed grains, that there are good fats and bad fats, that lean meat is better for you than meat with a high fat content, that complex carbohydrates are better than simple carbs. In this chapter, I'll explain what all that means.

If you eat well, you reduce your risk for many diseases. And if you do not have excess pounds on you, you also reduce your risk for developing many health problems. Also, as we get older, we begin to have more physical problems than we did when we were young. Many of these conditions, such as high blood pressure, diabetes, acid reflux and other digestive problems, and heart disease, are affected by diet. It really pays to eat right. You'll feel better and look better and live longer. It's hard to argue with that! In this chapter, I'll talk about eating for health and to lose excess weight, because both contribute to good health.

A GOOD DIET FOR LIFE

There is a great deal of research that supports the advantages of adopting a healthier way of eating. The Nurses' Health Study, a study of eighty-four thousand women, showed that women who ate 5 percent more saturated fat had a 17 percent increased risk of heart attack than those who ate less fat.[1] It also showed that those women who ate at least five servings of vegetables per day had a 25 percent lower risk of heart attack and stroke. The conclusion seems obvious: eat less meat and more vegetables.

The normal American diet of high-fat, salty, processed meats and saturated fats is a prescription for health problems. I am a great fan of the Mediterranean-style diet, which highlights the whole grains, vegetables, and fish eaten in countries on the Mediterranean, such as Italy and Greece. Although the countries have different cuisines, they do share some characteristics: lots of fruits, vegetables, grains, and nuts; the use of olive oil as a primary fat source; moderate amounts of fish and poultry; very little red meat; and moderate amounts of wine accompanying the meal. Although the Mediterranean diet is not a weight-loss diet, it is healthy, and by monitoring calories it can also be used to lose weight.

> **HEALTH PROBLEMS ASSOCIATED WITH BEING OVERWEIGHT**
>
> - Acid reflux
> - Breast cancer
> - Colon cancer
> - Diabetes
> - Endometrial cancer
> - Heart disease
> - High blood pressure
> - Joint problems
> - Shorter life span
> - Sleep apnea
> - Stroke

A study published in 1999 showed that men and women who followed a Mediterranean diet had a 70 percent improvement in survival rates after a heart attack.[2] The telling point of why I think this eating plan has staying power was that 95 percent of the people who started in the study said after 5 years that the diet was not only lifesaving but also tasty. This eating plan is excellent for people with heart disease, but it is also easy to live with and good for everyone. You can eat well, enjoy what you eat, and take care of your health all at the same time.

HEALTHY DIET RECOMMENDATIONS

HOW TO EAT

Slow down! When you eat on the run, not only do you tend to ignore portion sizes, but you can eat so fast that you don't give your brain enough time to realize that you've had enough to eat. There are several scientific studies showing that women who take more time to eat their meals consume fewer calories.[3,4] Also, there is evidence that the famously slim French generally consume fewer calories than Americans because they spend more time eating than Americans do.[5] So quit multitasking while you eat. Also, TV is bad for your diet. If you eat while watching TV, studies show that you will consume more calories and therefore gain weight.[6]

Eat smaller portions. Portions have been supersized over the last twenty years. Americans eat huge amounts of food compared to people from other countries. You'll find that if you reduce the portion size, you can eat what you want and not feel deprived, and yet you will lose weight. If you want a rule of thumb, or rather a rule of hand, use your palm to determine portion size. The palm of your hand is approximately the size of a three-ounce portion of meat, equal to one serving. I bet you have been having multiples of that, thinking you were eating one portion.

WHAT TO EAT

Eat fruits and vegetables. The Harvard School of Public Health recommends five to thirteen servings of fruit and vegetables daily, which translates into about five cups. If you are taking in about 2,000 calories a day, you should have about nine servings.

Whole grains are good sources of fiber and contain vitamins and other nutrients that are good for your heart, blood pressure, and general health. Whole grains include whole wheat, oatmeal, wild rice, brown rice, and bulgur. You can choose whole-grain bread over breads made with refined flour, and whole-wheat pasta and brown rice rather than regular or white. Oatmeal is better than sweetened cereals. You should try to have about three ounces of whole grains a day—that would be one slice of bread, one cup of cereal, and a half cup of pasta.

WHAT DOES THE "WHOLE" IN WHOLE GRAINS MEAN?

Everyone talks about whole grains, but how many of us understand what it means? Grains such as wheat, oats, and barley are composed of bran (the outer layer), the germ (the layer directly under the bran), and the endosperm (the inner part of the grain). As grains are processed and refined, the bran and germ are removed, taking the grain's fiber, vitamins, minerals, and antioxidants along with them. Whole grains are minimally processed and so have greater nutritional value because they retain all the parts of the grain.

You want your fats to come from polyunsaturated and monounsaturated sources, rather than trans fats or saturated fats (read the labels). Foods with good fats are fish and nuts; oils to choose include soybean, corn, canola, olive, and other vegetable oils.

Eat fish, especially oily fish such as sardines, mackerel, and salmon, because they are rich in omega-3 acids.

Eat chicken and turkey (no skin).

Eat low-fat dairy products such as skim milk, low-fat yogurt, and low-fat cheeses. You want to avoid the saturated fat, cholesterol, and calories in many whole-milk dairy products. Eating two to three servings a day of low-fat dairy will provide you with the health benefits of dairy, such as protein and calcium.

WHAT TO AVOID

White refined flour is typically found in white breads and cakes. White flour is a high-glycemic-index carbohydrate (see page 358), which means that its sugars break down quickly, causing more insulin to be released than needed, and resulting in the storage of fats.

Sugar is to be avoided if you want to maintain a healthy weight and a healthy diet. But it's not just the stuff in the sugar bowl (sucrose) that needs to be limited. There is sugar in fruit products (fructose), and in milk products (lactose), and of course in maple syrup, honey, molasses, and many other foods.

Limit red meat to no more than three ounces a week. Use leaner cuts, such as flank steak or sirloin.

Limit butter and cream. Olive oil and canola oil are better.

Limit alcohol intake to no more than one drink a day (a five-ounce glass of wine, twelve ounces of beer, or one and a half ounces of 80-proof alcohol). More than this amount of alcohol daily is associated with high blood pressure and increased risk of heart disease. Heavy alcohol intake is associated with a higher risk of breast cancer.

> **TRANS FATS**
>
> There is a great deal of media attention nowadays on the dangers of eating trans-fatty acids (a staple of fast food and packaged baked goods) because they raise LDL (bad) cholesterol, lower HDL (good) cholesterol, increase triglycerides, and raise the risk of type 2 diabetes, all associated with an increased risk of heart disease.[7]

ABOUT CAFFEINE

Caffeine is a stimulant, which is why you feel wide awake, are more alert, and concentrate better after drinking your morning coffee. Caffeine also improves muscle function. But there is a difference between being alert and being overstimulated, mentally and physically. If you have too much caffeine, your heart rate will increase, the acid produced in the stomach will increase, and the kidneys will increase urine production. You can wind up feeling anxious and jittery, with muscle twitches, dehydration, uncomfortable acid reflux, and palpitations.

You know you've had too much caffeine when you have:

- Palpitations
- Difficulty sleeping
- Dizziness
- Diarrhea

- Nausea

- Stomachache

- Acid taste in your mouth

- Dry mouth from dehydration

Most people know that colas, coffees, and teas contain caffeine. So if you need to cut back, of course start limiting the amount of caffeinated beverages you drink. But there are other sources of caffeine as well, such as over-the-counter headache medications and medications for menstrual cramps. Medications such as No-Doz also contain caffeine; the idea is to keep you awake. Over-the-counter decongestants contain stimulants such as pseudoephedrine and phenylephedrine. Energy drinks such as Red Bull contain caffeine. I recommend that you should not have more than 500 mg per day of caffeine from all sources.

Pregnant women should have no more than 300 mg of caffeine daily because high caffeine intake has been associated with miscarriage. That's about two cups of coffee.

WINNING THE BATTLE OF THE BULGE

Most of the women I know diet because they want to look thin, not because they want to be healthy. Even when I explain that being ten pounds overweight can result in significant harm, raising your blood pressure and cholesterol and putting you at increased risk for diabetes and other chronic diseases, it doesn't make an impression. The good news here is that if you lose weight, your health improves. We should all diet to preserve our lives, not for our vanity.

My friends wage a daily battle with their appetites and the scale. Guess which wins? Diets don't really work unless the diet is a lifestyle change, a way of eating that feels normal, not like deprivation. In a study of commercially available diets, researchers found that very-low-calorie commercial weight loss programs result in a 15–25 percent weight loss from baseline, although the first few pounds are from water loss. Sounds good, right? Wrong. The study also found that the participants gained back more than 50 percent of their weight loss within one to two years. You might also be surprised to learn that the average weight loss from these programs is only between three and five pounds.[8]

A recent study comparing the Atkins, Zone, LEARN, and Ornish diets showed that overweight and obese premenopausal women lost the most weight on the lowest-carbohydrate (Atkins) diet, five pounds, as compared with those on the other diets, who lost two to three pounds over the course of a year.[9] One of my patients called me after she heard about this study on the evening news and told me delightedly that she was running right out to have a bacon cheeseburger. No one knows what the long-term health effects are of such a high-protein, high-fat diet, although there have been suggestions that it could increase the risk for kidney stones and raise cholesterol levels.

One of my patients has tried everything to lose weight: personalized nutritional counseling, Weight Watchers, Jenny Craig, Optifast, and most recently a cookie diet. Knowing how I feel about diets, she was reluctant to share this information with me, but she did bring me the cookie package, which showed that the cookies contained fats, proteins, and carbohydrates. She was also drinking an eight-ounce glass of water with each cookie and eating only one real meal per day. I was worried that desperate as she was, she could become vitamin-deficient or anemic. Even if I sometimes have the impulse, I never yell at my patients. I try to work with them. I checked her blood for anemia and potential vitamin deficiencies and made a deal with her that if I found she was endangering her health, she would go off this diet.

Most medical professionals believe that there has to be a balance of nutrients, including carbohydrates, to maintain good health. Therefore, eating wisely and exercising regularly is a better idea for weight loss—and for general good health. Instead of a diet, I want you to think about an eating plan for a healthier life, one that makes you aware of what and how much you are eating.

More than dieting, the issue is getting started and sticking to a healthy eating regimen. I realize that healthy eating (and cooking) may not be easy to fit into your lifestyle. Not everyone can be like my mother, who worked all day and still managed to cook the family healthy dinners every night. Women today are balancing so much and working such demanding jobs that they find themselves working throughout lunch. In the evening fast foods seem convenient. Unfortunately they are not healthy and in fact are fattening as well. Since middle-aged women have a tendency to put on weight and keep it on, the extra pounds sit there.

It's a balance between calories in and calories out. If more come in than go out, you gain weight. If more go out than come in, you lose weight. It is not exactly rocket science that if you eat great gobs of high-calorie foods, you will gain weight. And if you don't exercise and eat great gobs of high-calorie foods or even healthy foods, you'll gain more weight. Similarly, if you work out vigorously several days a week, you may need to take in more calories to sustain a healthy weight.

I have a few friends who are very thin, and that's because they don't eat. They are not taking good care of their bodies, although they may think they are. If you live on diet sodas and not much else, your body will rebel and you'll develop health problems. You want to eat in a way that is satisfying and will keep you healthy and energized. You know perfectly well what a healthy diet consists of. We all do. You need to balance all the food groups and have protein, healthy carbohydrates, and fats in moderation. Yet the battle of the bulge continues.

THERE IS NO MAGIC PILL

Many of my patients think they can take pills to lower their cholesterol or their blood pressure and then eat whatever they want. Consequently I find myself raising the dose of their medications to combat their poor eating habits. The higher the drug dose, the more likely it is that my patients will have side effects. If there is a way to keep yourself healthy and on less rather than more medication, that is a good idea. You need to combine medication with a healthy eating program. It is not one or the other; it is both diet and medication.

Again, weight is about balancing calories in and calories out. You need a certain number of calories to live and be healthy. But if you take in more than you need, those calories go directly onto your hips, your waist, or wherever you least want to see fat accumulating. Therefore, if you want to lose weight, take in fewer calories or exercise more to burn more calories. Calorie recommendations depend on your age, height, weight, activity level, and metabolism. A moderately active woman needs between 1,600 and 2,000 calories a day to maintain weight and 1,200–1,500 calories daily to lose weight.

The more you move, the more calories you use. And I am not talking about going to the gym every day (although that's a great idea if you can do it). You can walk rather than ride, and you can use the stairs rather than an elevator. If it sounds as if I am lobbying against being a couch potato, I am! Also set reasonable goals for yourself. I know that sometimes losing weight can feel overwhelming. I had to help my patient Gwen set reasonable goals. She was fifty pounds overweight, and she said, "How will I ever lose even thirty pounds?" I told her to start with ten pounds at a time, and to give up wishing for a quick fix.

How Do You Know If You Need to Lose Weight?

Being overweight puts you at an increased risk for many medical problems, including diabetes and heart disease. Therefore, you want to know if you are overweight and should lose weight. The body mass index (BMI) is a better predictor of health than simply your weight in pounds or kilograms. Those charts that we all grew up with that matched height and weight have been replaced by the BMI index. It involves a calculation of your body weight in kilograms divided by the square of your height in meters. (Don't panic—see the chart below.) The resulting number reflects information about your body fat, with higher numbers showing higher risk for health problems.

Of course this is not an exact science, only an indicator. There are some obvious drawbacks. For example, the BMI does not distinguish between men and women. Generally, women have more body fat than men who have the same BMI, and older people have more fat than younger ones. Athletes may have a high BMI because of muscle weight rather than fatness.

BMI	Weight Status
Below 18.5	Underweight
18.5–24.9	Normal
25.0–29.9	Overweight
30.0 and above	Obese

BMI	19	20	21	22	23	24	25	26	27	28	29	30	31	32	33	34	35
Height (inches)							**Body Weight (pounds)**										
			Normal Range						Overweight						Obese		
58	91	96	100	105	110	115	119	124	129	134	138	143	148	153	158	162	167
59	94	99	104	109	114	119	124	128	133	138	143	148	153	158	163	168	173
60	97	102	107	112	118	123	128	133	138	143	148	153	158	163	168	174	179
61	100	106	111	116	122	129	132	137	143	148	153	158	164	169	174	180	185
62	104	109	115	120	126	131	136	142	147	153	158	164	169	175	180	186	191
63	107	113	118	124	130	135	141	146	152	158	163	169	175	180	186	191	197
64	110	116	122	128	134	140	145	151	157	163	169	174	180	186	192	197	204
65	114	120	126	132	138	144	150	156	162	168	174	180	186	192	198	204	210
66	118	124	130	136	142	148	155	161	167	173	179	186	192	198	204	210	216
67	121	127	134	140	146	153	159	166	172	178	185	191	198	204	211	217	223
68	125	131	138	144	151	158	164	171	177	184	190	197	203	210	216	223	230
69	128	135	142	149	155	162	169	176	182	189	196	203	209	216	223	230	236
70	132	139	146	153	160	167	174	181	188	195	202	209	216	222	229	236	243
71	136	143	150	157	165	172	179	186	193	200	208	215	222	229	236	243	250
72	140	147	154	162	169	177	184	191	199	206	213	221	228	235	242	250	258
73	144	151	159	166	174	182	189	197	204	212	219	227	235	242	250	257	265
74	148	155	163	171	179	186	194	202	210	218	225	233	241	249	256	264	272
75	152	160	168	176	184	192	200	208	216	224	232	240	248	256	264	272	279
76	156	164	172	180	189	197	205	213	221	230	238	246	254	263	271	279	287

One of the advantages of an electronic medical records system is that I can track my patients' BMI at every visit. Recently my patient Ilana came in for a follow-up visit. After six months of a dedicated diet and exercise program for weight loss, she'd gone from a BMI of 27 to 24. She went from overweight to normal, and by doing this she also lowered her risk from heart disease, heart attack, and stroke by 30 percent. Not to mention the thrill of a new dress size.

People store their body fat in different places. We have all seen women who seem to be very thick around the middle, with thin arms and legs, and others who seem to be very slim above the waist and have a lot of weight in the butt, hips, and thighs. Where you store your fat is also correlated to health, with apple-shaped women (weight stored around the middle) at greater risk for heart disease and diabetes than pear-shaped women.

Your waist-to-hip ratio reflects where you store your body fat and if you are at increased health risk. To calculate what your ratio is, put a tape measure around your waist at the level of your belly button. Then measure around your hips and divide your waist measurement by your hip measurement. Ideally you want the ratio to be under 0.8.

Women	Health Risk	Body Shape
0.8 or below	Low	Pear
0.81–0.85	Moderate	Avocado
0.85 and above	High	Apple

If your waist-to-hip ratio is more than 0.8, you are apple-shaped, and you should diet and exercise to try and get the weight off your middle. It takes work, though, because where you store your fat is genetically determined. However, if you do regular cardiovascular exercise and lose weight, you'll slim down all over and reduce your health risks.

How Much Weight Should You Lose?

Here's an example that may help you figure out how many calories to take in if you want to lose weight. If you weigh 150 pounds and you would like to weigh 140, 10 pounds less, then multiply 140 by 10, for 1,400. That's the number of calories you should take in daily in order to attain the weight loss. Of course, if you exercise a great deal, you can and should take in more calories. Generally, in order to lose one to two pounds per week, you need to reduce your caloric intake by 500–1,000 calories per week.

My patient Carla needed and wanted to lose weight. She would start a diet and lose a few pounds, but then she would feel so restricted by her low-calorie diet that she would start eating more, eventually gaining back more than she lost. I referred her to a certified dietician who recommended an eating plan that gave her choices (see page 339). Carla found the suggestions very helpful, particularly the snack suggestions, because having the three meals a day organized for her made food seem manageable. With the help of the dietician, she realized that her problem had been going four to five hours between meals without a snack, which left her starving. Now with the healthy snack suggestions, she is not hungry and stays within her calorie limits.

WHAT ABOUT LOW-FAT FOODS?

My advice is to count calories, not fat. Eating a diet low in fat is good for you, but if you are eating high-calorie foods, you won't take off weight. A diet of low-fat muffins and low-fat cookies will cause you to put on weight, not take it off. Check the labels so that you know how many calories you are eating.

Like Carla, some women need a great deal of structure to stick to a diet, but it has to be one that matches their lifestyle and their taste in food, in addition to their physical requirements. I recommend a consultation with a certified diet specialist. You usually don't need a great deal of advice, but some certainly helps.

HEALTH OR HYPE?

Every day there is a news story about a pleasurable food that can save your life. Don't believe it! Although it might sell newspapers, the wine-and-chocolate diet is a fantasy. Wait for science to establish the facts.

GREEN TEA

A long-term study of more than forty thousand green tea drinkers in Japan suggests that drinking five or more cups of green tea per day reduced the risk of cardiovascular death by 26 percent.[10] Before we know if this is true for American women, a similar research study would have to be done in the Unites States to confirm the protective role of green tea. These results seem promising, though, because of the large number of patients in the study. Be aware, however, that you can have too much of a good thing. Too much caffeine, even from tea, can cause palpitations and other problems (see page 341). Although green tea is lower in caffeine than black tea, you still need to be aware of your total caffeine intake. Remember that caffeine is a diuretic, so drinking iced tea is not a good way to hydrate. Drink water.

WALNUTS

Walnuts are good for your heart, according to a study reported in the *Journal of the American College of Cardiology*.[11] This small study of only four women and twenty men, sponsored by the California Walnut Board, showed that people who ate a high-fat meal (salami and cheese) followed by walnuts had less arterial inflammation and more flexible arteries than

DRUGS THAT CAUSE WEIGHT GAIN

Many of my patients don't realize what an uphill battle it is to lose weight or simply maintain their weight when they take certain medications. I always tell my patients when I prescribe something that may influence their weight. It doesn't seem fair not to warn them, although I know some doctors who never think of weight gain as a side effect of medication. But in my experience, some women become so frustrated with dieting and not losing weight that they stop taking their medication. If you stop without talking to your doctor, you might put yourself at risk medically, and a few pounds is not worth that. Never discontinue medication without discussing it with your doctor.

If you are on medication that causes weight gain, you may have to increase your exercise and decrease your calories just to maintain your weight. If you talk to your doctor, there may be options, such as lowering the dose (if that is safe for you) or choosing an alternative medication that doesn't cause weight gain. Communicate your concerns to your doctor. Common medications that are associated with weight gain include insulin, steroids, beta-blockers, SSRIs, and tricyclic antidepressants.

people who ate the same high-fat meal followed by bread soaked with olive oil. I still wouldn't recommend that you try this diet at home. This study, although publicized in a prestigious journal, is just preliminary work with very few participants. The participation of women was also very sparse. Walnuts have a favorable balance of good fats and alpha-linoleic acid; a handful makes a healthy snack, but be alert to their high calorie content.

SALT

Salt intake should be reduced to avoid hypertension, cardiovascular disease, and heart failure (see Chapter 8). Reducing salt intake is a first line of defense against these problems. The processed foods that we eat contain a tremendous amount of salt. Read the labels; you'll be shocked. Many health organizations, including the American Medical Association, recommend throwing out the salt shaker; they also want manufacturers to label the sodium content in foods and remove sodium from processed foods. The AMA is expected to recommend to the FDA that salt no longer be labeled as "safe." If that happens, then food manufacturers and processors would have to petition the FDA to approve salt as a food additive.

> ### DIET AND HEART DISEASE
>
> The way you live and the way you eat are associated with your risk for heart disease. A study involving more than eighty-four thousand women showed that women who didn't smoke, had a BMI under 25, engaged in a half hour a day of moderate exercise, and ate a diet high in fiber and low in trans fats had a very low risk of developing heart disease.[12]

A recent study published in the *Canadian Journal of Cardiology* concluded that if people cut their salt intake in half, from about 1½ tablespoons to ¾ tablespoon, more than a million people would not develop hypertension—and they believe that is a conservative estimate.[13]

FISH

The health benefits of eating fish have been confusing and controversial. There is the wild-versus-farmed debate, and the contaminants-versus-

HOW TO REDUCE YOUR SALT INTAKE

The first thing to do is to remove the salt shaker from the table. When you cook, don't prepare foods with salt. One of my patients is supposed to be on a salt-free diet and swears to me she never eats salt. She does, however, eat herring and salami and Chinese food! Avoid foods with salt, including condiments such as ketchup and soy sauce, which are particularly high in sodium. Read the labels for processed foods; they tend to be high in sodium. When you eat out, it's hard to control for salt because you are not involved in the food preparation. Try to order wisely. Even the best of plans can go awry, though. I remember going to a medical conference and was out to dinner with my colleagues. A few of them ordered steak. I ordered the salmon, theoretically a healthier choice. Unfortunately it was crusted with a layer of salt.

omega-3 debate. There is very little scientific evidence that either farmed or wild fish is better than the other from the nutritional or safety point of view (although some people think wild tastes better). However, the contaminant issue should be considered. For example, eating four or more portions of fish a week is good for your heart, with studies showing that modest fish intake decreases the rate of death from coronary heart disease by 25 percent. But the risk of mercury poisoning has made many people wary of exposure. It is difficult to know what to do.

Pregnant women, nursing women, and women of childbearing age are usually told to be cautious about eating fish. Recent reports indicate that eating more modest amounts—one or two servings a week—retains the health benefits and minimizes the risks. The Environmental Protection Agency says that these women should avoid swordfish, shark, bass, and mackerel and eat no more than six ounces of tuna a week.

Swordfish and shark are highest in mercury; oily fish, such as salmon, herring, and sardines are better than lean fish for lowering risk of heart disease. The best advice I can give you is to talk to your doctor and weigh the benefits of eating fish against the risks.

COCOA AND CHOCOLATE

Cocoa and chocolate contain flavonoids, an antioxidant compound known to have health benefits. Antioxidants help to protect cells against environmental contaminants (such as cigarette smoke) and help to reduce plaque in arteries. Flavonoids are also thought to increase blood vessel flexibility. They are found in such foods as cranberries, red wine, tea, peanuts, and chocolate. A recent study reported by the American Institute for Cancer Research compared single servings of cocoa, green tea, black tea, and red wine for health-promoting antioxidants. Cocoa scored higher than the others.

When my patients heard the news that there were health benefits to eating chocolate, they were delighted. However, there are a few things you should know. For example, not all chocolate has healthful properties. You want chocolate with a high cocoa content because the higher the cocoa content the more flavonoids there are; dark chocolate is higher in flavonoids and better for you than milk chocolate. White chocolate has no cocoa content at all. But don't start coating all your veggies with dark chocolate; chocolate is very high in calories. Fruits and vegetables are still your best bet if you want to eat foods with flavonoids.

BLUEBERRIES ARE GOOD FOR YOU

Blueberries are an excellent source of antioxidants. The substance responsible for the blue in blueberries, called anthocyanin, helps to reduce heart disease. Blueberries are also rich in fiber, iron, and vitamin C. The U.S. Department of Agriculture ranks blueberries as the number one antioxidant available through foods. Pomegranates are also a good source of antioxidants.

RESVERATROL

Many of my patients were as pleased as (red wine) punch when they heard that recent studies showed that resveratrol, a substance found in grapes, blueberries, peanuts, green tea, and some nuts, is good for your health. In fact, studies have shown that resveratrol can make obese mice live longer while reducing their risk of heart disease.[14] But the key word here is *mice*. There is no proof that resveratrol can help overweight or obese people live long and retain good health. Wouldn't it be nice if red wine turned out to be the elixir of youth? But for the moment, it's still all about diet and exercise. Sorry.

Antioxidants in Food Are Good for You

Antioxidants boost immunity and are generally good for you. They work by neutralizing unstable metabolic products called free radicals that can make cells vulnerable. Antioxidants also help to reduce oxidation of bad LDL cholesterol; oxidized LDL can increase the risk of heart attack. A diet rich in foods that contain antioxidants is good for your health. The American Heart Association has recommended that you get your antioxidants from foods rather than supplements because there is not enough scientific evidence available about supplements. Science does support a diet high in foods that have antioxidants. These foods include those with antioxidant vitamins:

- *Beta-carotene* is found in apricots, broccoli, cantaloupe, carrots, collard greens, kale, mango, peach, papaya, pumpkin, spinach, sweet potato, tomatoes, and winter squash.
- *Vitamin C* is found in blueberries, broccoli, cantaloupe, currants, grapefruit, kiwi, oranges, peppers, potatoes, strawberries, and tomatoes.
- *Vitamin E* is found in in whole grains, nuts, seeds, oils, dark green vegetables, avocado, and sweet potatoes.

Another antioxidant, lycopene, is found in tomatoes, where it's responsible for the red color. Cooked tomatoes are the best source for cancer-fighting lycopene because our bodies have difficulty extracting the lycopene from raw tomatoes. But include both in your diet because raw tomatoes have more vitamin C than cooked ones.

Foods with Vitamin B Are Good for Your Health

B vitamins, especially folic acid and vitamins B_6 and B_{12}, are good for your metabolism and for your heart. If you don't eat a diet rich in fruits, vegetables, and whole grains, you may not have sufficient folic acid or other B vitamins. Alcohol, coffee, and sugar, as well as oral contraceptives, smoking, and being a vegetarian, may cause you to be deficient in certain B vitamins as well.

Folic acid helps to lower homocysteine levels, which helps to reduce risk for stroke and heart disease (see page 299). A diet high in folic acid helps the arteries of the heart to dilate and therefore improves heart function—a good thing. Foods that are rich in folic acid include green leafy vegetables, beans, peas, peanuts, and citrus fruits.

Vitamin B_6 is important for the metabolism of carbohydrates, proteins, and lipids. If you don't have enough B_6, you could have elevated homocysteine levels and be at increased risk for blood clots. B_6 is also important for making the hemoglobin in red blood cells, and therefore a deficiency can lead to anemia. However, B_6 can be toxic if taken in large doses, causing nerve damage. It is difficult to overdose on B_6 from food; however, if you take it in the form of supplements, be aware of how much you are taking. You should not have more than 100 mg daily, according to the Institute of Medicine. Foods that are rich in B_6 are brown rice, peanuts, walnuts, soybeans, chicken, and fish.

B_{12} also lowers homocysteine levels and is good for the blood vessels. It is also necessary to maintain healthy nerve cells. Foods high in B_{12} are meat, fish, eggs, and milk. Vegetarians may take in insufficient amounts; a blood test will let you and your doctor know if supplements are necessary.

Niacin, another B vitamin (B_3), is good for your heart health, lowering your LDL (bad) cholesterol, raising your HDL (good) cholesterol, and lowering triglyceride and Lp(a) levels. Doctors prescribe niacin to promote good cholesterol, but like most cholesterol medications, it is metabolized in the liver, so your liver function should be checked regularly (see page 187). There may be side effects with niacin supplements, including nausea, diarrhea, headaches, flushing, and fatigue. Also, niacin has an impact on glycemic control, and so prediabetics and diabetics should not take it without discussing it with their doctor. Nor should people with gout.

GOOD FAT, BAD FAT

Not all fat is good for you, and not all fat is bad for you. It's important to understand the differences among fats so you can make wise choices for yourself. Good fats are monounsaturated fats, which are found in olive, canola, and peanut oils and avocados. Polyunsaturated fats are also good for you. These are found in nuts and fatty fish as well as safflower, sesame, sunflower, corn, and soybean oils. To keep cholesterol normal, the American Heart Association recommends using these fats rather than others.

Fatty fish, such as anchovies, Atlantic salmon, mackerel, sardines, tuna, and whitefish, are rich in omega-3 fatty acids, a good fat. Omega-3 fats have been shown to reduce triglycerides and lower blood pressure. For vegetarians, omega-3 fats can be found in soybeans, canola oil, nuts, and flaxseed.

It's no secret that trans fats are not good for you *at all*. Recently New York City adopted an ordinance requiring fast-food chains to change from trans fats to healthier ones. A diet high in trans-fatty acids can increase your risk of heart disease. Studies show that reducing your intake of trans fats can reduce the risk of heart disease.

In order to know what you are ingesting, you need to read the labels of the foods you buy. Hydrogenated or partially hydrogenated oils are high in trans fats. Avoid these foods. No more than 7 percent of your daily calories should be from saturated fats. These are found in red meat, cheese, cream, and coconut oil. Try to find foods made with monounsaturated or polyunsaturated fats.

IMPORTANT COMPONENTS FOR A HEALTHY WOMAN'S DIET

Fiber, especially as contained in fruits, vegetables, and grains, promotes heart and colon health. It's good for you. Fiber helps to lower cholesterol and blood pressure and relieves constipation. The NIH DASH (Dietary Approaches to Stop Hypertension) diet to lower blood pressure recommends seven to eight servings of grains a day and eight to ten servings of fruits and vegetables.

Fiber, which comes in soluble and insoluble forms, is not digested and therefore not absorbed by the body. Sometimes called "roughage," it is useful in maintaining healthy bowel habits, relieving constipation, and also helps to lower the risk of diabetes and heart disease. Soluble fiber turns into a gel; insoluble fiber moves through our intestines largely intact. Good sources of soluble fiber are grains such as oat bran and barley, flaxseed, nuts, dried beans, carrots, peas, and apples. Good sources of insoluble fiber include dark green leafy vegetables, fruit skins, whole wheat, seeds, and nuts.

The fiber in an average diet is about three-quarters insoluble and one-quarter soluble. But both are good and you shouldn't try and distinguish between them since many foods contain both. Five servings of fruits and vegetables and six servings of grains a day should achieve the recommended amount of 25 grams of fiber daily. And since fiber is not

UNDERSTANDING FOOD LABELS

Reading labels can be confusing. Often, in fact, I think they are designed to fool you. Manufacturers are trying to sell their products, not improve your health. That's up to you! When you see the labels, this is what it means:

If the label says . . .	It means that the product has . . .
Low-fat	Less than 3 grams of fat per serving
Low saturated fat	No more than 1 gram of saturated fat per serving
Reduced fat	At least 25 percent less fat per serving than the traditional product
Light	No more than 2 grams of fat or one-third the calories of the traditional product
Fat-free	2 grams of fat or less per serving

digestible, it helps to drink a lot of water when you eat fiber to help it pass through your digestive tract more easily.

Calcium is good for your bones and blood pressure (see Chapter 9). Dairy foods are a good source of calcium, but you want to remember to limit fats, so I recommend low-fat dairy products, which have the same amount of calcium as full-fat foods. Many of my patients are lactose-intolerant, which means they have trouble digesting dairy, and so I recommend other high-calcium foods, such as broccoli, sardines, tofu, mustard greens, and oranges. If they are still not getting enough calcium, I recommend calcium supplements (see Chapter 9).

Eliminate trans fats. You can easily spot foods containing trans fats if the label says "hydrogenated." If you see that, don't buy it. Trans fats raise LDL (bad) cholesterol and lower HDL (good) cholesterol—double whammy. A new law now requires food companies to label trans fats.

Reduce your intake of *saturated fat* to less than 7 percent of your daily calories. Saturated fats are found in meat, full-fat dairy products, lard, and butter.

Good fats are monounsaturated fats, such as in olive, peanut, and canola oils and avocados. They do not raise cholesterol. However, no more than 30 percent of your calories should come from fats.

Polyunsaturated fats also have health benefits and do not raise cholesterol; they are found in sunflower, corn, soybean, and sesame oils. Oils with the best balance of polyunsaturated and monounsaturated fats and also low in saturated fats include canola, corn, safflower, sunflower, flaxseed, olive, and soybean.

Omega-3 highly polyunsaturated fats are found in fatty fish, flaxseed, flaxseed oil, canola oil, soybean oil, and walnuts. Walnuts are high in alpha-linolenic acid. The U.S. Department of Agriculture recommends that women have a daily alpha-linolenic acid intake of 1.1 grams per day.

Choose low-fat protein alternatives, such as foods containing *soy*. Although soy has not been shown to reduce symptoms of menopause, it is a good low-fat protein alternative. Soy foods lower cholesterol and blood pressure.

Eat your antioxidants. A cup of tea (either green or black), a handful of almonds, and half a cup of broccoli will all provide you with the same amount of antioxidants. You can make choices based on your caloric intake for a given day.

Polyphenols, which are found in pomegranate juice, red wine, cranberry juice, and green tea, help prevent LDL cholesterol from oxidizing and potentially causing a heart attack. Since pomegranate juice has higher levels of these polyphenols than red wine or green tea, you don't need to increase your alcohol intake to have the health benefits of these important antioxidants.

Your *cholesterol* intake should be no more than 300 mg per day.

COMPLEX CARBOHYDRATES

Everyone needs carbohydrates in their diet because carbs provide the energy for the body and brain to work properly. Foods that contain carbohydrates are categorized as either simple or complex, depending on the number of sugars bonded together in the food; simple carbs have one or two sugars bonded together and complex carbs have more. Simple carbs are absorbed much more quickly than complex. Usually simple carbohydrates refer to sugar (table sugar, refined sugar, fruit sugars) and complex carohydrates to starches, such as whole-grain breads and cereals and starchy vegetables such as potatoes. Simple carbs have far less nutritional

---

THE GLYCEMIC INDEX

Let me tell you about the glycemic index. The glycemic index was developed as a research tool to show how quickly a carbohydrate triggers a rise in blood sugar. The higher the number, the faster the rise in sugar. There have been numerous research studies showing that diets with many foods high in the glycemic index are associated with greater weight gain. The glycemic load of a particular food is the amount of carbohydrate the food contains multiplied by the glycemic index of that food. An example is that whole fruit has a lower glycemic load than fruit juice. Women who ingested prepregnancy diets with a high glycemic load had a greater risk of gestational diabetes when pregnant. And even if you are not planning to be pregnant, a diet with low-glycemic-load foods is better for weight loss, triglycerides levels, blood pressure, and diabetes.

The chart below shows the glycemic loads of common foods.

GLYCEMIC LOAD OF COMMON FOODS

Food	Amount of Carbohydrates (gm)	Glycemic Index	Glycemic Load
Potato (1 baked)	37	1.21	45
White rice (½ cup)	35	0.81	28
White bread (2 slices)	24	1.00	22
Whole-wheat bread (2 slices)	24	0.64	15
Pasta, cooked (1 cup)	40	0.71	28
Popcorn, air popped (1 cup)	5	0.79	4
Lentils, cooked (½ cup)	20	0.60	16
Cornflakes (1 cup)	22	1.19	31
100% bran (1 cup)	24	0.60	14
Carrots, cooked (½ cup)	20	1.31	10

value than complex ones and also lead to weight gain. That is why low-carbohydrate diets are successful. But even those diets (for example, the South Beach diet) recommends complex carbohydrates. The NIH recommends that 40 to 60 percent of a person's daily caloric intake be from carbs. To be healthy and not gain weight, eat complex carbs, which are found in fruits and vegetables, whole grains, and legumes.

The bottom line on healthy eating for women is to keep it simple. Get over thinking that dietary supplements are going to save your life, and start a healthy eating plan by choosing good nutrients from all food groups. Also, remember that weight is about calories in and calories out. So either eat less or exercise more if you want to lose weight.

YOUR HEALTHY-EATING PLAN—FOR LIFE!

- Count calories.
- Eat slowly.
- Choose healthy fats.
- Choose low-glycemic-load carbs.
- Eat your antioxidants in their natural form as food.
- Throw out the salt shaker.

SEVENTEEN

You Really Do Need to Sleep

MANY OF THE WOMEN I SEE EACH DAY ARE IN A RUSH, FEELING pressured to fit extra hours into the day in order to manage their complicated lives. They hardly have any time to take care of themselves, being so busy taking care of others. Not surprisingly, many of these women report having trouble sleeping.

Most parents of small children can gauge very accurately the kind of day their child will have because it is so dependent on the kind of night's sleep the child has had. Disrupted or insufficient sleep leads to cranky children. Disrupted or insufficient sleep leads to more injuries and sicknesses. It's obvious that children *need* to sleep. It's less obvious, but nonetheless true, that adults need to sleep too. I remember all too well the sleep deprivation I experienced during my internship and residency. I always felt tired and had countless sore throats. My friend Mia, who is now an infectious disease specialist, used to tell me that once I finished my residency and could get more sleep, I would have fewer sore throats. She was right.

Although most of us have learned how to mask our crankiness better than the average four-year-old, it doesn't mean we don't need a good night's sleep to get through our day. Sleep is not just a time when you shut off and shut down. It is physiologically necessary to your well-being. In addition to feeling rested and energized, studies now suggest that sleep is necessary for retaining experience, making memories, improving the capacity to learn new information, and creative problem-solving. There is a reason people tell you to "sleep on it" when confronted by a big decision. There's wisdom in these folk sayings.

DIFFERENCES AND SIMILARITIES IN SLEEP PATTERNS

Some people say that they are very light sleepers and if the cat stretches in another room they hear it. Others say that they can sleep through a tremendous racket. There are people who can sleep standing up on a train and others who need to have the room, mattress, pillow, and sheets just so in order to sleep. Different people have different sleep habits and different sleep needs.

However, we all have an internal mechanism, sometimes called a biological clock, which refers to cells in the brain that are designed to respond to light and dark. In other words, the way we are built physiologically is to sleep when it gets dark and be awake when it is light. Night shift workers have difficulty staying awake because of natural sleepiness and may develop physical problems associated with lack of sleep, such as digestive disorders and even heart disease. Many of us have experienced jet lag, feeling disoriented and lethargic because our biological clock has been disturbed. The recommended "cure" for jet lag, among other things, is to be outside in the sunlight as much as possible. It resets the clock.

STAGES OF SLEEP

You are probably aware that there are different kinds of sleep—different cycles or stages. There is a stage of light sleep when you are easily awakened, akin to dozing; there is deep sleep, which is marked by slower brain waves than during light sleep; and there is REM (rapid eye movement) sleep, which is the stage you dream in, where your eyes move and your limbs are temporarily paralyzed. These cycles of sleep repeat during the night. All are necessary to good sleep—and good health.

WHY SLEEP IS IMPORTANT FOR YOUR HEALTH

If you get too little sleep, it can influence your response time and make it hard to focus. This makes driving dangerous and impairs your decision making. In addition to lowered mental facility, sleep-deprived people have poor hand-eye coordination, similar to being drunk. This is the reason the government regulates how long and often pilots can fly without a break. It's too risky to be tired and in control of so many lives. There are also great efforts from various advocacy groups to limit the number of hours medical residents work without a break. Residents who sometimes work up to a hundred hours a week make errors in the hospital or fall asleep when driving home. Lack of sleep also affects your mood; people who chronically don't sleep well are prone to becoming depressed.

There are physical issues associated with sleep problems as well. If you are a poor sleeper, you run a higher risk of developing diabetes, blood pressure problems, and heart disease.[1] When you sleep, you release hormones, including hormones that help to fight off infection. This is the reason why "get plenty of rest" is part of the prescription for overcoming a cold or other common infection.

SLEEP AND WEIGHT

There is a relationship between sleeping poorly and gaining weight, although it is not clearly understood. It used to be thought that if you didn't sleep well and were tired, you ate more carbs and sugars to give you more energy, and consequently you gained weight. However, research shows that women who slept less than five hours a night tended to become overweight or obese even though they actually ate less than women with better sleep patterns. Another theory was that the link between sleep and weight was due to lack of physical activity, which makes a kind of intuitive sense: if you are exhausted, you may be reluctant to move around and therefore burn fewer calories and put on weight. But that also does not seem to be the case. Although the link between sleep and weight is not clear, it is possible that people who sleep less than normal have a slower metabolic rate and higher levels of cortisol.

TYPES OF SLEEP PROBLEMS

According to the National Institute of Neurological Disorders and Stroke, about forty million Americans suffer from various chronic sleep disorders, and another twenty million suffer occasional sleeping problems. According to the National Heart, Lung, and Blood Institute, more than seventy million Americans suffer from sleep problems. Whichever number you choose, that's a lot of people not sleeping! It is estimated that by the year 2010, eighty million Americans will have a sleep problem and that the number will reach one hundred million by 2050. So if you have sleep problems, take comfort in the fact that you are not alone.

SLEEP PROBLEMS AND WOMEN

Many women have sleep problems that go ignored, undiagnosed, or untreated. For many, not sleeping becomes a "normal" way of life. But sleep problems can and should be addressed for good health and quality of life.

Many doctors fail to correctly diagnose sleep conditions in women because they don't fit the traditional—that is, male—clinical picture. For example, often sleep apnea (a condition where you stop breathing for short intervals repeatedly while you sleep) or sleep breathing disorders are not diagnosed correctly in women because the condition may not be accompanied by loud snoring, as it often is in men. Many women are incor-

---

CAUSES OF SLEEP PROBLEMS IN WOMEN

- High stress levels from having too much to do in too little time
- Hormonal fluctuations, especially during the menstrual cycle
- Hot flashes that disturb sleep due to decreased estrogen during perimenopause and menopause
- Lack of exercise
- Too much coffee or caffeine
- Depression
- Drinking alcohol
- Being overweight or obese

rectly diagnosed with chronic fatigue syndrome rather than sleep apnea or narcolepsy (a condition where you have a sudden and uncontrollable urge to sleep) because these conditions don't fit the classical (that is, male) pattern.

Women who sleep less than seven hours a night are at greater risk for high blood pressure and heart disease. Lack of sleep is also associated with increased cortisol (page 252) levels and type 2 diabetes (page 264). Poor sleep patterns, sleep problems, and abnormal breathing during sleep can have a negative impact on quality of life, leading not only to fatigue and lethargy but also to depression and various interpersonal and social problems.

INSOMNIA

Insomnia, which is defined as difficulty falling asleep or staying asleep, is the most common sleep disorder in women. I remember a friend telling me about a weekend celebration of someone's fiftieth birthday where a dozen women went together to a spa hotel. In the evening, when the group had gathered to plan the next day's activities, one of the women asked casually if anyone had an Ambien. Every single woman reached into her handbag to grab her bottle of this sleeping medication.

Insomnia can be caused by many factors, such as stress, trauma, or poor sleeping habits, but can also be due to an underlying illness such as thyroid disorders, arthritis, asthma, anxiety, or depression. As with any physical problem, it's a good idea to talk to your doctor.

WOMEN AND INSOMNIA

More than 50 percent of women between the ages of thirty and sixty have chronic or occasional insomnia. Hormones play a part in insomnia, so much so that sleep disorders are classified as menstrual-associated disorders, yet few doctors when evaluating sleep conditions relate them to menstrual status. In addition to menopause, other periods of hormonal fluctuations influence sleep patterns, such as pregnancy and menopause. Hot flashes and night sweats are associated with sleep problems. However, doctors should not be quick to write off sleep problems as a normal consequence of menopause. There could be underlying disorders such as sleep breathing disorders. Women with chronic insomnia are at a higher risk for depression. Hormone therapy (estrogen) used to be prescribed for sleep problems, especially for postmenopausal women, but recent studies show there is no significant advantage to taking HT for improving sleep.

TREATMENT FOR INSOMNIA

Insomnia is usually treated with medication, behavior modification techniques, or a combination of both. Most doctors believe that behavioral changes are better in the long run, and medication should be used for short-term problems. Over-the-counter medications, such as Nytol, are often antihistamines, which promote drowsiness and can help with falling asleep. However, antihistamines are not recommended for people with breathing problems or glaucoma, or if you are pregnant or nursing. Antidepressants, such as Zoloft or Prozac, are sometimes used to treat chronic insomnia, even for women who have no depression. They generally do not cause dependency, but they could cause dizziness.

> **TALK TO YOUR DOCTOR IF:**
>
> • It takes you up to an hour to fall asleep.
> • You wake up during the night and can't fall back asleep.
> • You are sleepy during the day.
> • You snore or have trouble breathing at night.
> • You have a feeling of crawling or prickling in your legs.

Other sleep medications, such as zolpidem (Ambien) and zaleplon (Sonata), can cause dependency. If you take any of these medications for more than two weeks, don't stop them suddenly. Talk to your doctor. And if you need to stay on medication longer, your doctor should supervise. Side effects of these sleep medications include headaches, drowsiness, and stomach upset. Sleep medications should not be combined with other sedatives.

Another class of drugs, called benzodiazepines—such as temazepam (Restoril), triazolam (Halcion), lorazepam (Ativan), and estazolam (ProSom)—are also prescribed for sleep problems. These drugs work on the brain and also help with anxiety. If you are over sixty-five, however, benzodiazepines have been associated with increased risk of hip fractures, due to side effects of drowsiness and lack of coordination. They are also habit-forming.

OBSTRUCTIVE SLEEP APNEA SYNDROME

Obstructive sleep apnea refers to the temporary and sporadic cessation of breathing that occurs during sleep. It's caused by tissue in the throat collapsing and blocking the airway. The sleeper actually stops breathing; the lack of oxygen causes a brief awakening, and then breathing resumes. This cycle can happen multiple times an hour, and usually the sleeper is unaware of stopping breathing or of waking up.

Sleep apnea is usually associated with snoring and with being overweight and can cause daytime sleepiness. Although millions of people have been diagnosed with sleep apnea, millions more are undiagnosed and untreated. Sometimes a partner complains of the loud snoring, or daytime sleepiness is so acute that the person thinks something is wrong and mentions it to the doctor. But sleep apnea is a very serious condition and should be treated.

How Do You Know If You Have Sleep Apnea?

The most reliable way to diagnose sleep apnea is to have a professional sleep study done. This all-night study can be done in a hospital sleep center or at home. A technician attaches sensors to your body and monitors your sleep all night. The sensors transmit data on how often you wake up and if there are any changes in your breathing patterns.

If you do have sleep apnea, it is important to treat it. There is a very effective—if not very sexy—treatment called a CPAP (continuous positive airway pressure) machine. Before you go to sleep you put on a mask that forces a continuous stream of air through your airway, which keeps an air passage open during sleep. The air ensures that your throat doesn't close and block the airflow. Also, if you are diagnosed with sleep apnea, it is very important to let your doctors know this, especially before undergoing a procedure that involves an anesthetic, because it might make a difference in how airflow is managed during surgery.

HEALTH RISKS FROM SLEEP APNEA

Untreated sleep apnea is associated with high blood pressure, coronary heart disease, heart attack, congestive heart failure, stroke, mental impairment, and injury from accidents, which is why it is extremely important to be properly diagnosed and treated. According to the National Commission on Sleep Disorders Research, the cardiovascular problems associated with sleep apnea result in approximately thirty-eight thousand deaths a year. Studies suggest that 40 percent of patients with high blood pressure also have sleep apnea, and when the sleep apnea is treated, hypertension is improved for many patients.

CLUES THAT YOU MAY HAVE SLEEP APNEA:

- If you are overweight or obese
- If you snore
- If your high blood pressure does not respond to treatment

Sleep apnea may also be implicated in increased risk for stroke because there is a decrease in blood flow to the brain during interrupted breathing. Because sleep apnea is known to increase after menopause and with age, there may be a connection between increased cardiovascular disease risk for postmenopausal women and sleep apnea.

Sleep apnea seems to be more prevalent in African Americans than in whites, especially for younger people. Hypertension is also more prevalent in African Americans, and there may be a connection, as yet poorly understood.

WOMEN AND SLEEP APNEA

Many of the women I see feel uncomfortable when I ask about snoring. They react as if it is a character flaw rather than a potentially serious medical issue. Since snoring is one of the symptoms of sleep apnea, the question should be asked and answered. It's also a good idea to have an evaluation by an ENT (ear, nose, and throat) specialist if you snore because sometimes the problem is caused by large tonsils that are obstructing the flow of air during sleep. This needs to be addressed.

Premenopausal women seem to suffer less from sleep apnea; after menopause the incidence of sleep apnea increases. Being overweight also increases the incidence of sleep apnea. Obese women with polycystic ovary syndrome are at increased risk of sleep apnea, and doctors should be alert to this association.

If there is any indication that you may have sleep apnea—for example, you find yourself unusually tired during the day, or a sleeping partner has told you that you snore or seem to stop breathing at night—you should have the overnight sleep test. If you are overweight and suffering from sleep apnea, losing weight and exercising are helpful. It's also a good idea to avoid sleeping on your back. If you have sleep apnea, you should avoid sleep medication because it might further suppress breathing as well as make it harder to wake up to kick-start your breathing.

RESTLESS LEG SYNDROME

Restless leg syndrome (RLS) is characterized by an almost irresistible urge to move your legs. Often there are sensations such as itching or a feeling of something crawling on your skin. Although the cause is unknown, it is thought to be a neurological condition. It can be very mild and hardly noticeable, or it can be severe.

The reason that RLS is considered a sleep problem is that the symptoms are usually exaggerated while lying down. Because there is relief of symptoms when you move your legs, people who have RLS move their legs during the night and may consequently suffer from insomnia. Some people find that increased walking, yoga, stretching, massage, and baths relieve the symptoms.

There is medication for restless leg syndrome, such as pramipexole (Mirapex), but it needs to be carefully monitored by a physician because of side effects such as dizziness, headaches, and nausea. Sometimes the medication can have psychological side effects as well, such as compulsive behavior and impulse control problems.

NARCOLEPSY

Narcolepsy is another neurological sleep condition caused by an inability of the brain to regulate the sleep-wake cycle. There seems to be a genetic component to who has it. Narcolepsy, which is characterized by

excessive and extreme sleepiness, is often misdiagnosed and can go untreated for many years. People who have narcolepsy fall asleep involun-
tarily for a few seconds or minutes during the day, sometimes in the
middle of a conversation, during an activity, while eating a meal, or driving a car. The condition can be disabling, embarrassing, and dangerous.
In addition to sleepiness, some people with narcolepsy have incidents of
hallucinations and muscle paralysis.

TIPS FOR BETTER SLEEP HABITS

- Put yourself on a regular schedule for going to sleep and waking up.
- Don't force yourself to go to bed before you are ready.
- Avoid eating large meals, drinking alcohol, or having caffeine before bed.
- Get daily exercise, but not right before bed.
- Avoid daytime naps that are longer than a half hour.
- Provide yourself with a good sleeping environment.
- If you are awake for more than a half hour at night, get up for a short while, do something relaxing, and try and get back to sleep after an hour.

Patients with narcolepsy are usually treated with stimulants, such as
methylphenidate (Ritalin) and various amphetamines. These medications, although effective, may have serious side effects, such as heart palpitations, and can also be addictive.

WHAT TO DO IF YOU HAVE SLEEP PROBLEMS

If you are having sleep disturbances, it is a good idea to keep a diary of
how much you sleep, when you wake up, how often during the night, and
so on, in order to assist your doctor in assessing your sleep-wake
rhythms. In any case, if you are having sleep problems, it's a good idea to
talk to your doctor. The doctor should take a careful history, do a physical examination, and ask you about your medications and your menstrual
and pregnancy history. Good health care should involve a sleep assess-

ment, especially for women who are overweight or obese, since there is an increased risk of sleep apnea. Don't medicate yourself for sleep problems without talking to your doctor.

ALCOHOL AND SLEEP

Many people are under the impression that alcohol helps to induce sleep. Indeed it may—*but* alcohol also disrupts sleep after a few hours. In other words, once the sleep-inducing effect is past, there is sleep disturbance associated with alcohol consumption. Even drinking as much as six hours before bedtime has been found to cause sleep disturbances. If you have trouble sleeping through the night, and in particular if you wake up after a few hours and then can't get back to sleep, try to avoid alcohol.

EIGHTEEN

Exercise for Good Health

I KNOW YOU HAVE HEARD IT ALL BEFORE. AND I KNOW YOU KNOW THAT exercise is good for you. You know you will be healthier, feel stronger, and look better if you exercise. The value of exercise is always being touted—it's hard to turn on the TV without seeing a dozen fitness shows, and the media are full of advertisements and information about exercise. So why is it so hard for so many of us to find the time, energy, and inspiration to get out there and move? Sometimes I think there is so much noise about exercise that we can't even hear it—like background music that no one listens to. I can't tell you how many times my patients tell me, "Dr. Goldberg, I really don't have the time!" But it is important that you make time. Get started. Stick with a program.

NO EXCUSE IS GOOD ENOUGH

I hear all kinds of rationalizations for not exercising. Every once in a while there is a news story about someone dying unexpectedly during exercise, and many of my patients tell me they are afraid of exercising because of this. In fact, this is an extremely rare event, especially for women—one death in thirty million hours of exercise. And all *you* need to do is three hours a week to maintain good health! So don't worry; the benefits of exercise far outweigh any risk.[1] No more excuses, please. The truth is that exercise is beneficial for many aspects of a woman's health; if it were a pill, everyone would be asking for it.

In this chapter I will share with you some practical tips to get you started, and tell you how to exercise safely and get the greatest benefits from

HEALTH BENEFITS OF EXERCISE

- Reduces the risk of heart attack
- Reduces the risk of stroke
- Lowers blood pressure
- Reduces the risk of developing type 2 diabetes
- Reduces the risk of breast cancer
- Helps to maintain good bone density
- Reduces depression
- Counteracts menopausal weight gain

your workout. Exercise programs for women should be based on your level of fitness and on whatever medical/physical situation is unique to you. If you are pregnant, if you have arthritis, if you are perfectly fit, if you have heart disease—there is an exercise program that is good for you.

GET CHECKED OUT BEFORE YOU START

Before you get started, see your doctor, particularly if you have never exercised before. It's a smart idea to be evaluated for orthopedic problems or physical weak spots so that you can design an appropriate exercise program for yourself. Some of my patients come to me thinking they are having heart problems because they have unexplained pain in their shoulder. By talking to them, I discover that they are golfers, and in fact are suffering from the repetitive motion of swinging the club. You and your doctor need to discuss your medical history and whether or not there are any risks to you with different types of exercise programs.

DEVISE YOUR OWN EXERCISE PROGRAM

Some of my patients resist the very idea of exercise, but I think that's because they imagine a regimented program at a gym. Or maybe it's because they remember those ugly gym suits we had to wear in junior high school. You can create your own exercise program. Make every effort to move around a lot each day. If you can do half an hour of exercise daily (maybe walk to work), that's great. Do what you like to do. That way you'll stick with it. If you have always wanted to dance and want to take lessons, that's terrific. Try to go a couple of times a week, and practice at home. If you like to swim, swim.

My friends have all sorts of exercise strategies. Chris has the kind of job where she finds it difficult to predict her free time. So she exercises to a video in her own bedroom several times a week; she also walks and does a strength-training routine with weights. As long as she can control what time she exercises, she finds that she is able to stick with the program.

> Before you exercise, you should be evaluated by a doctor to:
>
> - Check for existing medical conditions to help you design a healthy exercise program
> - Evaluate orthopedic limitations so as not to injure yourself
> - Assess whether your medications might affect your level of exercise
> - Set reasonable goals for yourself

Another friend, Hope, is retired from teaching and has time on her hands. She goes to an aquatics exercise class at her local Y every day. She likes the routine of having someplace to get up and go to and has made a group of friends who all exercise together. She also finds this type of exercise is less stressful to her arthritic knees.

My patient Debbie is recently divorced and looking to improve her social life. She joined a singles hiking club and walks every weekend. In order to stay in good shape for these hikes, she exercises at the gym during the week.

I participate in exercise classes at the 92nd Street Y in Manhattan. It works for me because it is just a few blocks from my office and I like classes. But I realize that what works for me may not be right for every woman. You need to pick activities you like; otherwise you won't stick with them. Make your exercise routine fit your lifestyle. We can each do something.

BEFORE YOU EXERCISE

Before you exercise, especially if you are doing strenuous or high-intensity exercise such as running, skiing, or tennis, make sure to warm up the muscles you will use for about five to ten minutes ahead of time, because otherwise you can damage yourself. Warming up means that you should use your muscles as you would use them during your exercise but at a much lower intensity. For example, a warm-up to running could be a gentle jog.

Avoid doing stretches where you hold a particular position for an extended time. It is unnecessary and could even be damaging to do static stretches before exercising. Latest studies show that doing gentle dynamic movement as part of your warm-up routine is more beneficial to your muscles. Examples of this type of movement are gentle arm circles or light marching in place.

Also, drink water to hydrate before exercise, about two or three cups. If you are doing long exercise, such as running a marathon, you'll need another two or three cups an hour. If the weather is especially hot or you sweat a great deal, you'll need to replenish your body's fluids with even more water.

It's important to eat before exercise, particularly in the morning, when your body is depleted of energy after a night's sleep. Many of my friends wake up and go jogging before breakfast. This is not a good idea. Make sure to eat breakfast before your morning workout. Don't think that you'll lose more weight if you exercise without eating. Exercising in such an energy-depleted condition actually tells your body to store more fat because it wants to redress its famished condition.

That said, your pre-exercise breakfast should not be pancakes with maple syrup and butter. I recommend a 300-calorie breakfast: a medium-size apple, pear, or banana or half a cup of dried fruit mixed with walnuts or almonds with low-fat yogurt. Or you can eat whole-grain cereal with low-fat milk and fruit. This meal keeps blood sugars stable through the workout. It is also rich in potassium, which helps muscles function.

One of my patients joined a gym so that she could exercise. She started on a rowing machine, but instead of warming up by performing the exercise at a low intensity, she accelerated at a vigorous pace. Is it any wonder she became short of breath? You don't want to jump into a too-heavy exercise program or to begin doing exercises incorrectly. You want to start slowly and gradually increase your pace.

Weekend warriors, as I like to call them, exercise primarily on Sundays because they find they are too busy other days. Not a good idea. It's too sporadic and you can injure yourself easily. The idea is to get frequent regular exercise, and once a week, although regular, is not enough.

WHEN NOT TO EXERCISE

Don't exercise if you have:

- Fever
- Anemia
- Uncontrolled high blood pressure
- Heart failure
- Chest pain
- Heart rhythm problems
- Dizziness
- Extreme fatigue

EQUIPMENT

If you can afford to have exercise equipment at home, that's great. And if you can afford a personal trainer and a gym membership, that's also great. But you don't really need them, and if you can't, you can and should still exercise. Instead of weights, you can lift bottles or cans. You can always walk; stairs provide very good exercise. My friend Dorothy lives on the fifteenth floor of her apartment building and uses the stairs instead of the elevator because she says it's the only exercise she gets. There is always some way to do what you need to do—if your heart is in it!

COMPONENTS OF AN EXERCISE PROGRAM

Everyone gets some benefit if they get off their behind and start moving. If you want to see the biggest health benefits from exercise, and improve the way you look and feel, you should do low-to-moderate-intensity exercise every day, including both aerobic and strength exercises. The four main components of any exercise program are type, frequency, intensity, and duration.

TYPE

There are two primary types of exercise, aerobic exercise and strength training. According to the American Academy of Sports Medicine, any activity that makes the heart and lungs work hard over a sustained period of time is considered to be aerobic. Aerobic exercise uses the large muscles of your body in repetitive movements without resistance. Aerobic activities include jumping rope, running, cross-country skiing, aerobic dancing, and swimming. Strength training involves resistance, usually with weights, to help strengthen muscles and bone. Both types of exercise are good for your health—and your weight.

> ### GET YOURSELF THE RIGHT SHOES
>
> We all know that the right shoes are very important. Buy shoes appropriate for your activity. If you are just starting out, cross-training shoes are good all-around exercise shoes. Make sure you have enough room in the toe box and that the ankles are supported.

Until recently, most research has focused on the cardiovascular benefits of aerobics. However, it has become clear that strength training is good for more than shaping up and balance. Strength-training exercise improves cholesterol and reduces body fat. Turning fat into muscle is a good thing; muscle is more metabolically active, and so you burn more calories.

FREQUENCY

You should aim to do aerobic activity almost every day, at least five times a week, and strength or resistance training at least twice a week.

INTENSITY

Aerobic exercise should be of moderate intensity. You don't get more value out of driving yourself too hard. There are two ways to measure intensity: monitoring your heart rate or using the modified exertions scale (opposite). If the intensity is too low, you won't get the benefits of the exercise, and if it is too high, you won't get extra benefit. You will merely build up lactic acid (a waste product) and get muscle cramps. What you want to do is to maintain a targeted range, one that you and your doctor agree is safe and will be most efficient for maximum health benefit.

Some of my patients find it very awkward to monitor their pulse while they exercise. They have found that buying a heart rate monitor watch at the local sporting goods store is a workable alternative.

HOW TO MONITOR INTENSITY

You can monitor your intensity for doing aerobic exercise by taking your heart rate during exercise. Your target heart rate is the range where you should be training to get the benefits of exercise. If you are a healthy woman without any cardiovascular problems and not taking medication that slows your heart rate, your ideal rate can be calculated as follows: subtract your age from 220, and then have your rate be 80–85 percent of that number.

For example, if you are a healthy fifty-year-old woman, subtract 50 from 220, which gives you a result of 170, and take 80 to 85 percent of that figure, which will give you a target range of 136–144 beats per minute. This is the heart rate range you want to achieve during your aerobic workout in order to obtain the maximum benefit.

If you have had a stress test, the target heart rate is calculated from your maximum heart rate during a stress test. Ask your doctor for your maximum heart rate, then take 80–85 percent of that number, and you will have your target heart rate range for exercise. It's best to discuss this with your doctor. Very often, I speak directly with the fitness instructors at various gyms about my patients so that I can be sure that the instructor understands any limitations on the exercise program.

Certain medications, such as beta-blockers and calcium channel blockers, are designed to slow down the heart rate. If you take those medications, the 220-minus-your-age calculation or the charts posted in the gym will be inaccurate because they are based on healthy individuals who are not on medication. Pregnancy is also another time where the heart rate method may be inaccurate, because during pregnancy your heart rate is faster than normal. Again, it's wise to check with your doctor.

An alternative way to gauge your intensity is to use the modified exertion scale. This scale connects your body and mind. Your goal is to feel that you are in the moderate intensity zone, between 5 and 7.

Modified Exertion Scale

1. Rest (sitting in a chair)
2. Very light exertion (just warming up)
3. Moderate exertion (starting to exercise)
4. Somewhat strong
5. Moderately strong (starting to huff and puff but still able to talk)
6. Strong (a little more difficult to talk but you can still do it)
7. Very strong
8. Outside your fitness zone
9. Exhaustion
10. Beyond exhaustion

HOW MUCH DO YOU SWEAT?

Some of my patients tell me they never work up a sweat and therefore think they are not working hard enough at their exercise program. Others tell me they know they are exercising to their maximum because of how much they sweat. They are all surprised when I tell them that sweat has nothing to do with anything. Different people sweat at different rates, and the only thing the level of sweat tells you about is simply how much you sweat.

As I said, you want your workout zone to be of moderate intensity because vigorous aerobic exercise with occasional or higher-intensity movements can lead to orthopedic injury. My patient Paulette decided to march up the stair climber at high intensity for fifteen minutes because she thought she would lose weight more quickly that way. Instead the only thing she did was to injure her knee, which prevented her from exercising at all. You need to start slow and build up intensity gradually. If you want to lose weight, increase the duration rather than the intensity of the exercise—you should do moderate-intensity exercise for sixty to ninety minutes. It's the longer duration rather than the intensity of aerobic exercise that burns more calories.

DURATION

You should do about thirty minutes of aerobic exercise a day for cardiovascular benefits and to reduce blood pressure. If you want to lose weight, lengthen the duration; don't increase the intensity. Doing sixty to ninety minutes a day is useful for weight loss. Strength or resistance training for balance and coordination should be done two or three times a week.

THE CARDIOVASCULAR BENEFITS OF EXERCISE

Aerobic exercise is good for your cardiovascular system because it improves HDL (good) cholesterol and reduces LDL (bad) cholesterol. It increases the amount of adrenaline in your body, which relaxes the blood vessels and thus lowers blood pressure. Aerobic exercise is not only good for your heart, it is good for your whole body, lowering your risk for getting diabetes, improving your blood glucose control if you have diabetes, and contributing to fitness and to weight loss.

STRENGTH TRAINING

Strength training involves slow movements while working against some resistance, such as weights, weight machines, or resistance bands. This kind of exercise is particularly useful for developing muscles and offsetting the 1.5 percent muscle mass loss that occurs naturally with menopause every year. Not only does strength training help strengthen muscles but it is also effective in decreasing body fat by helping to increase your metabolic rate. And it's also good for your heart and for your self-esteem.

My friend Susan is a computer scientist of some renown and travels all over the world giving lectures. She is very petite, under five feet. She told me that at age sixty she started to lift weights. When I asked why, she said that she was tired of asking men to hoist her carry-on bag into the overhead bins in airplanes. She was delighted to report that after only a few months, she could lift her suitcase over her head. (She does have to stand on the seat, however. But so do I.)

Women of all ages benefit from strength training. Many women, especially over the age of sixty-five, cannot lift or carry even ten pounds. Studies show that if those women have a short period of strength training, from three to six months, they improve their strength and endurance by between 25 percent and 100 percent.[2] My recommendation is to do at least one hour of strength or resistance training, for both upper and lower body, twice a week.

TYPES OF EXERCISE ACTIVITY

LOW INTENSITY

- Ballroom dancing
- Bowling
- Golf (with cart)
- Hatha yoga
- Slow water aerobics

MODERATE INTENSITY

- Ballroom dancing (fast)
- Bicycling
- Climbing stairs
- Gardening
- Golf (no cart)
- Low-impact aerobics
- Moderate swimming
- Walking

HIGH INTENSITY

- Cardio kick-boxing
- High-impact aerobics
- Hiking
- Jogging
- Rollerblading
- Soccer
- Spinning
- Tennis

PILATES

Pilates is an exercise technique developed in the mid-twentieth century by Joseph Pilates, who was a sickly child and became a gymnast who wanted to improve his performance. Born in Germany, he came to England and was interned as an enemy alien during World War I. While interned, he developed ways to use bedsprings for resistance and strength training for bedridden patients and used other available material to help maintain his body and those of the other internees. After the war, he and his wife moved to New York City, where they opened an exercise studio near the New York City Ballet. Many dancers, including George Balanchine and Martha Graham, used his methods to help maintain muscle strength and flexibility.

Pilates techniques and equipment are designed to strengthen the core or center of your body and are done on a mat or with equipment, most commonly a specialized table, known as a reformer, that is available at fitness facilities. The techniques require you to concentrate on small movements and on your breathing. In particular, these exercises strengthen your abdominal muscles, improve posture and balance, and help to reduce falls. You also get the extra benefit of a flatter abdomen.

DON'T FORGET TO BREATHE

It is very important to breathe during exercise, especially if you have high blood pressure and are doing strength-training exercise. Many people hold their breath. Don't. If you do, you will raise your blood pressure even higher. That's why so many fitness trainers talk about "breathe in" and "breathe out."

I was so excited when I heard that my patient Sabrina who is overweight and on blood pressure and cholesterol medication, inquired about the Pilates studio in my office building. I discovered this fact from the owner of the Pilates studio, who asked me if it was okay for Sabrina to participate. I said absolutely. Pilates is a great place for her to begin. Aerobic exercise will follow when she becomes more confident.

TAI CHI

Tai chi is a Chinese martial arts technique that has been practiced for more than three hundred years. Tai chi has been proven to improve balance, flexibility, and strength and can be done into one's old age. It also improves the quality of sleep and has been shown to reduce stress hormones by amounts similar to the reductions seen with moderate aerobic exercise.[3]

SOCIAL SUPPORT

One of the reasons I suggest that my patients join an exercise class or program is that there is evidence that social support encourages more active participation in and commitment to exercise.[4] My own research showed that women who exercised in an aerobics class had less anger, anxiety, and depression and a better quality of life compared to women who worked out on exercise machines (see page 40).

CHECK OUT YOUR HEART

You May Need a Stress Test

If you are over fifty and have never exercised before, it's a good idea to have a stress test to assess your heart function. The stress test gives information about your endurance. Exercise endurance is based on age, gender, and fitness level. Stress testing has been available for more than thirty years, but until 2005 doctors were calculating endurance levels for women based on research in men. In that year, Dr. Martha Gulati and her colleagues developed parameters to assess women's fitness. In a study of more than five thousand women, with and without heart disease, these researchers found that the length of time a woman could stay on the treadmill during a stress test predicted long-term survival. That is why I tell my patients that the longer they stay on the treadmill, the longer they are going to live.

> **BENEFITS OF WALKING**
>
> Studies show that walking twenty to thirty minutes daily improves bone density and can actually strengthen bones.[5]

If you recently have had a heart attack or heart surgery or if you have had stents placed recently, you should start with a monitored cardiac rehabilitation program. This is an organized program of exercise, nutritional counseling, and stress management. The exercise classes are usually for an hour, three times per week, and you will be supervised by a doctor, nurse, and exercise physiologist or physical therapist. These programs run six to twelve weeks, depending on your condition and your insurance coverage. Cardiac rehabilitation is usually covered by insurance if you are within six months of a heart attack, bypass surgery, or the placement of stents or if you have chronic angina (see Chapter 8).

If your doctor doesn't bring up exercise at your first visit after discharge from the hospital, bring it up with her. Studies show that women are less likely to be referred to cardiac rehabilitation compared to men.[6] I strongly encourage all women with heart disease to join a cardiac rehabilitation program.

CHECK OUT YOUR BLOOD PRESSURE

Blood pressure should be controlled before you start an exercise program because it naturally increases with exercise; if your blood pressure is high before you start, it will increase more than it should and can become dangerously high. Mary is forty-seven years old and scheduled a consultation with me because her primary care physician told her she had high blood pressure and he wanted to prescribe medication.

> ### INDICATIONS FOR HAVING A STRESS TEST BEFORE BEGINNING AN EXERCISE PROGRAM
>
> - Women over fifty who have not exercised before
> - Women of any age who have heart disease
> - Women who have symptoms of heart disease
> - Women with diabetes

Mary was reluctant to start medication. She hoped that with diet and an exercise program she would be able to lower her blood pressure. Talking with Mary about her medical history, I found out that she became out of breath when climbing a flight of steps or running for a bus. When I examined her, her blood pressure was 160/80, which is too high to try to lower with diet and exercise alone.

She was disappointed when I too recommended medication, but I explained to her that she needed medication to bring her blood pressure down to normal so that she could exercise safely. I do recommend diet and exercise without medication to women whose blood pressure is in the prehypertensive range or those with mild hypertension. Once Mary's blood pressure was controlled, she had a stress test to make sure her blood pressure increased appropriately with exercise. I also told her that if she maintains an exercise program, she might be able to reduce or even discontinue her medication.

EXERCISE FOR WOMEN WITH DIABETES

I always advise my diabetic patients to monitor their blood sugar before and after exercise. If their reading is below 100 either before or after, they should have a snack that has between 20 and 30 grams of carbohydrates (read the label). When you exercise, your sugar levels decrease. A nice benefit of regular exercise is that I am often able to reduce medications in many of my patients with type 2 diabetes because they have improved their sugar metabolism through exercise and weight loss.

EXERCISE IS GOOD FOR YOUR BONES

Exercise, especially weight-bearing exercise (exercise where you are upright so you put weight on the bones) strengthens the bones. Walking, dancing, racket sports, and so on all help to increase bone mass. Swimming is good exercise for sure, but it is not weight-bearing.

After age thirty-five or so, most women begin to lose bone mass at the rate of about 1 percent a year. After menopause that rate increases to about 3 percent a year. Therefore, you want to do whatever you can to improve your bone mass. Weight-bearing exercise is a prescription for better bones!

KNOW YOUR BONE DENSITY

It's a good idea to have a bone density test before you begin an exercise program. If you have osteoporosis, certain exercises should be avoided. The more you and your doctor know, the better care you can take of yourself.

The way it works is that weight-bearing exercise stimulates bone cells to make new bone. Women who do regular weight-bearing exercise can actually reverse bone loss and reduce their risk for osteoporosis. Also, since falling is a real problem for women as they age, having stronger bones can prevent hip fractures.

EXERCISE AND PREGNANCY

According to the American College of Obstetricians and Gynecologists, if there are no medical or obstetrical risks, pregnant women should do moderate exercise daily. Exercise that could cause abdominal trauma should be avoided, as should scuba diving, which can hurt the fetus. All sports and activities should be discussed with your doctor.[7]

Physically active moms-to-be are less likely to have gestational diabetes and preeclampsia. Remember that moderate exercise maintains the health of the mother, but too much exercise can be risky to the fetus.

Pregnant women have a faster basic heart rate; therefore, don't use the 220-minus-your-age equation to determine the intensity of your exercise. Use the modified exertion scale on page 379, or ask your doctor for a recommended heart rate.

Remember to stay very well hydrated and to dress ap-

> If you are pregnant, don't exercise if you have:
> - Uncontrolled high blood pressure
> - Preeclampsia
> - A high risk for premature labor
> - Persistent second- or third-trimester bleeding

propriately for the weather. If you exercise outdoors and it is very cold, you risk hypothermia. Exercising indoors will keep you from exposing yourself to extreme temperatures while you are physically active.

Your caloric requirement increases during pregnancy and lactation. Make sure you eat a carbohydrate snack before you exercise so that you don't risk hypoglycemia. Avoid exercise when you are lying down on your back after the first trimester because you can put yourself at risk for low blood pressure and symptoms of fainting. Avoid exercise that might put you at increased risk for falling, especially during the third trimester.

Menopausal Symptoms

The jury is still out on the role of exercise in relieving menopausal symptoms. A study in the *Annals of Behavioral Medicine* showed that menopausal women who exercised regularly in a walking program or participated in yoga reported a better quality of life and less anxiety and stress about their menopausal symptoms than those who didn't exercise.[8] Those who had the health benefits of exercise also reported a decrease in hot flashes. So exercise may not get rid of the hot flashes, but they probably won't bother you as much. And you'll feel better generally.

Benefits of Exercise for Women with Breast Cancer

Moderate exercise, such as walking three to five hours a week, has been found to improve survival in women with breast cancer, including women with hormone-responsive tumors, women with stage III cancer, and those women who have breast cancer and are also obese. Physical activity is also associated with improved quality of life.[9]

Keeping Your Mind in Good Shape

Alzheimer's disease affects three times as many women as men. Therefore, it should be regarded as a serious women's health issue. Exercise has been shown to be associated with a decreased risk of Alzheimer's, especially for postmenopausal women[10] and for older women who walked regularly.[11] In a study of women sixty-five and older, those women who did aerobic exercise for thirty minutes three times a week were found to have the most protection against Alzheimer's disease, reducing their risk by about 30 percent.

Shaping Up and Looking Good

The more muscles you build, the more metabolically active you will be. You want to convert fat to muscle for health and for weight loss. The exercises in this section are good for a resistance workout. Get yourself an elastic band from a local sporting goods store or use cans or hand weights. You want to start with about one to three pounds in each hand and work your way up to eight pounds.

All of the exercises help to improve posture and balance, thereby reducing the risk of falls. Strength training also helps to maintain muscle mass, which will enable you to do more physical activity. With firm muscles and reduced body fat, you will be able to move around without any difficulty. We all know women who begin panting as soon as they lift themselves off their seats. You don't want to be like that. You want to be able to walk upstairs and perform the normal tasks of living without any discomfort. No one is talking about turning you into a body builder, only into a fit and flexible woman who can do what she wants without injury. One of my good friends says her goal is to be able to hoist a case of wine into her van without relying on help from the store personnel.

THE STRENGTH-TRAINING STARTER PROGRAM

For the strength-training starter program, you will need an exercise mat, some light dumbbells, and ankle weights. The weight range should be between one and five pounds, depending on your level of training. If you have never done any strength-training exercise before, you should begin doing the exercises without any weights. Then add weight slowly and gradually. Start with a weight that you can use for eight repetitions of the exercise. When you can do about twelve to fifteen reps easily and comfortably, increase the weight. You don't want it to be too easy. If you don't have weights, you can use soda bottles or soup cans until you get them. No excuses!

No matter what your fitness level is, the way to do strength-training movements is to do them very slowly and with control. This is quite different from the rapid and repetitive movements involved in aerobic exercise.

What you are striving for is good form. Try the exercises without any weights the first time you do them so that you can concentrate on doing them correctly, getting the proper alignment for the exercise. Remember to breathe. Proper breathing means that you exhale when you perform the exertion or movement and inhale when you return to the resting or neutral position. This is important because when you hold your breath, which many people do when they strain, it raises the blood pressure. You don't want that.

Timing is everything. Count to ten slowly to get to the desired position, hold the position for a count of ten, then take another count of ten to return to the neutral or resting position. It may not sound slow, but it is. It's actually a challenge to have the control to move this slowly.

Since some of the exercises are done on the floor, an exercise mat should be used to avoid scraping your knees and to make yourself more comfortable. Here's an important warning: if you use a mat at a community gym, remember to wipe it down and cover it with a towel. You don't want your fitness program to be hampered by gym germs. Studies have shown that drug-resistant staph infections, which can be quite serious, have been acquired from shared gym mats and exercise equipment. The CDC recommends wiping down all equipment before and after use—and it's actually good gym manners. Mats are light and easy to find in stores, so you may want to bring your own.

The workout below is a combination of upper- and lower-body exercises adapted from a workout developed by my colleague Mirabai Holland, the director of fitness and wellness at the 92nd Street Y in New York City.

They start on the floor, so use your mat.

LEGS

The first two exercises are adduction and abduction exercises. *Adduction* means moving toward the middle of your body, and *abduction* means moving away from the body.

If you are using ankle weights, place them on your ankles before you start. You want strong legs because you want to be able to move and have the strength to exercise—not to mention having sleeker, nicely molded thighs.

OUTER THIGH/LEG ABDUCTION

Lie on your right side with the right knee bent and the left leg extended with the foot flexed at the ankle. Lift the left leg slowly to hip level. Remember to exhale when you life the leg. Do eight to twelve repetitions (remember to go slow) and then reverse to your left side and lift your right leg. Use weights up to five pounds to start.

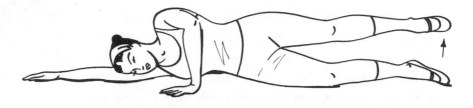

INNER THIGH/LEG ADDUCTION

Lying on the right side, bring the left leg across and in front of the extended right leg with the knee bent and left heel on the floor. (The right leg is on the bottom.) The right foot should be flexed at the ankle. Lift the right leg toward the left leg. Exhale as you lift the right leg up and inhale as you bring it down. Reverse and do the other side. Do eight to twelve repetitions for each side.

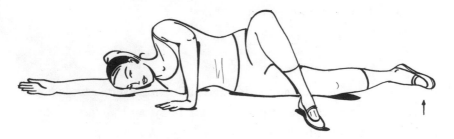

Buttocks Lift

This exercise strengthens the gluteus maximus, the muscles in your buttocks. No weights are used for this one. Lie on your back with your knees bent, heels on the floor. Exhale as you slowly lift hips off the floor, contracting your buttocks muscles. Do eight to twelve repetitions.

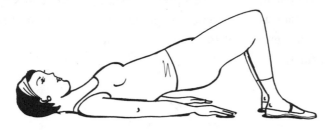

Abdominal Exercise

This exercise will help you get a flatter stomach. No weights are used. Lie on your back with your knees bent and your heels on the floor. Bring your hands behind your head, with elbows flared out to the sides. While contracting your abdomen, slowly bring the knees up to the chest as you lift the upper body. The exercise is for the upper and lower abdominal muscles. Try to do between ten and twenty repetitions. Remember to exhale as you contract your abdominal muscles and inhale as you relax. Avoid pulling on your neck; it will only feel sore.

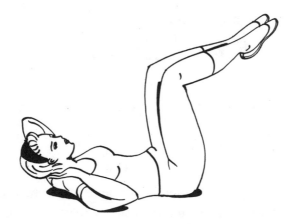

CHEST PRESS

For this exercise you want to use your hand weights. Not only does this exercise improve posture and balance, it is a natural breast lift because you are strengthening the muscles beneath the chest, giving them more support. Lie on your back, knees bent, heels on floor. Slowly lift arms in front of your chest, extending upward, making your hands meet. Remember to exhale as you extend your arms and inhale as you bring them down. I recommend eight to twelve repetitions with weights up to five pounds to start.

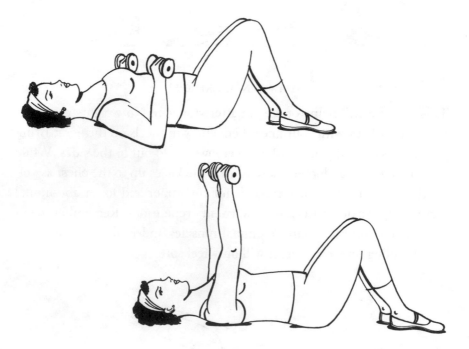

Now stand up. The next three exercises are done standing off the mat.

BACK EXERCISE

Not only is this exercise good for strengthening your back muscles and improving your posture, but you will also look better in a strapless dress or bathing suit. I very often have to wear formal gowns, and I learned from my trainer that if I exercise an hour before a gala, my arms and back look healthily muscled and sculpted. Nothing wrong with that—but to keep up the look you need to do the exercise regularly.

Use your hand weights. Begin by lunging forward, bringing your left leg forward, knee slightly bent. Bring the right arm in front of the body toward the left leg and exhale as you bend the elbow toward the back of your body, contracting the right back muscle. Do eight to twelve repetitions and then reverse to do the left back muscles.

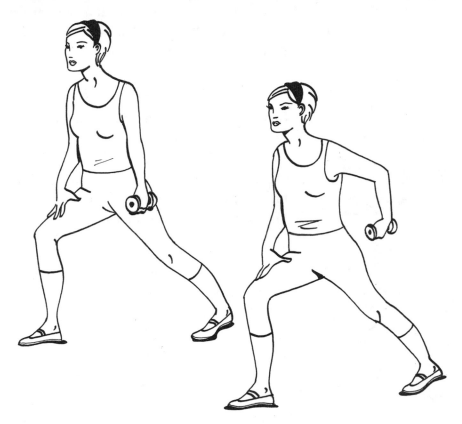

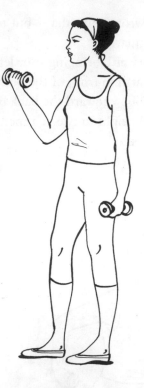

BICEPS CURLS

This exercise will allow you to lift packages with ease and look better wearing clothes that are sleeveless. Use your hand weights. Stand with your legs hip width apart, slightly bent at the knees. Exhale as you slowly bend the arms toward the shoulders, palms up. Inhale as you slowly bring the arms down. Do this for eight to twelve repetitions.

TRICEPS EXTENSIONS

Stand with your legs hip width apart. Weights are held in each arm. Bend your arms at the side ninety degrees and exhale as you slowly extend the arms in back of you. Inhale as you bring the weights back to the resting position. Do eight to twelve repetitions.

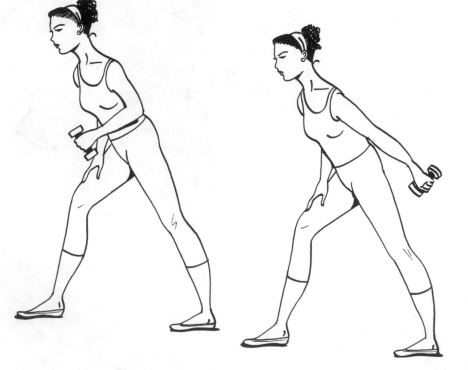

DON'T FORGET TO STRETCH

Stretching is an important part of any exercise regime. And it's the easy part, so think of it as your reward for your hard work.

The best way not to injure yourself is to stretch your muscles when they are warm. Do the following stretches to prevent aches and pains as well as muscle injury. Remember, don't bounce. The movements should be smooth.

LOW BACK STRETCH

Lie down on the mat and bring your knees to your chest. Hold the position for twenty seconds.

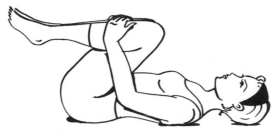

OUTER THIGH STRETCH

Lie on your back with your knees bent and your heels on the floor. Keep your left foot on the floor while you cross your right leg over the left thigh. You should feel the stretch on the outer right thigh. Hold the stretch for twenty seconds and relax. Reverse and stretch the left thigh.

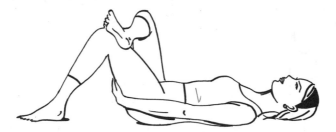

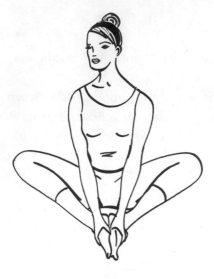

INNER THIGH STRETCH

Sit up and have your heels touch in a diamond shape, then bend slightly forward and hold the stretch for twenty seconds. You will feel the stretch on the inside of the thighs.

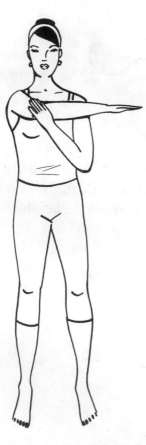

ARM AND SHOULDER STRETCH

Stand with your feet hip width apart, knees relaxed. Extend your right arm across the chest. Your right shoulder should be pressed down away from the ear. The right hand is relaxed. Use your left hand to press your right elbow into the chest. You will feel the stretch in the upper right shoulder. Hold the position for twenty seconds and then do the same for the left arm and shoulder.

CHEST AND BACK STRETCH

Raise your arms above your head and link your thumbs, forming a diamond-shaped pattern. Bring your arms back slightly. Hold the stretch for twenty seconds. You should feel the stretch in the chest and upper back. I like to do this stretch to reduce stress during the day.

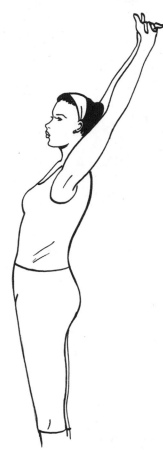

NINETEEN

A Six-Step Plan for Your Best Health

A FEW MONTHS AGO, JESSICA, MY MEDICAL ASSISTANT, WALKED INTO my office to tell me I had a very happy patient ready to be seen. Karen, forty-four, had been my patient for only three months. She had followed my recommendations to lose weight and exercise and had lost ten pounds. When I went into the exam room, Karen told me that I had changed her life. For me, having a patient follow my recommendations is like winning the Nobel Prize. I don't know who was more delighted, me or Karen.

I know how hard it is to motivate patients to diet and exercise; it takes commitment by both the doctor and the patient. My patients know that I believe in what I tell them. They see me at the gym and at the supermarket. One of my patients was impressed when she saw the healthy foods I had in my shopping cart. I think that seeing me practice what I preach helped me gain credibility with her. Another woman who is in my exercise class came running up to me to tell me that she'd seen me on a local news program talking about the benefits of exercise. My commitment to a healthy lifestyle seems to inspire my patients to take my recommendations seriously. By setting a good example, my patients know that I am involved in the same enterprise they are—being healthy. And they realize I understand how hard it is to get started and to stick with the program. After all, I can't expect you or my patients to exercise, eat right, quit smoking, and reduce stress all in one day. I know it takes planning, commitment, and time.

I developed a framework to help my patients get started on a healthy eating plan and regular exercise program. I know that it helps to have a simple program to get you started. Part of what I want you to do is to develop a healthier philosophy about eating and exercise, which is easy to do with a plan that is not overwhelming or too difficult to follow. I have created a plan of six steps that gradually integrates better food choices, exercise, and relaxation techniques into your daily life. I have found that when women decide they're going to make dramatic and sweeping changes in either their diet or exercise routines, it doesn't last very long, and soon they return to their old, unhealthy habits. Try this plan; it's gradual and manageable.

You start at week one and build up to week six, then use the new habits to continue your healthier lifestyle. These are relatively simple prescriptions that can make a very big difference in your health. Use the six-week plan to change your philosophy on health and carry it on for a lifetime.

WEEK ONE

Start Walking and Cut Down on Salt

Walking is easy to do—no equipment required. Most of us do some walking every day and don't think of it as exercise. But in fact walking is wonderful exercise, especially if you do it regularly. I recommend walking at a moderate pace, three miles per hour, for thirty minutes a day. Not only is it good for your health, but many of my friends and patients find that it's good for their mood too, and helps to reduce stress.

At the same time as you begin walking, reduce your daily salt intake. Start by noticing how much sodium is in your diet, and try to get it down to 2.3 grams (2,300 mg) per day. That's one teaspoon of salt. To help you lower your salt intake, I have listed the sodium content of some common foods. Get used to reading the labels of the foods you buy. Look out for words that contain *sodium*, such as:

- Monosodium glutamate—used for flavor enhancement
- Sodium nitrate—used to cure meats and sausages
- Sodium propionate—added to pasteurized foods, breads, and cakes to inhibit mold
- Sodium sulfite—used to preserve dried fruits

Portion Size	Food	Sodium Content
1 tablespoon	Soy sauce	914 mg
1 tablespoon	Ketchup	200 mg
1 teaspoon	Mustard	80 mg
1 teaspoon	Table salt	2,326 mg
1 ounce	Potato chips	186 mg
1 cup	Chicken noodle soup	1,100 mg
¾ cup	Canned tomato juice	825 mg
1 cup	Fresh tomatoes	9 mg
1 slice	Luncheon meat	575 mg
4 ounces	Cottage cheese	450 mg
3 ounces	Water-packed tuna	250–300 mg
3 ounces	Fresh chicken breast	58 mg
¼ cup	Raw almonds	0 mg
3	Green olives	720 mg

You can see from the chart that our diet is loaded with salt. If you begin your healthy life program by making careful sodium choices, you will be forced to phase out processed foods and to eat more fresh vegetables and fruits. For example, canned tomato sauce is high in sodium. You can choose low-sodium tomato sauce or, better yet, use a cup of fresh chopped tomatoes with basil and pepper. You'll find that you don't need to add salt. Lower-sodium choices also include lower-fat protein choices, such as white meat chicken. Eliminate processed luncheon meats, all of which are high in sodium. And by limiting sodium you also become more aware of portion control.

WEEK TWO

Begin Strength Training and Eat More Fruits and Vegetables

Continue to walk for thirty minutes a day and start strength-training exercises twice a week (see page 388). In addition, add more fruits and vegetables to your diet. In Chapter 16, I discussed the nutritional value of complex carbohydrates. Fruits and vegetables are complex carbohydrates. You want to eat five servings of vegetables and four servings of fruits per day. This may seem like a lot, but the following suggestions illustrate how you can do it.

Breakfast

4 ounces fruit juice

1 cup of whole-grain cereal with ½ cup blueberries *or* 6 ounces low-fat yogurt with ¼ cup dried fruits and nuts

Instead of the dried fruit and nut mixture, you can have a medium-sized apple, peach, or banana with your cereal. You have now had two fruits and your day is just starting!

Midmorning snack

1 cup of raw carrot sticks and/or celery sticks or 4 ounces vegetable juice

Lunch

Large salad with unlimited mixed salad greens and red, yellow, and green vegetables, such as colorful peppers, carrots, zucchini, or broccoli and a low-fat protein.

These vegetables are loaded with antioxidants and vitamins.

Afternoon snack

1 medium piece of fruit or 1 ounce walnuts and/or almonds

Eat the nuts up to three times per week. Although they count as a fruit, they are high in calories.

Dinner

> Salad to start
>
> 3 ounces grilled chicken, fish, or lean meat
>
> ½ cup cooked broccoli, spinach, or carrots
>
> ½ cup fresh fruit salad or ½ cup mixed berries

WEEK THREE

Relaxation and Transition from Simple to Complex Carbohydrates

You have spent the last two weeks incorporating walking and strength training into your routine. This week I want you to learn some relaxation techniques. You have reduced your sodium intake and increased your fruits and vegetables. This week I want you to phase out simple carbs.

Did you ever think that you would have to learn how to relax? But in today's stressful environments, we all do. Pull the plug for fifteen minutes a day to relax and have some private time to yourself. Disconnect from the grid. Get off the cell phone, BlackBerry, e-mail, computer, telephone. You need to find a quiet place without interruption for only fifteen minutes.

Some women I know find visualization a rewarding time-out period. Find a quiet space and visualize a peaceful scene, such as lying on the beach, listening to the sound of the waves and smelling sunscreen. You want to try to see, smell, and hear relaxing scenes. Remember a vacation that was relaxing. Become aware of your breathing as you visualize.

Another technique is meditation, where you can lie quietly and focus on your breathing or the silent repetition of a word. Whatever you choose, relaxation is an important step in your healthy lifestyle.

This week also, I want you to cut out simple carbohydrates. Usually simple carbs are associated with comfort food and therefore seem difficult to give up. Also, they give us a boost of energy, although it doesn't last long. You don't have to eliminate carbs from your diet; you just need to make better carb choices. Start by cutting back on sugar to five or fewer servings per week. You can have half a cup of sorbet as a healthy dessert; I sprinkle mine with strawberries. Try not to use more than a teaspoon of sugar or a tablespoon of jam a day. I recommend you buy products that say "no sugar added."

Choose complex carbs over simple ones—brown rice, not white; whole-wheat pasta; whole-grain breads. You don't have to give up carbs, just change their form.

Breakfast

1 cup whole-grain cereal *or* ½ cup cooked cereal such as oatmeal *or* 1 slice multigrain toast *or* ½ whole wheat bagel

Lunch

Small multigrain rolls with your salad

A sandwich on oat-bran bread

Dinner

No bread or crackers

Dinner salad—vegetables are complex carbs

½ cup cooked grains, bulgur, roasted buckwheat, or couscous to accompany your main course *or* ½ cup whole-wheat pasta with fresh tomatoes and broccoli as the main course

WEEK FOUR

Try Yoga, Tai Chi, or Pilates and Add Calcium to Your Diet

The activities of yoga, tai chi, and Pilates improve your balance. Look for classes at local community centers and gyms. The classes are usually an hour long. Try a class once this week. Even friends of mine who insist they have no time for exercise classes manage to find an hour and realize how much they enjoy it. Just try.

Calcium is important for our bones, and many women don't get enough calcium in their diet. See page 197 for calcium requirements. You want to get between 1,200 and 1,500 mg a day. One way to do that is through dairy products. I recommend three servings daily. If you are lactose-intolerant and can't eat dairy, there are many nondairy foods that contain calcium.

Portion Size	Food	Calcium Content
½ cup	Low-fat cottage cheese	70 mg
1 cup	1% milk	300 mg
1 cup	Whole milk	290 mg
1 cup	Nonfat plain yogurt	490 mg
½ cup	Cooked broccoli	45 mg
½ cup	Cooked green beans	100 mg
¾ cup	Mustard greens	156 mg
½ medium	Grapefruit	15 mg
3 ounces	Canned salmon with bones	180 mg

WEEK FIVE

Modify the Fats in Your Diet and Identify Dedicated Exercise Time

As I discussed in Chapter 16, you don't have to eliminate fats; you just need to choose good fats over bad fats. Less than 30 percent of your daily calories should be fat, and of that less than 7 percent should be saturated fat. So if you are eating a 1,800-calorie diet, that means that your fat calories for the day should be less than 540, and less than 38 of those calories should be saturated fat. The fat content of most foods is given in grams. Multiply the grams of fat by nine to get the fat calories. For prepared foods you need to read food labels.

Portion	Food	Fat Calories	Saturated Fat Calories
3 ounces	White meat chicken without skin, grilled	63	9
3 ounces	Dark meat poultry without skin	113	36
3 ounces	Baked cod	4	0

As you can see, cod is a better choice than the skinless chicken breast, and the skinless chicken breast is better than the dark meat chicken.

Lowering your fat intake is a step toward losing weight. You have been walking and doing strength-training and relaxing exercises. This week dedicate some time to more aerobic activity so you can burn more calories. A pound of fat is 3,500 calories. To lose that pound of fat you need to decrease your calories by 500 per day. I recommend you devote an hour to increasing your aerobic exercise.

The amount of calories you burn is related to how much you weigh, how long you exercise, and the intensity of your exercise activity. Just to give you an idea, women weighing between 130 and 150 pounds who swim leisurely for an hour burn about 400 calories; singles tennis uses about 500 calories; a moderate walk burns about 220 calories.

WEEK SIX

Decrease Caffeine and Identify Your Support Network

You don't need all that caffeine you drink. Sure, the first cup of coffee makes you feel alert, but by the sixth cup you are probably feeling jittery and your heart is racing. I want you to try to decrease your caffeine intake to below 500 mg daily. As a guide, here is a chart to help you count up your caffeine intake.

Portion	Food	Caffeine Content
5 ounces	Brewed coffee	100 mg
5 ounces	Brewed black tea	20–90 mg
8 ounces	Green tea	50 mg
2 ounces	Starbucks espresso	70 mg
12 ounces	Coke	46 mg
12 ounces	Diet Coke	46 mg
8.3 ounces	Red Bull	67 mg
1.5 ounces	Dark chocolate Hershey bar	31 mg

Dose	Drug	Caffeine Content
1 tablet	No-Doz	200 mg
1 tablet	Dexatrim	200 mg
1 tablet	Excedrin Migraine	65 mg
1 caplet	Midol	60 mg

If you have migraines and take a headache tablet or two, you need to decrease the amount of caffeine you take in from your beverages.

It's a good idea as you try to modify your diet and increase your exercise to identify and reach out to your support network. Call up a friend and ask her to walk with you. Talk about something other than work. Plan to have lunch together. In addition to having company while you continue your commitment to a healthier life, having the support of others has been shown to reduce stress and lengthen your life.

If you follow this six-week step-by-step plan, you will have gradually adopted a healthier way of life. It's manageable and reasonable. Doing any step on the plan will benefit you, and following the entire plan will make your fitter, healthier, stronger, and less stressed out. Stay on course and you will spend less time in the doctor's office because you are taking better care of yourself.

ACKNOWLEDGMENTS

The improvement of health for all women takes a team of dedicated, loyal, and supportive people working together, and I would like to acknowledge the support and encouragement of my family, friends, colleagues, and patients for this book.

Thanks to Dr. Judith Hochman, my teacher, my friend, and now my colleague at NYU, for pushing the women's health agenda through her research.

Thanks to Dr. Glenn Fishman for supporting a Women's Heart Program at NYU.

Thanks to Barnard College for giving a small woman the confidence to make big dreams a reality.

Special thanks to my friend Mirabai Holland, director of fitness and wellness at the 92nd Street Y, for keeping me sane and assisting me with the exercise chapter in this book.

Thanks to my friend Jane Chesnutt, editor in chief of *Woman's Day* magazine, who brings a healthier view of life to her readers, and also to her friends and colleagues, by sending them to the doctor for checkups.

Thanks to my colleagues at the NYU Heart and Vascular Center who help me take better care of my patients: Dr. Larry Chintz, Dr. Stephen Colvin, Dr. Frederick Feit, Dr. Aubrey Galloway, Dr. Jennifer Mieres, and Dr. Harmony Reynolds.

Special thanks to my colleagues and friends at the American Heart Association in New York City and at the The National Center.

Thanks to my staff—Colleen Landry RN, Fran Saponara, and Jessica Venture M.A.—for keeping the office together and making it a better place for me and my patients. Thanks to Martha McKitrick RD, for her assistance with the diet chapter.

Very special thanks to my girlfriends whose medical questions and commentary were the inspiration for this book: Denise Benmosche, Pamela Friedman, Elyse Feldman, Patti Kener, Amber King, Deborah Shapiro, Marcy Syms, Sandra Wilkin, and Susan Wolfson.

I cannot thank enough my family at the 92nd Street Y for their support of my work and keeping me healthy at the gym: Sol Adler, Stacey Eisler, Helaine Geismar-Katz, Cathy Marto, Marissa Scotti, David Schmeltzer, and my personal trainer, Rose Tirado.

Thanks to Dr. Richard A. Stein for teaching me that a good doctor is one who thinks about the whole patient, and for taking care of my patients so that I could take a vacation.

Very special thanks to Alice Greenwood for collaborating with me on this book. Alice is committed to improving not only women's health care but health care literacy for all. She also gave me encouragement and support as I transitioned to my new position at NYU. This project could not have happened without her.

Thanks to Bob Greenwood, Stephanie Greenwood, and Dara Greenwood for their encouragement and understanding, and a special thanks to David Greenwood, writer, editor, athlete, for giving his time and sharing his know-how.

Very big thanks to my agent, Flip Brophy, for enthusiastically supporting this project from the beginning and introducing me to Alice and to my editor, Caroline Sutton. Caroline's thoughtful editing and commitment that women have a clear message on how to take better care of themselves were invaluable.

Thanks to my parents, Minda and Leonard Goldberg, and to my mother-in-law, Leona Shapiro, for supporting me through this book and all of my professional endeavors.

From my heart, thanks to my husband, Robert, my life partner, whose love, support, and tolerance is the backbone of my success.

NOTES

CHAPTER FOUR

1. S. H. Ebrahim, R. L. Floyd, et al. "Trends in pregnancy-related smoking rates in the United States, 1987–1996." *Journal of the American Medical Association* 283:3 (2000), 361–366.

2. M. Saito, M. Hirata-Koizum, et al. "Undesirable effects of citrus juice on the pharmacokinetics of drugs: Focus on recent studies." *Drug Safety* 28:8 (2005), 677–694.

CHAPTER FIVE

1. A. Sura, J. Reefhuis, S. Rasmussen, et al. "Use of selective serotonin–reuptake inhibitors in pregnancy and the risk of birth defects." *New England Journal of Medicine* 356:26 (2007), 2684–2692.

2. A. Dunaif. "Hyperandrogenic anovulation (PCOS): A unique disorder of insulin action associated with an increased risk of non-insulin-dependent diabetes mellitus." *American Journal of Medicine* 98:1A (1995), 33S–39S.

3. R. L. Winer, J. P. Hughes, Q. Feng, et al. "Condom use and the risk of genital human papillomavirus infection in young women." *New England Journal of Medicine* 354:25 (2006), 2645–2654.

4. L. A. Wise, N. Krieger, S. Zierler, et al. "Lifetime socioeconomic position in relation to onset of perimenopause." *Journal of Epidemiology and Community Health* 56 (2002), 851–860.

5. B. L. Harlow, L. A. Wise, M. W. Otto, et al. "Depression and its influence on reproductive endocrine and menstrual cycle markers associated with perimenopause: The Harvard Study of Moods and Cycles." *Archives of General Psychiatry* 60:1 (2003), 29–36.

6. M. Ohayon. "Severe hot flashes are associated with chronic insomnia." *Archives of Internal Medicine* 166:12 (2006), 1262–1268.

7. J. Hsia, R. D. Langer, J. Manson, et al. "Conjugated equine estrogens and coronary

heart disease: The Women's Health Initiative." *Archives of Internal Medicine* 166:3 (2006), 357–365.

8. M. Stefanick, G. Anderson, K. L. Margolis, et al. "Effects of conjugated equine estrogens on breast cancer and mammography screening in postmenopausal women with hysterectomy." *Journal of the American Medical Association* 295:14 (2006), 1647–1657.

9. V. Beral, Million Women Study Collaborators, et al. "Ovarian cancer and hormone replacement therapy in the Million Women Study." *Lancet* 369 (2007), 1703–1710.

10. R. D. Jackson, A. Z. LaCroix, M. Gass, et al. "Calcium plus vitamin D supplementation and the risk of fractures." *New England Journal of Medicine* 354:7 (2006), 669–683.

CHAPTER SIX

1. D. A. Seehusen, D. R. Johnson, S. Earwood, et al. "Improving women's experience during speculum examinations at routine gynaecological visits: Randomised clinical trial." *British Medical Journal* 333 (2006), 158–159.

2. J. L. Melville, W. Katon, K. Delaney, and K. Newton. "Urinary incontinence in US women: A population-based study." *Archives of Internal Medicine* 165:5 (2005), 537–542.

3. A. D. McNaghten, D. L. Hanson, Z. Aponte, et al. "Gender disparity in HIV treatment and AIDS opportunistic illnesses (OI)." XV International Conference on AIDS, July 2004, Bangkok, Thailand.

4. D. Rozenman and E. Janssen. "Sexual function after hysterectomy." *Journal of the American Medical Association* 283:17 (2000), 2238–2239.

CHAPTER SEVEN

1. D. B. Thomas, D. L. Goa, R. M. Ray, et al. "Randomized trial of breast self-examination in Shanghai: final results." *Journal of the National Cancer Institute* 94:19 (2002), 1445–1457.

2. E. P. McCarthy, R. B. Burns, K. M. Freund, et al. "Mammography use, breast cancer stage at diagnosis, and survival among older women." *Journal of the American Geriatrics Society* 48:10 (2000), 1226–1233.

3. M. H. Gail, J. P. Costantino, et al. "Weighing the risks and benefits of tamoxifen treatment for preventing breast cancer." *Journal of the National Cancer Institute* 91:21 (1999), 1829–1846.

4. V. G. Vogel, J. P. Costantino, et al. "Effects of tamoxifen vs. raloxifene on the risk of developing invasive breast cancer and other disease outcomes." *Journal of the American Medical Association* 295:23 (2006), 2727–2741.

5. Z. Huang, S. E. Hankinson, et al. "Dual effects of weight and weight gain on breast cancer risk." *Journal of the American Medical Association* 278:17 (1997), 1407–1411.

6. F. Herrero, J. Balmer, et al. "Is cardiorespiratory fitness related to quality of life in survivors of breast cancer?" *Journal of Strength and Conditioning Research* 20:3 (2006), 535–540.

7. M. L. McCullough, C. Rodriguez, et al. "Dairy, calcium, and vitamin D intake and postmenopausal breast cancer risk in the cancer prevention study II nutrition cohort." *Cancer Epidemiology Biomarkers & Prevention* 14 (2005), 2898–2904.

8. A. H. Wu, P. Wan, et al. "Adolescent and adult soy intake and risk of breast cancer in Asian-Americans." *Carcinogenesis* 23:9 (2002), 1491–1496.

9. L. F. Degner, L. J. Kristjanson, et al. "Information needs and decisional preferences in women with breast cancer." *Journal of the American Medical Association* 277:18 (1997), 1485–1492.

CHAPTER EIGHT

1. K. Bønaa, I. Njølstad, P. M. Ueland, et al. "Homocysteine lowering and cardiovascular events after acute myocardial infarction." *New England Journal of Medicine* 354:15 (2006), 1578–1588.

2. P. M. Ridker, N. Rifai, M. A. Pfeffer, et al. "Long-term effects of pravastatin on plasma concentration of C-reactive protein. The Cholesterol and Recurrent Events (CARE) Investigators." *Circulation* 100:3 (1999), 230–235.

3. K. L. Margolis, J. E. Manson, P. Greenland, et al. "Leukocyte count as a predictor of cardiovascular events and mortality in postmenopausal women: The Women's Health Initiative Observational Study." *Archives of Internal Medicine.* 165:5 (2005), 500–508.

4. R. C. Christian, D. A. Dumesic, T. Behrenbeck, et al. "Prevalence and predictors of coronary artery calcification in women with polycystic ovary syndrome." *Journal of Clinical Endocrinology and Metabolism* 88:6 (2003), 2562–2568.

5. P. M. Ridker, N. R. Cook, et al. "A randomized trial of low-dose aspirin in the primary prevention of cardiovascular disease in women." *New England Journal of Medicine* 352:13 (2005), 1293–1304.

6. L. Mosca, N. B. Merz, R. Blumenthal, et al. "Opportunity to achieve American Heart Association guidelines for optimal lipid levels in high risk women in a managed care setting." *Circulation* 111:4 (2005), 488–493.

7. A. C. Goldberg. "A meta-analysis of randomized controlled studies on the effects of extended release niacin in women." *American Journal of Cardiology* 94:1 (2004), 121–124.

CHAPTER NINE

1. R. L. Prince, A. Devine, et al. "Effects of calcium supplementation on clinical fracture and bone structure: Results of a 5-year, double-blind, placebo-controlled trial in elderly women." *Archives of Internal Medicine* 166:8 (2006), 869–875.

2. Z. Yan, N. C. Lambert, M. Ostensen, et al. "Prospective study of fetal DNA in serum and disease activity during pregnancy in women with inflammatory arthritis." *Arthritis & Rheumatism* 54:7 (2006), 2069–2073.

3. M. Sinaki, E. Itoi, H. W. Wahner, et al. "Stronger back muscles reduce the incidence of vertebral fractures: A prospective 10 year follow-up of postmenopausal women." *Bone* 30:6 (2002), 836–841.

4. M. A. Fiatarone, E. C. Marks, N. D. Ryan, et al. "High-intensity strength training in nonagenarians. Effects on skeletal muscle." *Journal of the American Medical Association* 263:22 (1990), 3029–3034.

5. S. A. Brownstein. "American orthopaedic foot and ankle society women's shoe survey." *Foot Ankle* 14:5 (1993), 292–293.

6. E. M. Wojtys, L. J. Huston, et al. "The effect of the menstrual cycle on anterior cruciate ligament injuries in women as determined by hormone levels." *American Journal of Sports Medicine* 30:2 (2002), 182–188.

7. D. E. Gwinn, J. H. Wilckens, E. R. McDevitt, et al. "The relative incidence of

anterior cruciate ligament injury in men and women at the United States Naval Academy." *American Journal of Sports Medicine* 28:1 (2000), 98–102.

8. D. T. Felson, Y. Zhang, J. M. Anthony, et al. "Weight loss reduces the risk for symptomatic knee osteoarthritis in women. The Framingham Study." *Annals of Internal Medicine* 116:7 (1992), 535–539.

CHAPTER TEN

1. M. Nilsson, R. Johnsen, W. Ye, et al. "Obesity and estrogen as risk factors for gastroesophageal reflux symptoms." *Journal of the American Medical Association* 290 (2003), 66–72.

2. B. Jacobson, S. C. Somers, C. S. Fuchs, et al. "Body-mass index and symptoms of gastroesophageal reflux in women." *New England Journal of Medicine* 354:22 (2006), 2340–2348.

3. Y. X. Yang, J. D. Lewis, et al. "Long-term proton pump inhibitor therapy and risk of hip fracture." *Journal of the American Medical Association* 296 (2006), 2947–2953.

4. K. R. DeVault and D. O. Castell. "Updated guidelines for the diagnosis and treatment of gastroesophageal reflux disease." *American Journal of Gastroenterology* 100:1 (2005), 190–200.

5. K. M. Maclure, K. C. Hayes, G. A. Colditz, et al. "Weight, diet, and the risk of symptomatic gallstones in middle-aged women." *New England Journal of Medicine* 321:9 (1989), 563–569.

6. M. J. Stampfer, K. M. Maclure, et al. "Risk of symptomatic gallstones in women with severe obesity." *American Journal of Clinical Nutrition* 55 (1992), 652–658.

7. A. Emeran, B. D. Mayer, et al. "Stress and the gastrointestinal tract v. stress and irritable bowel syndrome." *American Journal of Physiology, Gastrointestinal and Liver Physiology* 280:4 (2001), G519–G524.

CHAPTER ELEVEN

1. J. J. Haggerty Jr. and A. J. Prange Jr. "Borderline hypothyroidism and depression." *Annual Review of Medicine* 46 (1995): 37–46.

2. A. E. Hak, A.P.H. Pols, T. J. Visser, et al. "Subclinical hypothyroidism is an independent risk factor for atherosclerosis and myocardial infarction in elderly women: The Rotterdam Study." *Annals of Internal Medicine* 132:4 (2000), 270–278.

3. D. Edelman, M. K. Olsen, T. K. Dudley, et al. "Utility of hemoglobin A1c in predicting diabetes risk," *Journal of General Internal Medicine* 19:12 (2004), 1175–1180.

4. R. J. Anderson, K. E. Freedland, et al. "The prevalence of comorbid depression in adults with diabetes: A meta-analysis diabetes care." *Diabetes Care* 24:6 (2001), 1069–1078.

5. H. Turhan, A. S. Yasar, et al. "High prevalence of metabolic syndrome among young women with premature coronary artery disease." *Coronary Artery Disease* 16:1 (2005), 37–40.

6. M. A. Birdsall, C. M. Farquhar, and H. D. White. "Association between polycystic ovaries and extent of coronary artery disease in women having cardiac catheterization." *Annals of Internal Medicine* 126:1 (1997), 32–35.

7. P. J. Hunt, E. M. Gurnell, et al. "Improvement in mood and fatigue after dehydroepiandrosterone replacement in Addison's disease in a randomized,

double blind trial." *Journal of Clinical Endocrinology & Metabolism* 85:12 (2000), 4650–4656.

8. W. K. Leung, J. C. Wu, S. M. Liang, et al. "Treatment of diarrhea-predominant irritable bowel syndrome with traditional Chinese herbal medication: a randomized placebo controlled trial. *American Journal of Gastroenterology.* 101:7 (2006), 1574–1560.

9. T. Fung, F. B. Hu, C. Fuchs, et al. "Major dietary patterns and the risk of colon cancer in women." *Archives of Internal Medicine* 163:3 (2003), 309–314.

CHAPTER TWELVE

1. K. M. Grewen, S. S. Girdler, J. Amico, and K. C. Light. "Effects of partner support on resting oxytocin, cortisol, norepinephrine, and blood pressure before and after warm partner contact." *Psychosomatic Medicine* 67 (2005), 531–538.

2. J. W. Kenney and A. Bhattacharjee. "Interactive model of women's stressors, personality traits and health problems." *Journal of Advanced Nursing* 32:1 (2000), 249–258.

3. K. Raikkonen, K. A. Matthews, K. Sutton-Tyrrell, and L. H. Kuller. "Trait anger and the metabolic syndrome predict progression of carotid atherosclerosis in healthy middle-aged women." *Psychosomatic Medicine* 66:6 (2004), 903–908.

4. K. A. Matthews, J. F. Owens, L. H. Kuller, et al. "Are hostility and anxiety associated with carotid atherosclerosis in healthy postmenopausal women?" *Psychosomatic Medicine* 60:5 (1998), 633–638.

5. R. A. Carels, A. Sherwood, R. Szczepanski, and J. A. Blumenthal. "Ambulatory blood pressure and marital distress in employed women." *Behavioral Medicine* 26:2 (2000), 80–85.

6. K. Orth-Gomer, S. P. Wamala, M. Horsten, et al. "Marital stress worsens prognosis in women with coronary heart disease: The Stockholm Female Coronary Risk Study." *Journal of the American Medical Association* 284:23 (2000), 3008–3014.

7. M. Malach, and P. J. Imperato. "Depression and acute myocardial infarction." *Preventive Cardiology* 7:2 (2004), 83–90.

8. M. R. Sable and D. S. Wilkinson. "Impact of perceived stress, major life events and pregnancy attitudes on low birth weight." *Family Planning Perspective* 32 (2000), 288–294.

9. T. Kurki, V. Hiilesmaa, R. Raitasalo, et al. "Depression and anxiety in early pregnancy and risk for preeclampsia." *Obstetrics and Gynecology* 95:4 (2000), 487–490.

10. M. Lobel, C. J. DeVincent, A. Kaminer, and B. A. Meyer. "The impact of prenatal maternal stress and optimistic disposition on birth outcomes in medically high-risk women." *Health Psychology* 19:6 (2000), 544–553.

11. K. S. Kendler, J. Myers, and C. A. Prescott. "Sex differences in the relationship between social support and risk for major depression: A longitudinal study of opposite-sex twin pairs." *American Journal of Psychiatry* 162:2 (2005), 250–256.

CHAPTER THIRTEEN

1. A. Fugh-Berman and A. Myers. "Citrus aurantium, an ingredient of dietary supplements marketed for weight loss: Current status of clinical and basic research." *Experimental Biology and Medicine* 229:8 (2004), 698–704.

2. S.F.L. Kirk, J. E. Cade, J. H. Barrett, and M. Conner. "Diet and lifestyle characteristics associated with dietary supplement use in women." *Public Health Nutrition* 2:1 (1999), 69–73.

3. K. M. Newton, S. D. Reed, A. Z. LaCroix, et al. "Treatment of vasomotor symptoms of menopause with black cohosh, multibotanicals, soy, hormone therapy, or placebo: A randomized trial." *Annals of Internal Medicine* 45:12 (2006), 869–879.

4. R. J. Baber, C. Templeman, T. Morton, et al. "Randomized placebo-controlled trial of an isoflavone supplement and menopausal symptoms in women." *Climacteric* 2:2 (1999), 85–92.

5. P. Albertazzi, F. Pansini, G. Bonaccorsi, et al. "The effect of dietary soy supplementation on hot flushes." *Obstetrics and Gynecology* 91 (1998), 6–11.

6. F. Kronenberg and A. Fugh-Berman. "Complementary and alternative medicine for menopausal symptoms: A review of randomized, controlled trials." *Annals of Internal Medicine* 137:10 (2002), 805–813.

7. E. B. Rimm, W. C. Willett, F. B. Hu, et al. "Folate and Vitamin B_6 from diet and supplements in relation to risk of coronary heart disease among women." *Journal of the American Medical Association* 279:5 (1998), 359–364.

8. K. H. Bonaa, I. Njolstad, P. M. Ueland, et al. "Homocysteine lowering and cardiovascular events after acute myocardial infarction." *New England Journal of Medicine* 354:15 (2006), 1578–1588.

9. S. Warshafsky, R. S. Kamer, and S. L. Sivak. "Effect of garlic on total serum cholesterol. A meta-analysis." *Annals of Internal Medicine* 119:7 (1993), 599–605.

10. S. Yusuf, G. Dagenais, J. Pogue, et al. "Vitamin E supplementation and cardiovascular events in high-risk patients. The Heart Outcomes Prevention Evaluation Study Investigators." *New England Journal of Medicine* 342:3 (2000), 154–160.

11. E. Giovannucci, M. J. Stampfer, G. A. Colditz, et al. "Multivitamin use, folate, and colon cancer in women in the Nurses' Health Study." *Annals of Internal Medicine* 129:7 (1998), 517–524.

12. M. C. Hochberg. "Nutritional supplements for knee osteoarthritis—still no resolution." *New England Journal of Medicine* 354:8 (2006), 858–860.

13. A. J. Norheim, E. J. Pedersen, V. Fønnebø, and L. Berge. "Acupressure treatment of morning sickness in pregnancy. A randomised, double-blind, placebo-controlled study." *Scandinavian Journal of Primary Health Care* 19:1 (2001), 43–47.

14. A. Aune, T. Alraek, H. LiHua, and A. Baerheim. "Acupuncture in the prophylaxis of recurrent lower urinary tract infection in adult women." *Scandinavian Journal of Primary Health Care* 16:1 (1998), 37–39.

15. K. Wedenberg, B. Moen, and A. Norling. "A prospective randomized study comparing acupuncture with physiotherapy for low-back and pelvic pain in pregnancy." *Acta Obstetricia et Gynecologica Scandinavica* 79:5 (2000), 331–335.

16. K. Ternov, M. Nilsson, and L. Lofberg. "Acupuncture for pain relief during childbirth." *Acupuncture & Electro-therapeutics Research* 23:1 (1998), 19–26.

17. Y. Wyon, R. Lindgren, T. Lundeberg, and M. Hammar. "Effects of acupuncture on climacteric vasomotor symptoms, quality of life, and urinary excretion of neuropeptides among postmenopausal women." *Menopause: The Journal of the North American Menopause Society* 2:1 (1995), 3–12.

18. D. C. Cherkin, R. A. Deyo, M. Battié, et al. "A comparison of physical therapy, chiropractic manipulation, and provision of an educational booklet for the treatment of patients with low back pain." *New England Journal of Medicine* 339:15 (1998), 1021–1029.

19. K. P. Lee, W. G. Carlini, G. F. McCormick, and G. W. Albers. "Neurologic complications following chiropractic manipulation: A survey of California neurologists." *Neurology* 45:6 (1995), 1213–1215.

CHAPTER FIFTEEN

1. N. J. Lowe. "An overview of ultraviolet radiation, sunscreens, and photo-induced dermatoses." *Dermatologic Clinics* 24 (2006), 9–17.

2. C. Castelo-Branco, F. Figuereras, et al. "Facial wrinkling in postmenopausal women. Effects of smoking status and hormone replacement therapy." *Maturitas* 29 (1998), 75–86.

3. B. Takkouche, M. Etminan, and A. Montes-Martínez. "Personal use of hair dyes and risk of cancer: A meta-analysis." *Journal of the American Medical Association* 293:20 (2005), 2516–2525.

CHAPTER SIXTEEN

1. F. B. Hu, M. J. Stampfer, J. E. Manson, et al. "Dietary fat intake and the risk of coronary heart disease in women." *New England Journal of Medicine* 337:21 (1997), 1491–1499.

2. M. De Lorgeril, P. Salen, J. L. Martin, et al. "Mediterranean diet, traditional risk factors, and the rate of cardiovascular complications after myocardial infarction: first report of the Lyon diet heart study." *Circulation* 99 (1999), 779–785.

3. S. Sasaki, A. Katagiri, T. Tsuji, et al. "Self-reported rate of eating correlates with body mass index in 18-year-old Japanese women." *International Journal of Obesity and Related Metabolic Disorders* 27:11 (2003),1405–1410.

4. R. Otsuka, K. Tamakoshi, H. Yatsuya, et al. "Eating fast leads to obesity: Findings based on self-administered questionnaires among middle-aged Japanese men and women." *Journal of Epidemiology* 16:3 (2006), 117–124.

5. P. Rozin, K. Kabnick, E. Pete, et al. "The ecology of eating: Smaller portion sizes in France than in the United States help explain the French paradox." *Psychological Science: A Journal of the American Psychological Society* 14:5 (2003), 450–454.

6. J. Salmon, A. Bauman, D. Crawford, et al. "The association between television viewing and overweight among Australian adults participating in varying levels of leisure-time physical activity." *International Journal of Obesity and Related Metabolic Disorders* 24:5 (2000), 600–606.

7. Q. Sun, J. Ma, et al. "A prospective study of *trans* fatty acids in erythrocytes and risk of coronary heart disease." *Circulation* 115:14 (2007), 1858–1865.

8. A. G. Tsai and T. A. Wadden. "Systematic review: An evaluation of major commercial weight loss programs in the United States." *Annals of Internal Medicine* 142 (2005), 56–66.

9. C. D. Gardner, A. Kiazand, et al. "Comparison of the Atkins, Zone, Ornish, and LEARN diets for change in weight and related risk factors among overweight premenopausal women." *Journal of the American Medical Association* 297:9 (2007), 969–977.

10. S. Kuriyama, T. Shimazu, K. Ohmori, et al. "Green tea consumption and mortality due to cardiovascular disease, cancer, and all causes in Japan: The Ohsaki Study." *Journal of the American Medical Association* 296:10 (2006), 1255–1265.

11. B. Cortes, I. Nunez, M. Cofan, et al. "Acute effects of high-fat meals enriched with walnuts or olive oil on postprandial endothelial function." *Journal of the American College of Cardiology* 48 (2006),1666–1671.

12. M. J. Stampfer, F. B. Hu, J. E. Manson, et al. "Primary prevention of coronary heart disease in women through diet and lifestyle." *New England Journal of Medicine* 343:1 (2000), 16–22.

13. S. B. Penner, N. R. Campbell, et al. "Dietary sodium and cardiovascular outcomes: A rational approach." *Canadian Journal of Cardiology* 23:7 (2007), 567–572.

14. J. A. Baur, K. J. Pearson, N. L. Price, et al. "Resveratrol improves health and survival of mice on a high-calorie diet." *Nature* 444:7117 (2006), 337–342.

CHAPTER SEVENTEEN

1. K. Spiegel, R. Leproult, and E. Van Cauter. "Impact of sleep debt on metabolic and endocrine function." *Lancet* 354:9188 (1999), 1435–1439.

CHAPTER EIGHTEEN

1. W. Wang, J. E. Manson, et al. "Physical exertion, exercise, and sudden cardiac death in women." *Journal of the American Medical Association* 295:12 (2006), 1399–1403.

2. C. M. Morganti, M. E. Nelson, M. A. Fiatarone, et al. "Strength improvements with one year of progressive resistance training in older women." *Medicine and Science in Sports ad Exercise* 27 (1995), 906–912.

3. F. Li, P. Harmer, et al. "An evaluation of the effects of tai chi exercise on physical function among older persons: A randomized controlled trial." *Annals of Behavioral Medicine* 23:2 (2001), 139–146.

4. A. E. Springer, S. H. Kelder, and D. M. Hoelscher. "Social support, physical activity and sedentary behavior among 6th-grade girls: A cross-sectional study." *International Journal of Behavioral Nutrition and Physical Activity* 3:8 (2006), published online.

5. M. E. Nelson, G. E. Dilmanian, et al. "A one-year walking program and increased dietary calcium in postmenopausal women: Effects on bone." *American Journal of Clinical Nutrition* 53 (1991), 1304–1311.

6. F. A. Spencer, B. Salami, et al. "Temporal trends and associated factors of inpatient cardiac rehabilitation in patients with acute myocardial infarction: A community-wide perspective." *Journal of Cardiopulmonary Rehabilitation* 21:6 (2001), 377–384.

7. ACOG Committee opinion. "Exercise during pregnancy and the postpartum period." *Obstetrics and Gynecology* 99:1 (2002), 171–173.

8. S. Elavsky. *Annals of Behavioral Medicine,* April 2007; online edition.

9. M. D. Holmes, W. Y. Chen, et al. "Physical activity and survival after breast cancer diagnosis." *Journal of the American Medical Association* 293:20 (2005), 2479–2486.

10. R. D. Brinton. "A women's health issue: Alzheimer's disease and strategies for maintaining cognitive health." *International Journal of Fertility and Women's Medicine* 44:4 (1999), 174–185.

11. K. Yaffe, D. Barnes, et al. "A prospective study of physical activity and cognitive decline in elderly women: Women who walk." *Archives of Internal Medicine* 161:4 (2001), 1703–1708.

Abdominal hysterectomy: the surgical removal of the uterus through the abdomen

ACE inhibitors (angiotensin-converting enzyme inhibitors): a class of medications used to lower blood pressure and treat heart failure

Acne rosacea: a skin disease that causes persistent redness on the face

Acupuncture: traditional Chinese method of reducing pain and enhancing health by inserting thin wire needles at particular points in the skin

Aerobic exercise: a form of physical activity that makes increased demands on the heart and lungs and is recommended for cardiovascular health

Alpha hydroxy acids (AHAs): organic fruit acids that are used for chemical peels

Angina (angina pectoris): chest discomfort due to decreased blood flow to the heart muscle, caused by atherosclerosis

Angioplasty (coronary angioplasty): a procedure that uses a balloon to open up a coronary artery without surgery and that usually inserts a stent to keep the artery open

Angiotensin receptor blockers (ARBs): medications used to lower blood pressure and treat congestive heart failure

Antacids: drugs that help to absorb stomach acid

Antiplatelet medication: medications that inhibit blood clotting cells (platelets) from sticking together to form blood clots; aspirin and clopidogrel are antiplatelet medications

Aortic regurgitation: the incomplete closing of the aortic valve, which causes the blood to leak backward into the left ventricle, also called aortic insufficiency

Aortic stenosis: a narrowing of the aortic valve, which obstructs the flow of blood from the left ventricle to the aorta

Arrhythmias: a deviation from the regular heartbeat; arrhythmias range from very slow to abnormally fast or irregular

Atherosclerosis: the narrowing of arteries due to the buildup of cholesterol

Atrial fibrillation: an arrhythmia that originates in the heart's upper chambers and impairs the normal emptying of blood from the atria into the ventricles

Autoimmune disease: a group of diseases that are characterized by the immune system producing antibodies against the body's own cells

Automatic implantable cardio defibrillator (AICD): a device that continuously monitors the heart for rapid or irregular rhythm and supplies therapy automatically if it detects an arrhythmia

Barium enema: a procedure used to examine the colon/bowel that uses X-rays after barium sulfite is inserted into the colon via enema

Benzodiazepines: a group of drugs used to treat anxiety and insomnia

Beta-blockers: a class of medication used to treat high blood pressure, symptoms of coronary artery disease, and certain arrhythmias; beta-blockers slow the heart rate and lower blood pressure

Biofeedback: a process by which a person learns how to monitor and control specific bodily functions

Bioidentical hormones: manufactured hormones that have exactly the same biological structure as your own hormones

Bisphosphonates: a class of drugs that increases bone density by preventing bone breakdown

Blood thinners: a class of medications used to reduce blood clotting

Botox: a bacterial toxin used to relax facial wrinkles

BRCA1/BRCA2: genes that indicate a predisposition to breast cancer

Broken heart syndrome: a condition where intense emotional stress can cause severe heart muscle weakness

CA-125 assay: a blood test for CA-125, a tumor marker, especially for ovarian cancer

Calcium channel blockers: a class of medications that lower blood pressure, slow heart rate, and treat arrhythmias

Carbohydrates: a food group that includes cereals, starches, sugars, fruits, and vegetables and is a source of energy for the body

Cardiac catheterization: a dye study (angiogram) to evaluate the coronary arteries and the pumping chamber of the heart

Cardiac rehabilitation program: a supervised program of exercise and education for patients who have had heart attack, heart surgery, stents, or angina

Cardiovascular disease: any disease of the heart, heart valves, blood vessels, and arteries, including stroke, hypertension, rheumatic fever, and heart attack

Chemical peels: a method that uses a chemical solution to improve wrinkles and sun damage to the skin

Chiropractic therapy: a therapeutic process that involves manipulation of the spinal column

Chlamydia: a common sexually transmitted infection caused by bacteria

Cholesterol: a waxy, fatlike substance found in the blood that helps produce hormones and cell structures necessary for the body to function normally; elevated cholesterol is a risk factor for heart disease and stroke

Chronic insomnia: persistent sleeplessness that lasts more than three weeks

Colonoscopy: a procedure that uses a flexible tube to examine the colon

Colposcope: a magnifying instrument used to examine the cervix and vagina

Complementary and alternative medicine: medical practices that are not considered part of traditional medicine

Complex carbohydrates: a group of foods characterized by complex sugar molecules that do not cause sharp rises in insulin

Coronary artery bypass surgery (CABG): open-heart surgery that uses arteries and veins from elsewhere in the body to go around obstructions in the coronary arteries to improve blood flow to the heart muscle

COX-2 inhibitor: a class of nonsteroidal anti-inflammatory drugs that target the enzyme (COX-2) responsible for pain and inflammation; used for arthritis

C-reactive protein: a protein that is increased in the blood in response to inflammation; a marker of heart disease risk

CT (computerized tomography) angiography: a diagnostic study that uses dye to image the coronary arteries with a scanner and does not require hospitalization

CT pulmonary angiogram: an imaging diagnostic procedure to assess for pulmonary embolism

CT scan: an imaging procedure that uses X-rays to examine the internal structures of the body

Dermabrasion: a procedure to remove scars and other skin imperfections by using revolving brushes or sandpaper

DEXA (dual energy X-ray absorptiometry) scan: a diagnostic imaging procedure used to measure bone density

DHEA (Dehydroepiandrosterone): a steroid hormone that is converted to testosterone and estrogen

Diabetes insipidus: an uncommon condition caused by pituitary abnormalities, head trauma, and brain tumors that affect the kidneys' ability to retain water; symptoms are frequent urination and increased thirst

Diabetes mellitus: a disease caused by elevated blood sugar; in type 1 diabetes, the cause is undersecretion of insulin, while in type 2, insulin is underproduced or underutilized and the body's cells are inadequately responsive to it

Diuretics: a class of medication commonly used to treat elevated blood pressure and to reduce fluid accumulation in heart failure

Diverticulitis: a condition of the intestine characterized by inflammation of small sacs (diverticula) that line the intestine

Diverticulosis: a condition of the intestine where small sacs develop along the intestinal wall

Echocardiogram: a diagnostic test that uses an ultrasound probe (sound waves) to produce images of the heart showing the shape, texture, and movement of the valves and allowing measurement of the size of the heart and its chambers; also assesses heart function

Electrocardiogram (ECG): a diagnostic test that records electrical currents to detect abnormal heart rhythm

Endometriosis: a condition where the tissue that usually lines the walls of the uterus occurs outside the uterine walls

Endoscopy: a diagnostic procedure using a flexible lighted device (endoscope) to see inside the body

Estrogen: a hormone that promotes female sexual characteristics

Event monitor: a device that is worn (usually for a month) to monitor heart rhythm; usually used for palpitations and arrhythmias

Exercise electrocardiogram (ECG stress test): a diagnostic test for the evaluation of coronary heart disease; an ECG monitors your heart during exercise (usually on a treadmill) for changes that indicate narrowed arteries

Fiber: the part of fruits and vegetables that cannot be digested

Fibric acid derivatives: a class of cholesterol-lowering medications that work primarily to reduce triglycerides and increase HDL cholesterol

Fibrinogen: a protein found in blood that helps with clotting

Fibroadenoma of the breast: a common benign breast lump

Fibroids: benign tumors usually found in or around the uterus

Flavonoids: naturally found plant compounds that function as antioxidants

Follicle-stimulating hormone (FSH): a hormone produced in the pituitary gland that stimulates egg development in the ovaries

Gastritis: inflammation of the stomach

Genital herpes: an infection, usually sexually transmitted, caused by the herpes virus; characterized by genital blisters

GERD (gastroesophageal reflux disease): a condition in which gastric juices back up from the stomach into the esophagus, causing burning and pain

Gestational diabetes: the impaired ability to efficiently metabolize carbohydrates caused by insulin resistance that occurs during pregnancy; may lead to type 2 diabetes in midlife

Gestational hypertension: high blood pressure that occurs during pregnancy and usually returns to normal after delivery

Glycemic index: a numerical system of measuring how fast a carbohydrate triggers a rise in circulating blood sugar; the higher the number, the faster the blood sugar response

Goiter: an enlargement of the thyroid gland

Gonorrhea: a common sexually transmitted bacterial infection

Graves' disease: hyperthyroidism associated with an enlarged thyroid

H. pylori: bacteria that can cause inflammation of the stomach

H$_2$ antagonists: a class of drugs used to decrease stomach acid

Hashimoto's disease: an autoimmune disease that affects the thyroid gland and often leads to hypothyroidism

HDL cholesterol: high-density lipoprotein or "good" cholesterol

Heart disease: collectively the diseases of the heart muscle, the heart valves, and the coronary arteries

Heart failure: a condition where the heart is unable to pump sufficient blood to meet the body's needs

Hiatal hernia: a small tear in the diaphragm that allows the stomach to move into the chest, commonly causing heartburn

HIPAA (Health Insurance Portability and Accountability Act): government standards for the security and privacy of health data

Histamine-2 receptor blockers: *see* H_2 antagonists

Holter monitor: a device worn for 24–48 hours that continuously records heart rhythms

Homocysteine: an amino acid derived from the metabolism of methionine, an essential amino acid predominant in animal protein; at high levels, homocysteine may damage artery walls

Hormone: a chemical substance produced by one part of the body that regulates the function of another part

Hormone therapy (HT): therapy that uses estrogen or estrogen combined with progestin (for women who have a uterus) to treat menopausal symptoms and osteoporosis

Hospitalists: physicians who specialize in providing for care for hospitalized patients

Human papillomavirus (HPV): a virus that causes genital warts

Hypertension (high blood pressure): higher than normal pressure in the arteries; a risk factor for heart disease and stroke

Hyperthyroidism: a condition characterized by an overactive thyroid gland

Hypnosis: a trancelike state that increases suggestibility, used to reduce pain

Hypothyroidism: a condition characterized by decreased function of the thyroid gland

Hysterectomy: the surgical removal of the uterus through the abdomen or vagina

Inflammatory bowel disease: disorders characterized by inflammation of the bowel, such as Crohn's disease or ulcerative colitis

Insomnia: chronic sleeplessness

Insulin resistance: a lack of responsiveness by the body to the actions of insulin; despite high levels of insulin, blood sugar levels rise and can lead to type 2 diabetes

Intrauterine device (IUD): a contraceptive device implanted in the uterus

Irritable bowel syndrome (IBS): an intestinal disorder associated with a change in bowel function

LDL cholesterol: low-density lipoprotein or "bad" cholesterol

Lipid panel: a blood test that measures lipids, which are blood fats, including total cholesterol, HDL cholesterol, LDL cholesterol, and triglycerides

Lipoprotein (a) (Lp[a]): a substance that is structurally similar to a blood clotting protein and LDL cholesterol

Liposuction: a technique for removing body fat with a suction device

Lower esophageal sphincter (LES): a valve in the lower esophagus that keeps stomach acid from backing up into the esophagus

Lumpectomy: the surgical removal of a tumor without removing large amounts of other tissue

Lupus: an autoimmune disease characterized by inflammation of connective tissue

Lycopene: a chemical substance found in tomatoes and other red fruits and vegetables

Mammography: an imaging test of the breast using X-rays to identify breast abnormalities

Mastectomy: the surgical removal of the breast

Mastitis: an inflammation of the breast usually caused by a bacterial infection

Menopause: when the menstrual period has not occurred for one year

Metabolic syndrome: a group of symptoms associated with an increased risk of heart disease and diabetes

Microvascular angina: a type of angina that causes chest pain because small blood vessels in the heart are not working properly

Mitral regurgitation: leakage of the mitral valve, where the blood is pumped backward into the left atrium; also called mitral valve insufficiency

Mitral valve prolapse: a common heart disorder when the valve connecting the left atrium and left ventricle doesn't close properly

Mitral valve stenosis: a condition where the heart's mitral valve is narrowed and therefore blood flow is obstructed

Monounsaturated fat: a fat that comes from plant foods that are liquid at room temperature, such as canola, peanut, and olive oils, as well as avocados

MRI: an imaging test, using magnets and radio waves, to image all parts of the body

Narcolepsy: a condition of uncontrollable sleeping

Niacin: a B vitamin sometimes used to lower cholesterol levels

Nitroglycerine: a medication that dilates or widens the blood vessels, including the coronary arteries, and is used to treat symptoms from obstructed coronary arteries

Nonsteroidal anti-inflammatory drugs (NSAIDs): a group of drugs used to help reduce inflammation and pain

Nuclear stress test: an imaging test of the heart that uses electrocardiogram and where a radioactive substance is injected into the body in order to measure your heart function during rest and exercise

Omega-3 fats: highly unsaturated fats found in certain fatty fish (tuna, mackerel, salmon), flaxseed oil, nuts, canola oil, and soybean oil

Osteoarthritis: a form of arthritis that affects the joints

Osteopenia: a condition of a loss of bone density

Osteoporosis: a condition characterized by abnormally low bone density

Oxytocin: a drug used to stimulate uterine contractions

Pap test: a method of testing cervical cells for abnormalities

Partial hysterectomy: the surgical removal of the uterus, leaving the cervix and ovaries intact

Pelvic inflammatory disease (PID): an infection or inflammation of the reproductive organs

Peptic ulcers: open sores that occur in the lining of the stomach, upper small intestine, or esophagus

Pericarditis: an inflammation of the sac surrounding the heart

Perimenopause: the years preceding menopause, characterized by a decline in estrogen and irregular menstrual cycles

Peripartum cardiomyopathy: a rare disorder of pregnancy and the months following delivery characterized by a weakened heart muscle

Peripheral artery disease (PAD): a common circulatory problem characterized by decreased blood flow to the limbs, usually caused by atherosclerosis

Pilates: a low-impact exercise program that tones, stretches, and strengthens the body

Polycystic ovary syndrome: an endocrine disorder characterized by irregular menstrual periods, often accompanied by multiple cysts on the ovaries and increased hair growth

Polyunsaturated fat: a fat that is liquid at room temperature, including from plant foods, nuts, seeds, and some seafoods, and sunflower, corn, soybean, safflower, and sesame oils; polyunsaturated fats can help to get rid of newly formed cholesterol and reduce cholesterol deposits in the arteries

Post-traumatic stress disorder (PTSD): a psychological disorder characterized by intense emotional reactions to severe emotional or physical stress

Preeclampsia: a condition characterized by high blood pressure; occurs after the 24th week of pregnancy

Prehypertension: slightly elevated blood pressure that, if untreated, could lead to hypertension

Premature menopause: menopause that occurs before the age of 40

Premature supraventricular contraction: early heartbeat from the upper chamber of the heart that causes fast heart rhythms

Premenopause: *see* Perimenopause

Progesterone: a hormone that affects menstruation, pregnancy, and conception

Protein pump inhibitors: a group of drugs used to reduce stomach acid

Pulmonary embolism: a potentially dangerous condition characterized by blood clots that block the flow of blood to the lungs

REM (rapid eye movement) sleep: one of the stages of sleep, characterized by rapid eye movements

Restless leg syndrome: a condition of itching and tiredness in the legs, accompanied by twitching and sometimes pain

Resveratrol: an antioxidant plant compound found in the skin of red grapes, blueberries, other fruits and in peanuts

Rheumatoid arthritis: a chronic autoimmune disease characterized by inflammation and swelling of the joints

Rhinoplasty: a plastic surgery procedure to reshape the nose

Sarcopenia: the age-related loss of muscle mass associated with reduced muscle strength

Selective estrogen receptor modulators (SERMs): a class of medications, such as raloxifene and tamoxifen, that are used to build bone in osteoporosis

Selective serotonin reuptake inhibitors (SSRIs): a class of antidepressant drugs used to treat depression and anxiety

Sexually transmitted infections: a group of infections, caused by bacteria, parasites, or viruses, transmitted through sexual contact

Sick sinus syndrome: heart arrhythmias that arise from poor functioning of the heart's natural pacemaker

Sleep apnea: a sleep disorder characterized by frequent short periods of stopping breathing

Spermicide: a substance that kills sperm, usually used as a contraceptive

Statins: a class of cholesterol-lowering medications

Stent: a tiny wire mesh that is inserted into an artery after it has been opened by angioplasty

Strength exercises: exercise designed to increase muscle mass and strength, usually done with weights

Stress (exercise) echocardiogram: a diagnostic test that evaluates for coronary artery obstruction, using ultrasound to image the heart during exercise

Stress incontinence: an involuntary loss of urine that occurs during physical exertion

Stroke: brain tissue damage due to blood vessel disease

Surgical menopause: menopause that occurs when the ovaries are removed before natural menopause

Tachycardia: a rapid heart rate that exceeds 100 beats per minute

Tai chi: a Chinese exercise characterized by gentle movements that is used to improve balance and reduce stress

Testosterone: a hormone, secreted by the testes in males and the ovaries in females, that promotes male sexual characteristics and plays an important role in health and well-being

Therapeutic touch: a healing method designed to balance the body's energy

Tissue plasminogen activator (tPA): a medication used to quickly dissolve blood clots in victims of stroke

Total hysterectomy: surgical removal of the uterus and cervix, through the abdomen or vagina

Trans fats: fats that are produced commercially by hardening liquid vegetable oils into shortening and margarine; increase levels of LDL (bad) cholesterol and decrease HDL (good) cholesterol

Transcendental meditation: a stress management technique using meditation

Transdermal patch: a medicated pad placed on the skin that delivers medications to the bloodstream

Transient ischemic attack (TIA): a little stroke or "ministroke"—temporary loss of brain function

Triglycerides: a type of blood fat that increases atherosclerosis

Ultrasound: a diagnostic imaging technique that uses high-frequency sound waves to create images of the organs of the body

Urinary incontinence: loss of bladder control

Uterine prolapse: a condition where the uterus falls from the pelvis into the vagina

UVA rays/UVB rays: ultraviolet rays from the sun that are harmful to the skin

Vaginal hysterectomy: a surgical procedure where the uterus is removed through the vagina

Ventricular fibrillation: a life-threatening rapid and disordered heart rhythm from the lower heart chambers

Ventricular tachycardia: a rapid heartbeat originating in the lower chambers of the heart, associated with fainting and sudden death

Virtual colonoscopy: a diagnostic imaging test that uses X-rays and computers to visualize the colon

Weight-bearing exercise: exercise where the skeleton carries the body's weight, such as walking, running, dancing

Women's Health Initiative (WHI): a long-term large national study that focuses on research on women's health issues

Wolff-Parkinson-White syndrome: episodes of rapid heart rate caused by abnormal electrical activity of the heart

Yoga: ancient Indian practice of mental and physical exercise involving meditation and movement

RESOURCES

RELIABLE WEBSITES

www.acg.gi.org (American College of Gastroenterology)

www.acog.org (American College of Obstetricians and Gynecologists)

www.ahrq.gov (Agency for Healthcare Research and Quality)

www.americanheart.org (American Heart Association)

www.apa.org (American Psychological Association)

www.cancer.gov (National Cancer Institute)

www.cdc.gov (Centers for Disease Control and Prevention)

www.diabetes.org (American Diabetes Association)

www.fda.gov (U.S. Food and Drug Administration)

www.goredforwomen.org

www.healthology.com

www.komen.org

www.MayoClinic.org

www.movingfree.com

www.nccam.nih.gov (National Center for Complementary and Alternative Medicine)

www.niddk.nih.gov (National Institute of Diabetes and Digestive and Kidney Diseases)

www.nimh.nih.gov (National Institute of Mental Health)

www.nlm.nih.gov (National Library of Medicine—National Institutes of Health)

www.nof.org (National Osteoporosis Foundation)

www.sistertosister.org

www.webmd.com

www.womenheart.org

ORGANIZATIONS

Agency for Healthcare Research and Quality

American College of Gastroenterology

American College of Obstetricians and Gynecologists

American Heart Association

American Society of Colon and Rectal Surgeons

National Center for Complementary and Alternative Medicine

VIDEOS BY MIRABAI HOLLAND, MFA, CREATOR OF
MOVING FREE® EXERCISE TECHNIQUE

Fabulous Forever® Trilogy: Easy Strength, Easy Stretch, and Easy Aerobics

Moving Free® Longevity Series

Skeletal Fitness®: A Workout for Your Bones

ABOUT THE AUTHORS

Nieca Goldberg, M.D., is an associate professor of medicine and the medical director of New York University's Women's Heart Program, the co-medical director of the 92nd Street Y's Cardio Rehabilitation Program, and a national spokesperson for the American Heart Association's "Go Red" campaign. She is the former chief of women's cardiac care at Lenox Hill Hospital. Dr. Goldberg has appeared on many shows, including *Today*, *The View*, and *Good Morning America*, and her articles have appeared in many publications, including *The Wall Street Journal*, *The New York Times*, and *Fitness* magazine. She is the recipient of numerous awards, including the American Heart Association/NYC affiliate Dr. with Heart Award. She lives and works in New York City.

Alice Greenwood, Ph.D., is a sociolinguist who has worked in health care for many years. She specializes in research and writing about gender differences in communication styles. She has written and edited numerous professional and popular articles and books on various health care issues. She lives with her family in New Jersey and New York.

ABOUT THE TYPE

This book was set in Ehrhardt, a typeface based on the original design of Nicholas Kis, a seventeenth-century Hungarian type designer. Ehrhardt was first released in 1937 by the Monotype Corporation of London.